RESTORING THE SPIRIT

Restoring the Spirit

THE BEGINNINGS OF OCCUPATIONAL THERAPY
IN CANADA, 1890–1930

Judith Friedland

McGILL-QUEEN'S UNIVERSITY PRESS

MONTREAL & KINGSTON • LONDON • ITHACA

© McGill-Queen's University Press 2011
ISBN 978-0-7735-3912-9 (cloth)
ISBN 978-0-7735-3922-8 (paper)

Legal deposit third quarter 2011
Bibliothèque nationale du Québec

Printed in Canada on acid-free paper that is 100% ancient forest free
(100% post-consumer recycled), processed chlorine free

This book has been published with the help of a grant from the
Ontario Society of Occupational Therapists.

McGill-Queen's University Press acknowledges the support of the
Canada Council for the Arts for our publishing program. We also
acknowledge the financial support of the Government of Canada
through the Canadian Book Fund for our publishing activities.

Library and Archives Canada Cataloguing in Publication

Friedland, Judith, 1939–
Restoring the spirit : the beginnings of occupational therapy in
Canada, 1890–1930 / Judith Friedland.

Includes bibliographical references and index.
ISBN 978-0-7735-3912-9 (bound).
ISBN 978-0-7735-3922-8 (pbk.)

1. Occupational therapy – Canada – History.   I. Title.

RM699.3.C3F75 2011   615.8'5150971   C2011-903533-2

Set in 10.5/13 Goudy Oldstyle with Gotham
Book design & typesetting by Garet Markvoort, zijn digital

CONTENTS

PART THREE   Building a Profession

We at the Ontario Society of Occupational Therapists (OSOT) are delighted and honoured to offer a foreword to this important new book, a work that contributes comprehensive and uniquely Canadian perspectives to existing historical accounts of occupational therapy. Judith Friedland, the author, is superbly qualified to describe the conditions, the beliefs, and the personal commitments that gave rise to our profession.

This year, 2011, marks several "birthdays" for the profession of occupational therapy in Canada. Both the Canadian Association of Occupational Therapists (CAOT) and the Department of Occupational Science and Occupational Therapy at the University of Toronto turn eighty-five. Our own association, OSOT, is celebrating a vibrant ninety years of active service to our members with a commitment to "Honouring Our Past – Advancing Our Future." But our past has been sparsely documented and often obscured by more dominant histories. This book serves to close that knowledge gap by providing the first comprehensive history of the early decades of occupational therapy in Canada. Only with this knowledge and from these perspectives can we confidently and proactively plan for our profession's future.

Writing a book is no small undertaking, but the task is even more challenging for a book such as this, which required many hundreds of hours of sifting through the literature and archival records. Others have previously attempted to compile this history, and Judith benefited from their work. Her achievement is to be lauded, and we are indebted to her for her determination, passion, and tenacity in making this text available to all of us.

Of course, Judith is accomplished both inside and outside the world of occupational therapy, and we would be remiss not to highlight a few of her contributions and accomplishments. In 1988, she received a doctorate in education. She is currently professor emerita in the Department of Occupational Science and Occupational Therapy at the University of Toronto, having served as chair of the department for ten years. She has been included in *Canadian Who's Who* and *Who's Who of Canadian Women* since 1995, and she won the University of Toronto's Alumni

Achievement Award in 2000. In 2003, Judith's peers in the Canadian Association of Occupational Therapists honoured her with the prestigious Muriel Driver Lectureship Award.

Judith focuses on the early years of occupational therapy in Canada. In looking at its beginnings, at its growing knowledge and developing theory, and at some inspired practical initiatives, she explores four decades of tremendous change within the young profession, decades that also saw tremendous social change in Canada. As we read the book, we learn about the social and political climates that influenced the growth and direction of the profession between 1890 and 1930. While discovering our past, we also find many themes that resonate with our present.

In this second decade of the twenty-first century, we too live in dynamic times that challenge us to ensure that our practice keeps stride with Canada's changing social and cultural tapestry, with advances in medicine and technology, with an aging population, and with the demand for evidence-based practice. Informed and inspired by the stories that come to life in these pages, we will be better able to build on the lessons of our past as we too seek to survive and thrive in a climate of constant change.

We are part of the living history of our profession. Judith's vivid account enables us to celebrate the tenacity, vision, and accomplishments of our forebears, those early pioneers who carved a niche for our treasured profession by focusing on restoring the spirit. This unique book honours their memory and will inspire us to imagine and enact a vibrant future.

Christie Brenchley, executive director, OSOT
Gail Teachman, president, Board of Directors, OSOT

Occupational therapists often have difficulty explaining their work. The people they work with, the settings in which they work, and the interventions they use vary widely. They work with all age groups, from children through to the elderly; with people with physical illness and disability; and with those who have mental health problems. They work in prevention and health promotion programs, in hospitals and in the community, in the private and the public sectors, and within different governmental spheres such as health and long-term care, social services, labour, immigration, housing, education, and corrections. The interventions they use range from supportive counselling, through making a hand splint or adapting a kitchen, to the teaching of very specific skills, such as handwriting.

A recent Canadian definition of occupational therapy attests to the ongoing broad scope of the field. Occupational therapy "is the art and science of enabling engagement in everyday living, through occupation; of enabling people to perform the occupations that foster health and well-being; and of enabling a just and inclusive society so that all people may participate to their potential in the daily occupations of life."[1] This definition harkens back to the very essence of the profession and to the power of occupation, and now it applies to society as a whole.

The work of early occupational therapists was derived from several social, political, and artistic movements. The mental hygiene movement, the arts and crafts movement, the settlement house movement, and educational reform each played a part in determining the interventions used. At the beginning of the twentieth century, crafts were the primary means of treatment in occupational therapy. While many other interventions were added over the years, crafts of some sort remained, albeit in an ever-diminishing form.

During my occupational therapy education, I enjoyed learning how to do specific crafts, but I knew nothing of where this notion of "doing" had come from.[2] Later, as a graduate practising in mental hospitals,[3] I still did not fully understand why I was using crafts with patients on the ward or in the department, nor did I know why I was taking patients on outings, teaching homemaking skills or work skills, or placing them in situations where particular social skills were required.

When I came back to work after a time at home with my three children, I worked as an occupational therapist in the community. Now I could use an even broader range of skills: I could help my clients (as patients were now called) to find appropriate work or schooling, link them with community resources, or adapt their homes to accommodate their physical limitations. In every instance, what I was doing as an occupational therapist seemed to be useful and was always appreciated by my clients; but again, I had no sense of where my extensive kit bag came from. At times, it seemed almost inappropriate that I should be venturing into so many different areas.

Later still, as a faculty member at the University of Toronto, I often struggled with students who questioned their role and indeed their very identity as soon-to-be health professionals. Why was the role so broad and seemingly ill-defined? How could they explain it to the interdisciplinary teams of which they were a part – let alone to their own families and friends? While they generally had a theoretical rationale for what they were doing, they did not have the comfort of knowing where the original ideas came from and why they developed as they did. Very little had been written on the history of occupational therapy in Canada before 2000.[4] Students did not have a foundation upon which to build their knowledge. I was not able to help them as much as I would have liked, and this awareness made me uncomfortable.

Most likely, it was this feeling of not being able to help my students adequately that motivated me to explore the early history of occupational therapy in Canada, at first through a series of articles and now with this book. Thus, a personal goal of this research was to provide a knowledge of the past: to satisfy my own curiosity, to help other faculty members introduce their students to the discipline, and, of course, to help the students themselves. "The best teachers," writes historian Ken Bain, "have an unusually keen sense of the histories of their disciplines, including the controversies that have swirled within them, and that understanding seems to help them reflect deeply on the nature of thinking within their own fields."[5] This book is intended to increase awareness of the histories of occupational therapy, the controversies that existed in the early years, and the paths that were and were not taken.

Reflecting on the nature of thinking in occupational therapy can, however, have much broader consequences, and here lies a major reason for my having written the book. It is to share the unique perspective held by occupational therapy on health and well-being: the idea, implicit in the discipline, that being engaged in occupations is, in effect, a determinant of health. Across all the settings and populations within which occupational therapists work, this unvarying theme is evident.

Although none of the movements that contributed to the underlying philosophy of occupational therapy was medical in nature, the profession made its home within the health care system. And while occupational therapy does not fit comfortably within the definition of the medical model, it is in a position to help broaden the medical model. Critics have suggested for some time that a broader, biopsychosocial approach is needed,[6] that health must be seen as more than the absence of disease. Thus, there remains an unrealized potential for occupational therapy to help medicine take a more holistic approach.

Therefore, this book is addressed well beyond the members of the profession of occupational therapy. It is addressed to educators and policymakers who deal with the health and well-being of those who have suffered injuries and illnesses (work related and otherwise) and to people who are homeless, who are in prison, who are new immigrants, or who are among the aging population. It is an exercise in history recovered and tells a story that has never been told. While the profession has evolved in several countries with some similarity, this book tells the Canadian story.

ACKNOWLEDGMENTS

I probably caught the history bug from an article by Ruth Levine Schemm published in the *American Journal of Occupational Therapy* in 1987, entitled "The Influence of the Arts-and-Crafts Movement on the Professional Status of Occupational Therapy."[7] The article opened doors to new knowledge for me and started me on a new path of inquiry. Articles I published in 1988 and 1998 reflected on our history, but it was not until I was asked to deliver the Muriel Driver Lecture in 2003 that I became fully engaged in this area of research.[8] My lecture was entitled "Why Crafts? Influences on the Development of Occupational Therapy in Canada from 1890–1930." It was well received, and as it seemed to stimulate an interest within the audience to learn more about their history, I felt encouraged to continue. Parts of this book build upon my earlier work that was published in the *American Journal of Occupational Therapy* 49, no. 9 (1988); 52, no. 5 (1998); and 62, no. 3 (2008); and in the *Canadian Journal of Occupational Therapy* 68, no. 5 (2001); 70, no. 4 (2003); 72, no. 3 (2005); and 74, no. 1 (2007).

I had great support from the late Isobel Robinson, a former teacher of mine at the University of Toronto and a long-time friend. She headed the Archives Committee for the Canadian Association of Occupational Therapists and was deeply interested in the history of the profession. She kept excellent records for many years, and gathered and catalogued much material. Isobel was the recipient of a draft manuscript for a book on the history of occupational therapy that Helen LeVesconte, the director of the Department of Occupational Therapy at the University of Toronto from 1933 to 1967, had written but unfortunately not completed. Isobel tried to carry on with the work, but it proved too large a task. LeVesconte's manuscript, annotated by Isobel, came to me in 2006 when Isobel's health began to decline.[9] I have found the work a very helpful resource in my research.

I have had help from many research assistants over the years and also from some final-year occupational therapy students who did their major research projects with me in this area. All provided great help, each in his or her own way. Pamela Albrecht MacLaren, a social worker with an undergraduate degree in history, saw me through my Muriel Driver Lecture. Jennifer Silva, Sarah Sang Tran, Naomi Davids-Brumer, Hadassah Rais, Christina Gallucci, Victrine Tseung, Marianne Sofronas Griezis, Sarane Poon, and Meisan Brown-Lum have worked on my history-related projects over the years. Most recently, Jennifer McBrearty, Taryn Bolt, and Jonathan Ding have been of tremendous help during the preparation of this manuscript.

I am also most indebted to the families of the various people I have written about: Thomas Kidner's descendants, various relatives of Ina Matthews, and Dr Alexander Primrose's granddaughter Clare Coulter were all helpful. Margaret Reid talked to me about her father, Norman Burnette, and Ann Kerr-Linden shared her mother's first-hand report, providing a glimpse of how the Spanish flu affected ward aides' training.

A small group of Canadian academics in occupational therapy has provided support and stimulation. Sue Baptiste (McMaster), Liz Townsend (Dalhousie), Brenda Head (Memorial), Barry Trentham and Lynn Cockburn (U of T), and I have worked together to bring history to the Canadian Association of Occupational Therapy annual conference for several years. Brenda and I have also collaborated on our own projects on Jessie Luther. MaryAnn McColl's recognition of and enthusiasm for my historical work has been of great help over the years. Staff at the American Occupational Therapy Association Archives have been most helpful: Mary Binderman, who was followed by Mindy Hecker, provided assistance during my visits and by email at other times. My colleagues in the Department of Occupational Science and Occupational Therapy at the University of Toronto have all provided support and encouragement. A special mention should be made of John Court, archivist at the Centre for Addiction and Mental Health in Toronto. John has been a great fount of information and has given generously of his time. Harold Averill and others at the University of Toronto Archives have also been most helpful.

I have been fortunate to hold grants from the Associated Medical Services–Hannah Fund for the History of Medicine and the Social Sciences and Humanities Research Council (SSHRC) to support my research. I have had wonderful support from McGill-Queen's University Press; Mark Abley shepherded me through the early and crucial stages that led to the acceptance of the manuscript, Judith Turnbull helped make it more readable, and Joan McGilvray kept everything on track. The Ontario Society of Occupational Therapists has been particularly helpful throughout the research process and I am most grateful for their recent support of the publication of this book.

Finally, I owe a great debt to my husband, Marty Friedland. I have watched him write many books over many years. They were concerned primarily with the law in some form except for his major historical research on the University of Toronto.[10] He has had to walk a fine line between offering advice and sitting back and letting me do it my way, knowing that being told what to do would never work for me. He has been a great support as well as a very inexpensive and most accomplished research assistant on many of my visits to libraries and archives outside of Toronto. My children, Tom, Jenny, and Nancy, and their partners have encouraged me and tolerated my preoccupation. My eight grandchildren (Michael, David, Elliott, Daisy, Cecilia, Tillie, Levi, and Nate) don't seem to know that the book has kept me from spending more time with them, but I vow to make up for that now.

INTRODUCTION

There is currently no comprehensive history of occupational therapy in Canada. Given that occupational therapy is as old in Canada as anywhere else in the world, the lack of a written history leaves a major gap for the profession and, it is argued, for health care in general. To help close this gap, I have chosen the period from 1890 to 1930 as a frame for my work. This was the time when occupational therapy began to take shape as a profession; when individual women worked with those in need, used occupations to raise morale and self-esteem, and taught skills for daily living; and when a cohesive discipline emerged from the work done by these women scattered across the country. It was also a time of many concrete achievements, when the first training programs, professional associations, university-based educational program, and professional journal were established.

The years from 1890 to 1930 marked a time of great change in Canadian society with new approaches to social reform, the movement of populations to new locations, high levels of immigration, political upheaval brought on by a world war, a greatly increased number of injured young men, and, perhaps most significantly for the purposes of this book, a changing role for women. All of these factors played a part in the emergence of the new profession of occupational therapy in Canada.

HISTORIOGRAPHY

Internationally, the history of occupational therapy is defined by a fairly circumscribed world. Three major books have been written in English: one for the United Kingdom, one for the United States, and one for Australia. The most ambitious work is the two-volume UK history by Ann Wilcock, *Occupation for Health*, published in 2001–02.[1] It is a comprehensive intellectual history, covering a very wide period, and many of the references to the philosophical underpinnings of the profession have a broad application. However, the focus is on the history of the profession in the United Kingdom, and there are few direct references to Canada. The American book by Virginia Metaxis Quiroga, *Occupational Therapy:*

The First 30 Years, 1900–1930, was published in 1995.[2] It covers much the same ground as my book but refers only to the United States. For example, it mentions Thomas Kidner (the vocational secretary to the Military Hospitals Commission of Canada in World War I) but only in connection with his role as a founding member of the American Occupational Therapy Association and his activities after he left Canada. Yet it was the work that Kidner did in Canada that prepared him for the contributions he would make in the United States. As occupational therapy in Australia was only established after World War II, Anderson's *Occupational Therapy: Its Place in Australia's History* does not add to our understanding of the formative period of interest here in Canada.

A number of articles on the history occupational therapy in Canada have appeared in the *Canadian Journal of Occupational Therapy* from time to time,[3] and the national practice magazine, OT *Now*, published a series of historical articles to celebrate the seventy-fifth and eighty-fifth anniversaries of the Canadian Association of Occupational Therapists. A column entitled "OT Then" was a feature in the practice magazine designed to encourage interest in history,[4] and some articles that refer to the history of Canadian occupational therapy have been published elsewhere.[5] However, all of these articles have been stand-alone pieces. No publication has integrated the parts to provide a comprehensive whole.

Although there have been no professional histories of occupational therapy in Canada, many professional histories intersect with that of occupational therapy. For example, the considerable body of work that examines "the allied health professions" provides an important context for my work. However, occupational therapy's place within allied health has not been adequately taken into account, in part because its contributions are not yet fully known. Thus, the material in this book will complement the histories of allied health professions such as nursing, social work, vocational rehabilitation, and physical therapy.[6]

The growing literature on women's professions describes and analyses many of the issues that influenced women at this time.[7] Here, too, the story of the women who entered into occupational therapy complements existing perspectives. Many of the women who became occupational therapists were artistic, enjoyed the creative process, and liked to teach. They wanted to help those who were disadvantaged by poverty, illness, or disability to become productive members of society. However, their stories, most of which have never been told before, are unique to occupational therapy and help to expand the broader narrative on women entering into professions. The role played by male physicians in the development of occupational therapy, which was then – and remains – a largely female profession, is of interest in the context of health professions in general.[8]

Much has been written on the plight of the injured soldier, the treatment received, and the outcomes of various interventions. Work in the field of disability studies informs this literature and sheds light on the difficulties of helping soldiers take up useful lives after World War I. With the most prevalent prior experience of work with "crippled children" being of little relevance for these young men, society was desperate to find new approaches to treatment.[9] One of these approaches was that provided by the ward aides (as occupational therapists were originally known).

Another professional history that intersects with occupational therapy is that of education. The experience of establishing a female profession within a university-based program offers insights into the workings of academia at the time. The roles played by men in facilitating the entry of the program into the university and overseeing its implementation shed light on this phase of women's development. That the program found a place at the University of Toronto in 1926 is itself of interest. The content of the curriculum reflected, in some measure, the lives of women of the day; it was concerned with caring, understanding human development, illness, fostering the skills then needed for everyday living, and craftwork. This content was not the usual fare to be found within the more common – and more highly regarded – liberal arts education of the day.

This book explores the issues and events that called forth occupational therapy as a response from society, and from women in particular, to illness and other difficult circumstances. It asks a number of questions: Why did occupational therapy come about when it did? What prompted an increased sense of societal responsibility for people living in poverty or with illness and disability? What made it more acceptable for women to pursue careers in general and in occupational therapy in particular? Who were the women who were drawn to this fledgling profession? What helped or hindered the profession's growth and development?

As the first book to examine the early history of occupational therapy in Canada, this work focuses on "recovering history."[10] Perspectives (e.g., feminist) that might have shed more light on particular issues have only been hinted at, and there is a place for professional historians to apply a particular theoretical lens to the analysis and interpretation of the material in the future.

SOURCES

Primary sources have come from various collections, including Library and Archives Canada, the Archives of the Canadian Association of Occupational Therapists, the Archives of the American Occupational Therapy Association, and provincial, municipal, and university archives across the country. News clippings, articles, and books that deal with the period helped provide context for matters such as the place of women, the development of allied health professions, and the progress of health care.

A valuable source of primary information has been the families of several of the people about whom I have written. While tracking down relatives and asking them to dig deep for memories of or connections with deceased family members and hunt for relevant material has been difficult, gathering these private family papers and artifacts has been most rewarding in terms of both the information found and the relationships forged.

I encountered great difficulty when I used finding aids in collections not directly related to occupational therapy. Rarely is the term "occupational therapy" used in those collections. Neither are the names of people important to this profession readily found. In part, this is because many of the people involved directly in the work – especially the women and their families – did not think enough of it (or of their role in it) to preserve any records they may have had. The work has been made even harder because in those days a woman always changed her name upon marriage. This difficulty in uncovering records for women is not new or unique to occupational therapy. For example, the historians Ruby Heap and Meryn Stuart found it necessary to explore a wide array of primary sources and to re-examine many conventional sources to find pertinent information on nursing and physiotherapy in Canada at a similar period.[11] As with any research of this type, the records that do exist must be considered in light of why they were made, who made them, and who preserved them.

There are, of course, limitations to the work I have produced. I knew from the outset that I would have to limit the content of the book in order to make any contribution at all. I naively thought I was doing that by restricting the period of interest, but even so, many aspects of the profession have been left unexplored, as have many parts of the country. In particular, I have told almost nothing of the origins of occupational therapy in French Canada. My excuse here is straightforward: my language skills are regrettably not up to the task. Further, the structure for occupational therapy in French Canada was not set until almost the end of the period of my focus (e.g., the founding in 1928 of the Quebec Society of Occupational Therapy). But best of all, I have francophone colleagues (Elisabeth Dutil and Francine Ferland) who are telling that story (at least for Quebec) and will do a much better job of it than I could possibly do.[12]

ORGANIZATION OF THE BOOK

This book unfolds within three broad sections and over fifteen chapters. Part 1 sets out the context within which the story is told. It also reflects what I see as the major premise of occupational therapy and therefore the basic unit of interest – that is, mental health and the connection between engagement in occupations and well-being. The idea of using occupations to raise morale, build self-esteem, and develop skills lies at the heart of occupational therapy. And this idea was rooted in the moral treatment era and developed with the mental hygiene movement. Three chapters delineate the other movements that directly influenced the profession: the settlement house movement, with its efforts to help immigrant and poor populations improve their lot; the arts and crafts movement, with its celebration of art and the making of objects to nourish the soul; and educational reform, which stressed manual training and its role in learning through doing. The last chapter in this section describes the work of three women who took on occupational therapy–like roles prior to the World War I: Jessie Luther at the Grenfell Mission in Newfoundland and Labrador; Alice Peck of the Canadian Handicrafts Guild in Montreal, Quebec; and the almost anonymous "Miss Scott" at the Homewood Asylum in Guelph, Ontario.

Part 2 centres on the war and the use of occupations to treat injured soldiers. World War I is seen as the signal event that led to the beginnings of occupational therapy as a profession in Canada. The rationale for occupations as treatment during World War I becomes defined: to support injured soldiers through the lengthy period of their convalescence and to begin to prepare them for an eventual return to work. It is in this work that the psychological, social, artistic, and educational influences of the movements described in the first section of the book begin to coalesce. The program for retraining injured soldiers started with the work done by ward aides (as occupational therapists were then called) at the bedside and in the workshop. Their primary role was to "rehabilitate the spirit," to bring hope to men who had lived through the horrors of war and seen their lives changed. Chapter 8 describes the work of three women who worked as ward aides in the early years of the war: Ina Matthews, who helped design the soldiers' retraining program that the federal government adopted; Cybel Lighthall, a former kindergarten teacher who supervised other ward aides in Montreal; and Hilda Goodman, a handicrafts teacher in Alberta. A new phase of the ward aides' work came with the increased number of wounded returning to Canada and the decision to train and pay women specifically for this role. Chapter 9 describes the training courses established at the University of Toronto and McGill University, while chapter 10 tells the stories of a number of graduates from those courses.

Part 3 deals with the formalization of the profession. Chapter 11 heralds the beginnings of occupational therapy as a profession and deals with the work of organizing provincial societies and establishing curative workshops, a national association, and a professional journal. Establishing the educational program at the University of Toronto in 1926 is the focus of chapter 12. This chapter also includes a section on Helen LeVesconte, a graduate of the first diploma program who was to be a major force in the profession for the next forty years. The role of several male supporters of the profession is discussed in chapter 13. These men (Dr Alexander Primrose, Sir Robert Falconer, Thomas Bessell Kidner, and Dr Goldwin Howland) were keen enthusiasts and, given their social status, able to promote the work of occupational therapists in important circles. Implications of their volunteer role are analysed in terms of their influence on the leadership of the profession and the effect of that role on the membership. Chapter 14 examines the conceptual conflicts that were evident from the beginnings of the profession (e.g., between the vocational idea and the medical model) and considers the relationships between occupational therapy and other disciplines such as nursing, social work, and physical therapy. Chapter 15 first focuses on the values that have endured since the profession began and then considers some of the challenges and opportunities that face the profession in the twenty-first century.

Looking back over the century that has passed since what was to become occupational therapy began to emerge, one sees many significant changes. While occupational therapy was shaped initially as a gendered profession, men have taken their place and helped broaden the profession, if – regretfully – remaining a small minority. Populated at first by middle-class women who worked for the public good, occupational therapy is now diverse in terms of its members' racial and ethnic background and socio-economic composition. Meanwhile, war is still with us, and the soldiers returning from Afghanistan face many of the same issues as those injured in World War I. There remains a need to raise morale, build self-esteem, and teach skills to these soldiers, to new immigrants, to the homeless, and to those with illness and disability. There also remains a need to convince society of the significance of engagement in occupations for health and well-being.

PART ONE

Context and Foundations

Social and Political Context

POPULATION

In the 1890s, Canada was still a young country. Seven provinces (Ontario, Quebec, Nova Scotia, New Brunswick, Manitoba, Prince Edward Island, and British Columbia) and the Northwest Territories had joined Confederation by that time, with Yukon joining in 1898 and Saskatchewan and Alberta in 1905. The total population of Canada was just under five million. Ontario and Quebec were the most populated provinces, followed by Nova Scotia, New Brunswick, and Manitoba.[1] Until 1911, those of British ancestry made up 55.5 per cent of Canada's population. "Other European" comprised 41.7 per cent, with two-thirds of this group being French; the Asian population was 0.6 per cent; and "Other" was 2.2 per cent.[2] Immigration was high, the number doubling roughly every three years between 1896 and 1907. As the Victorian era drew to a close, Canada remained deeply tied to Great Britain, retaining many of its customs and traditions. While Canada managed its own internal affairs, it was under the control of Great Britain for all of its external dealings. This fact would become very meaningful with the outbreak of World War I and Canada's immediate involvement owing to its status as a British colony.

Canada also had close relations with the United States, and people and ideas moved freely across the border between the two countries. Communication was primarily by surface mail or telegram, and travel was by train and measured in days. By the 1890s, hydroelectric power had been harnessed at Niagara Falls for almost a decade, the gold rush was about to end, and what was soon to be the Ford Motor Company had produced its first car. The West was a great expanse of agricultural production, and mining and forestry were growing rapidly. From that largely agricultural base, the country was beginning to shift to a more urban society. Although 68 per cent of the population was rural and 32 per cent urban in 1891, the proportions became equal by 1921.[3]

SOCIAL CONDITIONS, POVERTY, AND UNEMPLOYMENT

Poverty was widespread in Canada, especially in the cities. Emigration from the United Kingdom and Europe was successful for some but resulted in poverty for many. Indeed, emigration to the "colony" of Canada was considered a solution to problems in countries like England where assisted-immigrant programs paid for the removal of their poorer citizens, including children.[4] In the early 1900s, large numbers of immigrants from eastern Europe began to arrive. They came with hopes of a better life, but many encountered difficulties finding work. Unemployment compounded the problems of adjusting to the customs of a new country and learning its language.

There was also unemployment among Canadians who moved from rural areas to the cities, believing they could easily exchange farm work for factory work. However, the industrial revolution had created a surplus of workers in the cities, and unemployment increased accordingly. Poverty meant poor housing and overcrowding, conditions that bred illness, disease, and injury. Slum areas expanded in the cities, and homelessness was common. Residents in these areas needed help just to exist. They needed to learn new skills to improve their lot.

In Canada's cities – as elsewhere in the Western world where the industrial age had taken hold – factory workers worked long hours at boring tasks under dreadful conditions. Work was often mechanical and repetitive with little connection to the end product. Workers were paid according to the number of items produced, not on the basis of an hourly wage. The pay was not enough to sustain families, and some women entered the workforce to supplement their husband's income. Factories looking for cheap sources of labour found it among women, children, migrants from rural areas, and immigrants.[5]

It came to be recognized that more than just the means of production had changed, and a certain longing and malaise set in. People felt they had lost touch with the natural environment, which had grounded them previously, and felt that their souls had suffered in the process. The arts and crafts movement had made its way from the United Kingdom to North America and was seen as an antidote to the negative changes brought about by the industrial revolution (see chapter 3). Activities that could help people reconnect spiritually with themselves and with the environment became popular; horticulture and pottery were seen as particularly beneficial, as these activities helped people to reconnect with nature through the very earth itself.

Throughout Canada, craftwork held a special place: not only could it provide some of the necessities of daily life (e.g., weaving homespun or sewing for the family's clothing), but it might even turn a profit. Handcrafted articles were prized and exhibited at competitions across the country. Articles made by Native people were gathered up and brought to market by groups like the Women's Art Association of Canada (WAAC).

According to the philosophy expounded by the arts and crafts movement, craftwork was uplifting to the spirit and could ameliorate stress. There was an idea that health and art or creativity were somehow connected and that using one's hands had healing properties.[6] Within a few decades, Canadian occupational therapists would take up the idea that the connection of mind and hand in activity could improve mental and physical health.[7]

There was a growing awareness that unsuitable employment could affect health and frequent unemployment resulted in stress. Craft and labour unions were becoming established, and more attention was being paid to working conditions and injuries sustained at work.

ILLNESS AND HEALTH CARE

There were no standards for clean water in the 1890s, and proper sanitation existed only for the wealthy. Public health measures were just being introduced to deal with sewage, sanitation, and the sterilization of milk. Women were expected to keep their homes clean and free of disease. Conversely, the appearance of illness and disease was seen as the result of a woman's negligence in maintaining her home.[8] Lack of clean water meant that epidemics of typhoid or cholera were always threatening. Smallpox remained a major concern, with Montreal experiencing a major outbreak in 1885. Other threats to health included scarlet fever, measles, whooping cough, and diphtheria. Diphtheria alone was responsible for the deaths of thirty-six thousand children in Ontario between 1880 and 1929.[9]

The discovery of the germ theory of disease came in the 1860s, but infection still killed until the discovery of penicillin almost six decades later. Venereal disease was prevalent and incurable until 1908, when a drug to treat syphilis was discovered. The use of this drug soon became widespread despite public concern that a cure for the disease would foster sexual promiscuity. The new treatment for syphilis opened the door to the development of antibiotics and the discovery of penicillin in 1928.[10] With these medical breakthroughs yet to come, many of those who were physically ill were considered incurable.

Tuberculosis (TB) was the primary cause of adult death in Canada as in much of the world. The bacterial cause of TB was discovered in 1882; however, the first effective treatment for the disease did not come until 1944. Until then, those with TB could only be treated with rest and fresh air. As the work of occupational therapists became known, graded activities were introduced, bringing functional improvement and hope to those having to endure a lengthy convalescence.

There was concern over appropriate treatment and care for those who were blind, deaf, or in some way "crippled." However, for the most part, these individuals were hidden away and considered unable to lead productive lives.

While the science of medicine progressed and was marked by many important discoveries, the "art" of medicine was being established by the great Canadian physician Sir William Osler.[11] From McGill University, where he had been head pathologist, Osler moved to the United States to take up posts at the University of Pennsylvania and Johns Hopkins. Osler soon gained pre-eminence as a healer and as a leader in medical education worldwide. Banting and Best, along with Macleod and Collip, developed insulin to treat diabetes in 1921, and Canada's pioneering reputation in health care grew along with its pride.[12]

Hospitals gradually appeared across the country. From a time when people with means chose to be treated at home and only the poor were seen in hospitals, the situation began to reverse itself. Not-for-profit groups, including government and religious organizations, established hospitals, and their number grew such that there were some fifty hospitals in Ontario by 1900. Those who were able to pay, like the urban middle class, were charged fees for health care.[13] Amounts were set to accommodate the patient's ability to pay for varying degrees of luxury.

Asylums were built to house people with mental illness, although, once admitted, patients often stayed for the remainder of their lives. Many who were not mentally ill were also placed in asylums as a means of removing them from the family home or from other institutions. Thus, asylum residents might include the poor, criminals, and those termed "imbeciles," alongside those with mental illness. Though housed in buildings that were architecturally beautiful, patients were often physically restrained. They were left untreated except, perhaps, with alcohol as a sedative or with an assortment of surgical experiments, the latter used particularly with women.[14] For the most part, patients remained isolated and idle and left to suffer. Some medical superintendents, familiar with the ideas of the moral treatment era that had been popular earlier in the nineteenth century, realized that when their patients were engaged in occupations, the use of restraints could be decreased or even eliminated.[15] The occupations often came in the form of work that was of use to the institution. The mental hygiene movement (see chapter 2), established early in the twentieth century, brought important changes in the approach to the treatment of those suffering from mental illness. Occupational therapists were to play a key role in the new treatment regime.[16]

The health of people in rural areas was of great concern, as medical care for them was generally lacking. One attempt to deal with the situation was made in Newfoundland in 1893 when Dr Wilfred Grenfell established a medical mission at St Anthony. He took his hospital ship along the coast of Newfoundland and Labrador, and while providing medical help, he also attended to economic problems that enabled diseases like tuberculosis to flourish.[17] In 1906, he brought Jessie Luther (later to be considered an occupational therapist) to the mission so that she could help members of these communities develop skills to enhance their productivity.[18] Appreciating the link between economic conditions and health at both the community and the individual level was an important step toward prevention; however, then as now, the approach was not widely supported.

HELPING THE SICK AND THE POOR

As the state did little for the welfare of its citizens, care for those who were poor or ill was left to members of religious groups who saw the need to preach a more relevant social message. Christian teachings turned to a "social gospel," which promoted the importance of working to build the Kingdom of God on earth through reforms that would bring social justice for all.[19] The movement was seen by some more as a reaction against prevailing political views that seemed to favour more individualistic behaviours than as an ideology of its own.

The central belief of the social gospel movement was that God's work was in social change. This belief was in some measure a response to the evils of industrial capitalism as well as a reaction to the role of the church and the clergy in dealing with social issues of the day.[20] The movement was influential in Canada from the 1890s to the 1930s, taking on a variety of issues affecting the working classes, such as the increasing urbanization of the population, industrialization, and immigration. It became well established in the cities, where it tried to address problems through collective social action. It contributed to the establishment of several church-run settlement houses and city missions.[21] Protestant clergy tried to promote social justice for the poor but found themselves in competition with the Roman Catholic Church, which was more popular with immigrant groups. Jewish groups, newly immigrated and relatively small in number, cared for their sick, their orphans and elderly, and ultimately their dead. Their charitable acts were seen in the context of justice and righteousness, with the acts most highly thought of being those that enabled a recipient to become self-reliant.[22]

The settlement house movement began in London, England, with the establishment of Toynbee Hall in 1884, flourished at Hull House in Chicago, and was soon found in Canada. Settlement houses – similar to modern-day community centres – were established by concerned groups to address social problems resulting from poverty, industrial expansion, poor living conditions, and the growing number of immigrants (see chapter 4). They provided a place for people to gather and attend classes in an environment where those who were helping and those who were being helped were meant to learn from one another. Settlement house ideology promoted the idea that rather than giving alms to the poor, society should provide friendship and opportunities for learning.[23]

THE NEED FOR SOCIAL CHANGE

By the end of the nineteenth century, it was becoming clear that political action needed to be taken to address social concerns. Political activists sought reforms that would provide ethical and effective governance, and would address poverty, disease, and illiteracy. The Liberals, who had come to power in 1896 with Wilfrid Laurier as prime minister, created a department of labour, signifying some acceptance of the need for oversight in the welfare of workers.[24] Socialist ideology, which claimed its relevance to many issues, including poverty and unemployment, was present in Canada but was not strong. The Social Democratic Party of Canada was founded in 1911, but social welfare policies were a long way off. Ideas of reform became secondary as a worldwide economic depression took hold in 1912. Although World War I initially exacerbated Canada's financial situation, exports of wheat, timber, and munitions soon contributed to economic growth and stability.[25]

Everyone saw the need for change, but they saw it for different reasons: religious groups sought social justice as a component of their faith; businessmen thought social justice would improve the economy; and the working class and ethnic minorities thought it would make for a better life. Many citizens were ready to take matters into their own hands and did not want to wait for government.[26] With no ideas about what a social safety net might look like, people recognized nonetheless that illness and poverty could no longer be ignored. Not only was it their moral obligation to be their brother's keeper, but it was also to their advantage to control conditions that ultimately threatened everyone's health and well-being.

The politics of the progressive era in the United States brought an enthusiasm for reform and social justice that was also apparent in Canada. Journalists drew attention to the various social ills they saw, and vocal groups of middle-class Canadians sought wide-ranging reforms. They advocated changes across a host of conditions: in city government; in child labour laws; for sewage and sanitation; for housing, parks, and schools; and for the suppression of prostitution and illegal alcohol sales.[27]

One "solution" to the social ills that plagued Canada was offered by the supporters of the eugenics movement. Mendel's discovery of the laws of heredity in the middle of the nineteenth century and Galton's ideas of social Darwinism and the "survival of the fittest" had prepared the way for a "scientific" response.[28] The eugenics movement sought to rid the country of most of its ills – poverty, crime, alcoholism, prostitution, and mental illness. The "unfit" would be prevented from entering the country and those already here could be prevented from reproducing through enforced sterilization.[29] A more subtle solution to the perceived ills in society – the "Canadianization" of the immigrant population – became a focus of voluntary groups, including the Imperial Order of the Daughters of the Empire (IODE).

The educational system was also undergoing a profound change during this time. People were beginning to question the results of schooling and to consider changing their methods. Reformers in Europe and North America asked if there were better ways for children to learn than solely through books and by rote. John Dewey (1859–1952), an American philosopher and educator, advanced the concept that learning by doing was superior to rote learning and that the hand and the head must work together.[30] Courses in manual training were a practical expression of his pragmatist philosophy.

Children from kindergarten onwards were to be given creative and artistic tasks. Craftwork was thought to lead to disciplined coordination of hand and eye, accuracy, clarity of thought, and industriousness – all of which were integral to learning. Thomas Bessell Kidner was brought from England in 1900 to develop manual training programs in Nova Scotia, and he later became a key figure in the development of occupational therapy first in Canada and then in the United States.[31] Much of the new philosophy of education, with its emphasis on manual training, became incorporated in programs that occupational therapists offered to injured soldiers during World War I.

WOMEN'S ROLES

Around the turn of the twentieth century, role expectations for Canadian women varied greatly according to class and marital status. Wives of men successful in business, politics, or the professions were expected to become members of philanthropic organizations such as the IODE.[32] Married women who were less financially secure worked to augment the income of their households, often taking in boarders or making and selling hand-crafted items.[33] When single women did go out to work, they earned lower pay than men, especially for jobs that were considered "women's work," such as cleaning.[34] In 1911, women made up 13 per cent of the total paid labour force, their primary employment being in what the census termed "personal and recreational services" – which meant domestic service, primarily. The next most popular work for women was in retail and wholesale trade (textiles and clothing), followed by education and health and welfare services.[35] In these latter two categories, women outnumbered the men. Women were more likely to enter the paid labour force if they lived in urban centres such as Toronto and Montreal. Women who lacked formal education or did not speak English well tended to work in factories.

Domestic service was considered respectable work for women because it was carried out in a family setting and prepared a woman to become a housewife.[36] Teaching was also a large employer of women, but it was not highly respected at the time. Girls and young women might work for families, helping with the care of children and being responsible for some of their education. Teaching was seen as a stage in life prior to marriage; a girl might live at home and teach in the local school, or she might move from school to school and board with local families, before eventually marrying and having her own children.[37] Still other women worked at jobs that involved the protection of women; for example, they served as police officers on "morality squads," with the purpose of protecting single women workers – especially women factory workers.[38]

During World War I, women were hired to make munitions and were better paid than women in traditionally female jobs, but their pay was still 20–30 per cent lower than a man's for the same work.[39] They also worked in other traditionally male-dominated domains – in offices and banks and in the transportation sector – taking on jobs that they would generally be forced to give up when the war ended and the men returned home.[40] While the patterns of employment and the numbers of women employed changed during World War I, the changes did not last and women would not work outside the home in great numbers for decades yet to come. Many women felt unfulfilled; they yearned to be more involved in the wider world and to be challenged. Existing employment options were no longer adequate.

In these years, women were seen as morally superior to men. This assumption helped them to enter the public arena but only in certain areas. The idea was that they would bring to society what they brought to their own homes. Middle- and upper-class women were expected to do good works as purveyors of culture, as educators, and as fundraisers. Women's organizations also became involved with the direct, hands-on care of those in need. Class generally determined which women would find new roles as rescuers or reformers and which would be the objects of philanthropic concern.[41]

It was thought that social activism came to women in their role as housekeepers of society and also as part of their religious faith. Conversely, they were not welcome in broader political circles because the political environment was thought to be morally degrading. The Women's Christian Temperance Union (the WCTU), established in Owen Sound, Ontario, in 1874, was an example of that unworkable arrangement. It lobbied on moral grounds to prohibit alcohol, but realizing that it could not change the law without women having the ability to vote, it soon became a base for the suffragist movement and greater equity for women in general.

The right to vote was both a federal and a provincial matter. After much lobbying, female citizens aged twenty-one and over finally became eligible to vote federally in 1918. The right to vote provincially was given to women in Nova Scotia, New Brunswick, and Prince Edward Island soon thereafter. However, other provinces lagged behind considerably on this issue, with Quebec not achieving suffrage until 1940. Similarly, women were given the right to stand for office federally and provincially at different times, with their appointment to the Senate not being permitted until after the *Persons* case of 1929.[42] Although it was recognized that democratic principles were involved, the strongest support for women's suffrage was thought to have come from their exemplary work during the war.

In 1893, the National Council of Women of Canada (NCWC) was formed with the express purpose of denouncing liquor, divorce, prostitution, profiteering, and self-indulgence. The council also had issues specific to women; for example, it raised concerns about the age of consent and about their working hours, safety, and overall health. By 1895, all major urban centres had a local council that was a collaborative association of local societies. The NCWC then became an "association of associations," offering a political and social network of women across Canada, inclusive of many groups.[43]

Another women's group founded in this same period was to have a very direct connection to occupational therapy within a few decades. The Women's Art Association of Canada, established in 1896, was dedicated to supporting female artists. The Canadian Handicrafts Guild (CHG) formed in 1905 as an offshoot of the Montreal Branch of the WAAC. Combining social welfare concerns with artistic interests, the CHG focused on celebrating and preserving the arts and crafts of immigrant and Native Canadians and promoting home industries as a means of enabling women to contribute. Their goal of helping people to help themselves was congruent with the emerging ideas about the role of occupational therapy.[44]

The years from 1890 to 1930 are now thought to be within the period referred to as first-wave feminism. It was a time of considerable ambiguity and confusion for the women most directly involved. Most women saw their goal as doing better with what existed rather than as initiating a new social order; that is, they wanted reform, not revolution.[45] Women wanted to be separate but equal. Some were concerned that if they had equal opportunity – to jobs, for example – they might become the same as men and unable to celebrate their difference. Meanwhile, the Catholic Church continued to pressure women to remain in their roles as wives and mothers. Some physicians voiced concern for women's physical frailty lest they try to do too much.[46]

Women began to attend university and earn degrees, first at Mount Allison, in New Brunswick, in 1872.[47] Few women were prepared to challenge the system by attempting to enter the new professions of medicine or law; most middle-class women entered the fields of teaching, nursing, or some form of social service, professions that were considered more appropriate for women and supportive of what was thought to be their ultimate role of wife and mother.[48] Many women trained at "normal school" (later to be known as "teachers' college"), while others enrolled in art colleges both in Canada and in the United States. Nursing training in Canada was first established in St Catharine's, Ontario, at the General and Marine Hospital in 1874.[49] Before long, nurses were expected to take on a variety of helping roles in addition to providing direct patient care. They assumed roles that resembled what would soon be known as "social work," and they also provided occupations and gave massages, activities that would eventually be identified with occupational therapy and physical therapy, respectively.

By the early years of the twentieth century, middle-class women had become more than ready to take on more challenging roles. Charitable and philanthropic work had given them leadership skills, and their formal and informal routes to education had further prepared them. By the time of World War I, they had the confidence and the skills to venture into the new areas that were suddenly open to them. Society desperately needed their contributions and they were ready.

Within this background and context, the three social movements referred to – the mental hygiene movement, the arts and crafts movement, and the settlement house movement – set the scene for the development of occupational therapy. Each movement employed occupations in some way to address individual, community, and societal needs. Concepts drawn from these movements, along with the new philosophy driving education reform, combined to develop the interventions used in early occupational therapy.

2

Mental Illness and Mental Hygiene

Undoubtedly occupation adapted to the habits and condition of the patient is the most valuable of all curative agents.

Dr Maurice Bucke, London Asylum, 1889[1]

FIRST PREMISES: OCCUPATIONS AND MENTAL HEALTH

The beginnings of occupational therapy are most clearly seen in treatments for mental illness. Occupations have been provided for those with mental illness for centuries. From biblical times to the present, being engaged in some form of activity has been found to be helpful. However, not all of the reasons for providing occupations were altruistic. Occupations were used to control patients' behaviour or, through the patients' labour, to benefit the institution financially. Only occasionally were they used as a direct form of treatment for the individual.

OCCUPATIONS TO CONTROL PATIENTS' BEHAVIOUR

It was apparent to many of those responsible for the care of people with mental illness that when patients were engaged in an activity, their behaviour was more easily controlled. Physical and chemical restraints could be reduced or even eliminated if patients were kept occupied. That was the simple and expedient reason for providing activities – often in the form of work – to "mental" patients in the nineteenth and early twentieth centuries.

The idea that mental patients could be more easily managed if kept occupied first took hold during the moral treatment era, which extended from about 1792 to 1850. This benevolent regime – first described by the psychiatrist Philippe Pinel at the Bicêtre and Salpêtrière hospitals in Paris in 1795 and by the Tuke family at their retreat in York, England, at the very same time (but unknown to one another) – is considered a signal event in the history of treatment for those with mental illness. Pinel's approach took a scientific direction and included careful histories and observations of the patients, while the Tuke family, who were Quakers, used moral treatment because they thought it humane and it met their religious values.[2]

Bockoven explains that the term "moral" in the name of the movement was not laden with modern-day meanings but referred instead to emotional or psychological factors. Within that perspective, there were four meanings attached to the idea of moral treatment: the first dealt with "morale" and the need for treatment to instil hope and confidence; the second, with a way of living that could bring a sense of order that was otherwise lacking; the third, with the idea that those who were mentally ill were not responsible for their acts and therefore warranted assistance; and the fourth, with the idea that it was right for those who were more fortunate to provide compassionate and understanding treatment – even to those whose illness might be considered wilful.[3] Although the movement did not last much beyond the middle of the nineteenth century, its philosophy has continued to inspire. Indeed, many would consider the moral treatment era to be the major influence on the development of occupational therapy.

The philosophy of moral treatment was given expression at the Toronto Lunatic Asylum by Dr Joseph Workman (1805–1894), who had been appointed as the first medical superintendent in 1854. Workman advocated kindness, was against restraints, and provided occupations in the form of work, employing large numbers of patients in agricultural work on the grounds.[4] In his effort to provide a caring environment in the asylum, Workman regularly spent time talking with patients on the wards in the evening, finding some topic of interest to divert them from their morbid thoughts.

This new humanitarian approach was in great contrast to the oppressive conditions generally found in asylums at the time. Not only was patients' behaviour difficult to control in these asylums, but the behaviour of the staff in charge had also become an issue. Now, a caring attitude replaced the otherwise harsh and punitive treatment generally given to those living in insane asylums. Friendship was offered; time was managed and filled with activity.[5]

By the late 1800s, occupations were being used in many asylums in Canada to a greater or lesser degree. They were a major component of daily life at the London Insane Asylum, where Dr Maurice Bucke was superintendent. His regime, which extended from 1877 to 1902 and saw an increase in the use of occupations and a decrease in the use of physical restraints, became something of a model.[6] Bucke had not seen the harm in mechanical restraints when he first began work at the asylum. However, after visiting institutions in the United States that practised non-restraint, his views began to change. In his report for 1884, he comments, "It is not simply that we have disused mechanical restraint and seclusion, but we have revolutionized at the same time the whole morale of the institution, the disuse of restraint and seclusion being only a small part of the revolution. The central element in the change to which I refer is undoubtedly the employment of the patients."[7]

In his report for 1885, Bucke notes that of the 1,018 patients in residence at the time, an average of more than eight hundred were employed each day at some kind of useful labour. While he thought that amusement, proper feeding, and "medical treatment" by drugs were all beneficial, he found occupation the most valuable of curative agents.[8] Included among the activities provided at the London Asylum were work on the premises, workshop activities, opportunities for music and dance, and sports. Bucke's use of the social environment as a means of raising morale extended to employing a female attendant in a male ward for the first time in 1883. In his report for that year, he notes, "[S]ince this lady's coming to the Asylum, a greater tidiness in person, a greater activity in employment, and a general brightening of the condition of those in the male wards is perceptible."[9] The changes Bucke made were prompted not only by his growing awareness of reforms in the treatment of mental illness, but also by his own spiritual awakening and the very strong influence on him of his friend and mentor, the American poet and philosopher Walt Whitman.[10]

Another physician who valued the therapeutic use of occupations was Dr C.K. Clarke, the medical superintendent of Rockwood Asylum in Kingston, Ontario.[11] Clarke had been influenced by Joseph Workman, who had employed him as a clinical assistant in 1874 when he was only seventeen and who had later taught him when he was a medical student.[12] Clarke brought Workman's treatment philosophy with him to his work at Rockwood in 1885 and also followed the example set by Bucke at the London Asylum. He established a myriad of crafts and other occupations, including music and drama. One short-lived but highly successful venture was brush making. In an early example of a sheltered workshop, the brush-making enterprise employed about twenty patients and realized a profit. However, labour groups complained, and the operation was soon shut down by the inspector of asylums.[13]

Whether it was because of the occupations themselves or because of their ability to reduce the need for physical restraints, Clarke became a strong proponent of occupations. Looking back on his time at Rockwood, he recalled, "No one comforted himself with the belief that occupation was a panacea for all the ills that the mind is heir to, but we did realize that intelligently supervised occupation was a tremendous factor not only in aiding cure in recent cases, but in making happy and improving the most unfortunate class in our community."[14]

Clarke advocated the use of occupations to academic audiences abroad as well as at home. In his Maudsley Lecture in London, England, in 1923, he reported that occupational therapy was not only a substitute for restraint but also a "promising addition to the routine treatment of some acute and many chronic cases of mental disease. The results were striking and nearly every patient at Rockwood was occupied daily."[15] Not only were occupations being seen as the best option for managing patients' behaviour, they were now being considered as a unique form of treatment.

Asylums, such as the ones in London and Kingston, were meant to be places of refuge where patients could be protected while they recovered. They were to have decent living conditions in keeping with the "asylum movement" begun by the American Dorothea Dix (1802–1887).[16] Built on the Kirkbride plan, asylums were intended to be therapeutic by design, situated on large tracts of land and offering good light, adequate air, and space for workshops.[17] Dix had been something of a catalyst in the building of several asylums in what would become Canada, including one in New Brunswick in 1855 and one in Nova Scotia in 1857.[18]

While the asylum movement had the best of intentions, before long asylums were severely overcrowded and once again custodial care was all that could be managed. Conditions deteriorated and the ideas of moral treatment began to erode. Some modern critics, such as Michel Foucault, have argued that so-called moral treatment was itself a punishing form of control meant to bring patients to a point of weakness where they would admit to madness.[19] A recent analysis by Charland stresses the fact that

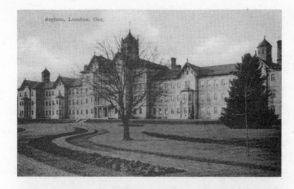

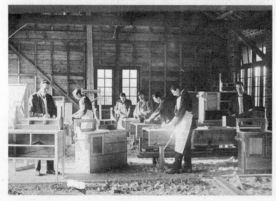

ABOVE London Asylum, c. 1900, where Dr R.M. Bucke established the widespread use of occupations for patients. In Daniel J. Brock, *Best Wishes from London, Canada*; BELOW Male patients at work in an asylum carpentry shop, c. 1910. Courtesy of Sanofi-Pasteur Limited (Connaught Campus), Toronto.

Tuke's moral treatment was a lay movement with its roots in the Quaker religion. Seeing moral treatment as far from a means of control, he argues that benevolent theory provides an ethical and affective explanation for the success of moral treatment and promotes an acceptance of people with mental illness. Of particular interest for occupational therapy is Charland's discussion of the centrality of self-esteem to moral treatment: in his analysis, occupations that build self-esteem lead to respect for self, which leads to self-restraint and control.[20]

OCCUPATIONS AS WORK

With mental illness (and physical illness) still seen in society as a punishment for wrongdoing, there was a sense that mental patients *should* be doing something. At the root of much of the thinking behind activities for patients in psychiatric facilities was the continuing theme from earliest Greek and Roman times that to not be working – and certainly to be idle – was evil. Not only might the devil have caused the mental illness in the first instance, but to be safe from the devil in the future, one must not be idle. Backing up this thinking were pronouncements from the great Greek physician Hippocrates (460–377 BC), who said, "Idleness and lack of occupation tend – nay are dragged – towards evil." Centuries later, the Roman theologian and religious leader St Jerome (347–420 AD) warned his followers: "Keep doing some kind of work that the devil may always find you employed."

The idea that being engaged in occupations could make reparations for any wrongdoing and provide ongoing protection would have been part of the thinking of nineteenth-century asylum administrators, who saw it as their duty to look after their patients' souls as well as their bodies. The family was a common metaphor for life within asylums, with the superintendant as the father. This image was supported by the fact that the superintendent (and his family) generally lived on the hospital grounds along with the other staff. The superintendent therefore would have felt that it was his responsibility to protect his "family" from the evil brought on by idleness and would want to keep them occupied.

Descriptions of the occupations for mental patients at the turn of the last century suggest that most were in the form of work for the asylum, such as agricultural work on the grounds or cleaning jobs on the wards. These occupations would obviously have defrayed the expenses of the institution. The question of whether the work should be of therapeutic benefit to the patient or of financial benefit to the institution was highly controversial over the decades.

In an early example of work as therapy, the American physician Benjamin Rush (1745–1813) supported a moral treatment approach toward institutionalized patients and emphasized its work-related aspects. He writes, "It has been remarked, that the maniacs of the male sex in all hospitals, who assist in cutting wood, making fires, and digging in a garden, and the females who are employed in washing, ironing, and scrubbing floors, often recover, while persons, whose rank exempts them from performing such services, languish away their lives within the walls of the hospital."[21] The list of activities Rush refers to reflects the (gendered) type of work that needed to be done in an asylum: keeping the institution and its inhabitants warm and clean and tending the grounds. In assigning jobs to patients capable of working, the staff made no explicit attempts to use work to interest the patients or develop their skills. Activities were not selected with a specific patient's treatment needs in mind.

Around the turn of the twentieth century, the use of work as treatment for mental patients was challenged by labour groups who saw their livelihood threatened by this cheap – if not free – labour. There were good grounds for their concerns. In his report for 1893, Clarke described how a group of patients built a new hospital building (Beach Grove, at Rockwood), noting that "the cost of the structure has been reduced and pleasant occupation furnished for many of the inmates."[22] At the Brockville Ontario Hospital for the Insane, some 50–75 per cent of patients were employed at tasks that supported the institution. The medical superintendent, T.J. Moher, justified this practice, saying that no remuneration should be given to patients on the grounds that the institution could not pay patients for their work at a fair rate and to do otherwise would be inappropriate. In an effort to appear more altruistic, Moher noted that paying for the work would make the occupations seem more related to the needs of the institution than to the needs of the patients.[23]

More recently, the rationale for patients' work in asylums has been challenged on the grounds of exploitation. Reaume examined hospital records at the Toronto Hospital for the Insane during the period from 1870 to 1940. He noted that while it was undeniable that the work was beneficial for some patients' self-esteem and gave them a sense of self-worth, the work was often "more intense than any light duties that the architects of moral reform had envisioned."[24] The value of the work was not recognized despite the fact that it clearly benefited the institution.

In his 1835 treatise that supported work as treatment, Rush had pointed out an issue that would haunt mental institutions for more than a century. While it was seen as appropriate for public patients to do work, this was not the case for private patients who paid for their treatment.[25] As the notion of work as treatment took hold, private patients were seen, somewhat ironically, to be disadvantaged; if private patients could not be asked to work, they could not benefit from these presumably restorative activities. Families and friends of private patients became increasingly concerned that their relatives had nothing to do during convalescence and that the prescribed "rest cure" was not enough.[26]

To fill the need for activity, craft-oriented occupations were provided; they were less like work and were more acceptable to this moneyed class of patients. Crafts such as weaving, carpentry, and basketry were introduced into asylums, and special spaces were set aside to house these activities. In addition, as the philosophy of the arts and crafts movement (see chapter 3) became more widely known – that doing things with one's hands promoted health and might have a spiritual healing power – crafts came to be seen as therapeutic.

In addition to the private patients who were not asked to perform work-related occupations, there were also patients whose mental state was such that they could not work for the institution. Yet, their need for occupations was also recognized. In 1912, the American Medico-Psychological Association held a symposium on the diversional occupation of the insane.[27] They noted that it was not difficult to occupy a small – and presumably capable – number of patients who performed routine duties on the ward, on the farm, in the kitchen, or in the laundry. However, it was more difficult to occupy the larger number of patients who were not able to carry on such work and remained "idle, noisy and destructive." For these patients, the answer appeared to lie in diversional occupations – or re-educational classes, as they were also called.[28]

It should be noted that craftwork, like work for the institution, was not without its own problems with respect to potential remuneration for the sale of the crafts. Should the institution recoup the costs of materials? If there were profits to be made, should they go towards defraying hospital expenses or should they go to the patients (private or not) who had made the items?

The term "occupational therapy" was becoming synonymous with "work" in its broadest terms and applicable to almost all patients. By 1919, a magazine article on conditions in various asylums referred to the widespread use of occupations, quoting C.K. Clarke as saying, "You may search Cobourg [Psychiatric Hospital] from top to bottom without finding any such [chronic patients who are vegetating], even the patients in bed are at work. Occupational therapy is no sham here, industry is the gospel preached by every official, and even the introspective patients have their attention diverted from their insane thoughts by all sorts of well-devised methods of treatment."[29] The many virtues of work were celebrated more generally by the Canadian physician Sir William Osler, who considered work the "open sesame to every portal, the great equalizer in the world, the true philosopher's stone, which transmutes all the base metal of humanity into gold."[30]

While providing occupations to those with mental illness was considered the right thing to do and was seen as helpful both in terms of controlling patients' behaviour and contributing financially to the institution, by the early twentieth century it was beginning to be understood that occupations could be used as treatment. There were two suppositions involved: first, that occupations could build confidence and self-esteem, which in turn would enhance the learning of needed skills; and second, that occupations used as diversion would improve one's mental state more generally.

OCCUPATIONS THAT BUILD CONFIDENCE AND SELF-ESTEEM

In the nineteenth century, educators and psychologists examined the role of volition, particularly in relation to the development of the child.[31] In 1910, the workings of "the will" and the role played by successful engagement in occupations more generally were described by Narziss Ach (1871–1946), a noted German psychologist. Ach theorized that the feelings accompanying successful occupation frequently included "a state of pride, of victory, especially when substantial obstacles have been overcome."[32] He described the reaction that accompanies achievement of a goal in the face of obstacles, noting an overflow effect in all areas of life: "The psychological and physiological consequences of success in conjunction with an increase in self-confidence (the awareness 'I can') and independence represent very significant consequent effects of volition: they bring about an increase in overall life-activity."[33]

Ach went on to describe what might now be considered the central mechanism at work in occupational therapy whereby hope is instilled. He said, "[T]hrough the success and through the knowledge that 'I am the cause of this success,' the awareness of ability, i.e., the knowledge that 'I have accomplished this through my volition, I can do this' emerges. After repeated energetic acts of will accompanied by success, one realizes that 'I have the strength, the power, to carry out whatever I will. I can (do) whatever I will.'"[34] In a footnote to this statement, Ach refers to occupational therapy as follows: "It appears that very important information for the therapy of manifold pathological conditions, especially of neuroses, can be found in this consequent effect – a fact that is receiving more and more notice in the so-called occupation therapy."[35]

Decades later, when the Canadian-born psychologist Albert Bandura built his learning theory, he used many of the same principles involving the successful performance of an activity (as well as limited failures) to build the important coping skill of self-efficacy.[36] Researchers in the field of occupational therapy have worked within this same paradigm to establish the significance of successful occupational performance in daily life.[37]

OCCUPATIONS AS DIVERSION

The idea of diversion as treatment recognized the possibility that occupations could be used to change pathological thinking. The value of diverting attention from "insane thoughts" had been described in 1862 by the American physician Edward Jarvis. In his report of a visit to the United

Kingdom, Jarvis explained what he had seen as the benefit of occupations for patients: "[W]hile they are thus engaged, their minds are brought back from their wandering, or down from their exaltations, or raised up from their groveling, to the common level and course, and applied to the active and sober realities of things which their hands more or less effect, and for which they feel some responsibility, and consequently their disturbing emotions are, at least for the time, quieted and easy."[38] He went on to provide a rationale for why occupations could produce such results:

> As no two particles of matter can occupy the same point in space at the same moment, so no two absorbing thoughts or emotions can occupy the mind or heart at the same instant of time. So long then, as those, whose minds are prone to wander in delusions, are engaged in mechanical or other employments, their thoughts must be given exclusively to the conduct and succession of natural events and real processes; and as the mind can not admit or be possessed by both the sane and the insane idea, the insane one must be excluded, and the sane one reign paramount; all the mental powers of the worker which are in action for the moment are sane, and the mental disorder is for the moment, or that succession of moments, suspended.[39]

Until recently, there has been little explanation of how or if this phenomenon occurs. Two major, and somewhat intertwined explanations, have been offered for the two-thoughts hypothesis.

Diversion and Limits on Cognitive Processing

It had been assumed that the brain had a limited amount of "space" for thinking, and that if healthy thoughts – necessitated by the carrying out of an activity – were in place, then there would be no room for unhealthy thoughts, if only for that period of time during which the activity was taking place.[40] As the behaviours needed for the activity became habit, unhealthy thoughts would be kept away. In this way, the balance and rhythm of healthy life would gradually be re-established.[41]

The phenomenon of diversion continued to be of interest a century later within the field of cognitive science, where various dual task paradigms were explored.[42] Current research suggests that engaging in a diversional activity that is appropriately complex requires controlled processing, which, in turn, prevents "mind wandering." Controlled processing is generally associated with the intentional pursuit of a goal, while mind wandering often happens without intention.[43] Tasks that rely heavily on controlled processing leave few working-memory resources available for mind wandering.[44] Experimental evidence confirms that mind wandering increases when a task is well practised, since working memory and the amount of controlled processing are reduced.[45] This explanation underscores the importance of monitoring the complexity of activities used for diversional purposes.[46] The features of an appropriately complex activity for any one individual correspond to the contemporary notion of an experience of "flow," proposed by Csikszentmihalyi.[47]

Whether current theories on mind wandering explain what Jarvis meant a century ago when he described his two-thoughts hypothesis cannot be known. While it can no longer be stated in such simple terms that two thoughts cannot be held at the same time, it is nevertheless still clear that processing is affected when attention is distracted.

Diversion and Psychological Theories of Mental Illness

In the early 1900s, diversional activity was given an important place in Adolf Meyer's psychobiological approach to the treatment of mental illness. Meyer, a prominent psychiatrist and often considered the father of occupational therapy in the United States, was not concerned about an activity's ability to simulate work; rather, he suggested that the leading principle in selecting activities should simply be that the activities provide helpful enjoyment.[48]

Psychobiological theory saw mental illness as primarily stress induced. Anyone could be more or less biologically predisposed to respond poorly to stress, but socio-environmental forces caused the disequilibrium that resulted in mental illness. To recover, the individual needed to be protected both physically and mentally from the stressors. Physically, this could be accomplished with the help of a supportive family and rest at home or by admission to a hospital; but mentally, this protection could only be achieved – in the days before medication – by activities that engaged the mind.

A scientific explanation of how stress could be relieved through activity came with the Canadian endocrinologist Hans Selye's discovery that most stressors result in the same stress reaction. The "general adaptation syndrome" refers to the body's attempt to restore itself to its former state of homeostasis. The body produces the same biochemical changes irrespective of the origin of the stressors.[49]

Selye recommended relaxation and/or diversion to deal with stress and to help the body achieve homeostasis. Activating the whole body through exercise or relaxation or focusing on some other problem through diversion so that the source of worry automatically seemed less important in proportion was essential to achieving homeostasis. Selye's prescription was simple: "[Y]ou must find something to put in the place of the worrying thoughts to chase them away."[50]

Cognitive therapy, first described by Beck, has spawned a number of similar approaches, including mindfulness-based cognitive behavioural therapy (MCBT). Cognitive therapy placed great importance on what an individual felt about an event. The goal of identifying – and then refuting – intervening thoughts, which tended to be automatic and generally negative, required the patient to engage in activities that could then be used as evidence for contradicting the patient's negative thoughts. However, the activity had to first be capable of diverting the patient from perseverative, negative thinking. It also had to be carefully graded to ensure continued success and thus be capable of undermining the patient's belief that he or she is not capable. Beck and his colleagues thought that when patients learned to use diversion as a coping skill, they had gained an important sense of control.[51] The importance of diversional activity was again recognized during World War I when soldiers required long periods of convalescence and morale was low. However, despite the demonstrated value of diversional activities for over a century, their use by occupational therapists continues to attract negative comment.[52]

OCCUPATIONS AND THE MENTAL HYGIENE MOVEMENT

With the decline of the moral treatment era in the latter half of the nineteenth century, the idea of occupations as treatment lost some of its impetus. However, occupations were again promoted with the birth of the National Committee for Mental Hygiene (NCMH) in the United States in 1909 and, subsequently, with the committee's appearance in Canada a decade later.[53] The NCMH focused on the prevention of mental illness and the improvement of hospital care in general, and it showed particular concern for the daily activities – or lack thereof – for patients.

The formation of the mental hygiene movement was spurred on by former mental patient Clifford Beers, whose book, A Mind That Found Itself, was published in 1908. Beers writes about the dreadful conditions he had had to endure while confined to an asylum. He also tells of his relief when he had been occupied doing art and his appreciation of the value of trained occupation instructors.[54] No doubt Beers's success in spearheading the NCMH campaign owed something to his class and status in life. A graduate of Yale University and successful in business when he was well, he was able to draw the attention of those in positions of power and influence. Beers's efforts to establish a mental health reform movement in the United States had the support of social activists Jane Addams and Julia Lathrop, prominent psychologist William James, and leading psychiatrist Adolf Meyer. Their goal was "to create and carry forward a means effective to the end of promoting and conserving mental health and ameliorating the scourge of mental ill health."[55]

Julia Lathrop had seen the living conditions of mental patients and was determined to intervene. Educated at Vassar and Yale, Lathrop had toured the asylums in Illinois with Rabbi Emil Hirsch, a fellow member of the Illinois State Board of Control. She reported seeing "rows of cleanly dressed patients seated in absolute idleness for hours together, their attendants satisfied with supplying their bodily needs and making no effort to rouse and stimulate them." She described the work of the attendants: "It is a strenuous, joyless and singularly isolate life ... routine rules supreme, with all its warping and deadening influence."[56] Lathrop decided it would be best to intervene at the level of the hospital attendant.

Lathrop and Hirsch resigned from the Illinois Board of Control in protest of the conditions they had found. They then arranged for the Chicago School of Civics and Philanthropy to provide a summer course for attendants in "curative occupations and recreations" in order to try to remedy the situation.[57] The course emphasized the role of educational activities, as opposed to custodial care and discipline, in controlling behaviour.[58] Eleanor Clarke Slagle, soon to become a major figure in occupational therapy in the United States but at the time a social worker and committed social reformer, enrolled in the course in 1911 at age forty. In 1912, Slagle went to Johns Hopkins Hospital, where she worked closely with Adolf Meyer at the Phipps Psychiatric Clinic, developing her program of habit training. She returned to the Chicago School of Civics and Philanthropy in 1914 to give lectures on occupations and to start a workshop for the chronically unemployed. By 1915, she was ready to direct the Henry B. Favill School of Occupations, considered the first occupational therapy program in the world.[59]

Beers continued to influence the mental hygiene movement and in some measure helped to focus the content of occupational therapy programs. For example, in an article published in 1913 in the journal *The*

Playground, he recommended a schedule of instruction that included every hour of the day, and he noted the connections between play and work and recovery. He stressed the need for patients to learn to concentrate their attention and, by the use of their hands, to re-educate the brain in much the same way that the brain of the child is first educated. Beers noted that diversional occupations were the most important of these activities, as they could engage the attention of patients. He recognized the role of the instructor in engaging the patient in the first instance through the choice of occupation. That he wrote the article for a journal whose audience was primarily educators was consistent with his idea that the state should train teachers to work among the insane.[60]

The Canadian National Committee for Mental Hygiene was formed in 1918 by the psychiatrist Dr Clarence Hincks, with the help of Beers. Like Beers, Hincks had also suffered from mental illness and had been open in sharing his experiences. By this time, Hincks had established a mental hygiene clinic at the Toronto Juvenile Court and had collaborated with Clarke to provide out-patient care at the Toronto General Hospital.[61] Hincks proved to be a good organizer and fundraiser and was able to win the support of business and professional leaders in Ottawa, Montreal, and Toronto. He also engaged many female philanthropists in his cause, including Lady Eaton, wife of the wealthy department store owner Timothy Eaton.[62]

The American and Canadian Committees on Mental Hygiene shared goals and, at times, personnel. In 1924, Hincks became the medical director of the Canadian committee, and in 1930, he was appointed the medical director of the American National Committee for Mental Hygiene.[63] With their goals for patient care including occupations, it was not surprising that many members of the mental hygiene movement were also strong supporters of occupational therapy. Drs C.K. Clarke, C.B. Farrar, Ed Ryan, Goldwin Howland, and Hincks himself were all involved in helping to establish occupational therapy in Canada. Indeed, each of these physicians served in some capacity in the early years on the advisory board of the Ontario Society for Occupational Therapy, the board of the Canadian Association of Occupational Therapy (CAOT), or the editorial board of the *Canadian Journal of Occupational Therapy*.

By this time it was clear that a special instructor of occupations was needed, one who could interest not only the patients but also the staff, whose cooperation was necessary for such programs to succeed. It was essential to have someone who knew how to engage patients and when to vary activities to maintain interest. The need for a new type of health care worker, soon to be known as an occupational therapist, became apparent.[64]

Over a long and somewhat erratic history, occupations have been used as a treatment in mental illness. For much of the twentieth century, occupational therapy had a pride of place in mental health, and occupational therapists who worked in "psych" were well respected and thought to have interesting jobs.[65] However, in psychiatry's more modern history, occupational therapy's role changed greatly and, by some measures, decreased overall.[66] With the de-institutionalization of patients in the 1960s, mental health services moved to the community, but the funds provided were not adequate for the additional supports required. In recent years, home care programs in the community, assertive community treatment (ACT) teams, and the prominence of the recovery model have provided new environments for the work of occupational therapists. With the recognition of employment as a social determinant of health, there is a renewed focus on occupational therapy in mental health, one that harkens back a century and more. The old idea of work as therapy has been enhanced by supported employment schemes as well as by the addition of consumer/ mental health survivor-driven businesses.

The original concepts associated with occupational therapy in mental health continue to inform practice.[67] Occupational therapists have always tried to boost morale, improve self-esteem, and build competence and confidence – no matter their clients' clinical diagnoses. It is this ethos that lies at the heart of the profession and emanates from its early role in mental health.[68]

3

The Arts and Crafts Movement

It would be well if all of us were good handicraftsmen in some kind,
and the dishonour of manual labour done away with altogether.

John Ruskin[1]

Little is understood of how crafts came to be used as an intervention in
occupational therapy. With few exceptions,[2] the occupational therapy literature dismisses the use of crafts as having been appropriate only in the
time past and ignores any intrinsic meaning they may have had. There
are few references to the value attached to crafts by society – then or
now.[3] The assumptions about crafts and, to some extent, a whole range
of creative occupations (e.g., art, music, horticulture) are thus dismissed.
With that, much of the underlying philosophy – and uniqueness – of occupational therapy is ignored.[4]

In the last part of the nineteenth century, crafts provided occupations
for people with mental illness when work within the asylum buildings or
on the grounds was not an option. As discussed in chapter 2, some patients were too acutely ill to work and some of those who were chronically
ill could not manage the demands of work. Moreover, in those days private psychiatric patients paid for their hospitalization, making it difficult
to argue that work that benefited the institution financially was intended
primarily for the betterment of patients' health.[5] As well, labour unions
complained that patients were taking up the jobs that regular workers
would otherwise do.[6] In instances such as these, where work on the premises was not feasible, craftwork provided the much-needed occupations.
Crafts also found a place in occupational therapy because they were a

part of everyday life for many people – as a necessity to maintain life (e.g., spinning and weaving to make clothes for the family), as a skilled trade (e.g., woodwork or pottery), or as a form of leisure and amusement.

However, there was also a much more powerful reasoning at work regarding the use of crafts. *Doing* – and *creating* – seemed to have health-giving connotations. At the end of the nineteenth century, craftwork held a certain attraction for a population still suffering the malaise of post-industrialization. There was something about working with one's hands, mind, and heart that was thought to bring a special benefit – a new dimension to life that would enhance spiritual well-being. Further, when value was attached to work done with the hands, there was an opportunity to reduce inequities between the classes and promote social justice. These ideas gained popularity because of the arts and crafts movement.

THE ARTS AND CRAFTS MOVEMENT IN THE UNITED KINGDOM

The arts and crafts movement was born in the United Kingdom of both socialist and artistic ideologies. At one level, it was a socio-political response to the industrial age and the alienation felt by workers. People seemed to have lost their connection to nature, to their communities, to one another, and to themselves. There was particular concern for the plight of factory workers who could no longer take pride in a finished product at the end of their labours; instead, they became a part of an anonymous process that resulted in the mass production of inferior goods. Design, production, and marketing had all become separate functions, and workers generally did not see the final product of their labour.[7] Factory work was unfulfilling and conditions were unsafe; workers were overworked and poorly paid, their lives were often marked by poverty and discontent. The arts and crafts movement focused on these workers and endeavoured to improve their lot.

At another level, the arts and crafts movement was seen as a celebration of the beauty and significance of the artistic effort embodied in architecture and in everyday objects, and expressed through the use of one's hands. Such work was thought to benefit the individual and society. It connected people with nature and with the world around them. It also improved morale, drew people together, and appeared capable of restoring community life. The founders of the arts and crafts movement, John Ruskin and William Morris, each brought ideas about celebrating art and bettering society.

John Ruskin

John Ruskin (1819–1900) was said to be the most powerful and original thinker of the nineteenth century.[8] He was a painter, a poet, a philosopher, an art critic, and a philanthropist. Ruskin first came into the public eye with his critical writings on painting and architecture and his reverence for works of the Gothic period. Independently wealthy and widely travelled, he devoted the early part of his life to writing art criticism. However, by mid-life and under the influence of his friend and mentor Sir Thomas Carlyle (1795–1881), the Scottish historian and essayist, Ruskin became distressed about the inequities within society and the terrible conditions in which many people lived. He then attempted to effect social reform through his writings in books and newspapers.[9] His writings covered a wide spectrum of societal concerns – for the poor, for the aged, for women, for housing, for education, and for employment. While generous in his support to those in need, he was against giving money for charity indiscriminately and favoured teaching people useful skills. In 1868, he wrote a letter to the editor of the *Daily Telegraph* about the benefits of employment for those he termed the destitute poor and criminal classes: "That is the help beyond all others; find out how to make useless people useful, and let them earn their money instead of begging. Few are so feeble as to be incapable of all occupation, none so faultful but that occupation, well chosen, and kindly compelled, will be medicine for them in soul and body."[10]

For Ruskin, there were many routes to social reform, but he particularly believed in the power of art to improve society. He believed that good architecture contributed to mental health, that art was a means of educating and elevating the human spirit, and that beauty was as necessary to a person's survival as food, shelter, and a living wage.[11] And while his friend Carlyle spoke to the nobility of work, saying, "All work, even cotton-spinning, is noble; work alone is noble,"[12] Ruskin challenged the idea that all work was intrinsically good. For him, only work that was enjoyable and not degrading was to be valued.

Concerned about the plight of the worker and despairing of the appearance of industrially produced objects, Ruskin saw the decorative arts (which included crafts) as offering a way forward. He particularly valued workers who were true craftsmen, those who would both design and create their work and, having control over the entire process, would be invested in the objects produced.[13] He found the decorative arts par-

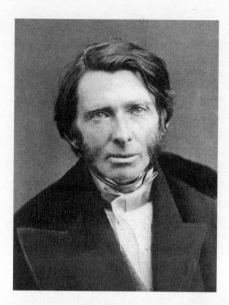

John Ruskin, painter, poet, philosopher, art critic, philanthropist, and founder of the arts and crafts movement.

ticularly praiseworthy because they combined manual and mental labour. In his words, "It is only by labour that thought can be made healthy, and only by thought that labour can be made happy, and the two cannot be separated with impunity. It would be well if all of us were good handicraftsmen in some kind, and the dishonour of manual labour done away with altogether."[14]

Ruskin thought that it did not matter whether the producer of art was considered an "artist," a "craftsman," or a "workman." The difference depended on experience, skill, and excellence of achievement.[15] While he wrote primarily for fellow intellectuals, he also wrote about the needs of the masses, drawing attention, for example, to the need for schools to teach artisan skills and stimulate what he called the "art spirit." The art spirit, educators thought, had the potential to liberate the individual, to unlock creativity, and in this way, to encourage freedom.[16]

Creating art was an activity that needed defending and celebrating. In *Fors Clavigera, Letters to the Workmen and Labourers of Great Britain*, Ruskin spoke about the doing of art, saying, "No one can teach you anything worth learning but through manual labour; the very bread of life can only be got out of the chaff of it by 'rubbing it in your hands.'"[17]

Ruskin was putting his thoughts directly into practice when he founded – and taught art at – the London Working Men's College in

1854. Prominent men gave their time to the college without pay, teaching a variety of subjects, including literature, mathematics, history, and art. In 1865, one of Ruskin's pupils, Frederick Brigden – a young man deaf since childhood from a bout of scarlet fever – was apprenticing to be an engraver. Brigden recalled that Ruskin gave him help, wrote careful criticisms of his work, and was generous in his praise. Brigden later emigrated with his wife and two sons to Toronto, where he became a successful illustrator and engraver.[18]

Ruskin supported craftsmanship as a means of uplifting the downtrodden and providing them with needed skills. In one such venture, he arranged for inmates from the House for Delinquent Girls to learn to weave. He was aware that women of a certain class often found handicrafts beneficial and noted that what "soothed the nerves of the upper middle-class woman, nervous from her relatively easy but empty life, surely would benefit the poor."[19] In celebrating the use of one's hands at a time when machine-made articles were becoming more highly valued, Ruskin was going against common practice. However, the fact that it was Ruskin who was extolling the virtues of craftsmanship greatly enhanced the popularity and respectability of manual activities among the public.

Ruskin's efforts to help the disadvantaged took on a new form in 1868 when he held discussions in his home that eventually led to the establishment of Toynbee Hall and the subsequent settlement house movement (see chapter 4). In a less concrete but perhaps more powerful contribution, Ruskin succeeded in establishing, through a lifetime of teaching and advocating, the idea that design and architecture were expressions of a way of life.[20] Thus, he is linked to occupational therapy because of the value he placed on art and craft and the use of one's hands. He highly valued the work of the skilled craftsman, but at the same time, he saw that craft skills could be taught to the working classes so as to better their lives.

Ruskin is also linked to occupational therapy through personal connections. He was a good friend of the social reformer Octavia Hill (1838–1912) and financially supported her Working Ladies' Guild, which trained and found employment for single women. He also supported Hill's housing projects for poor and immigrant populations in south London (see chapter 4).[21] One of Hill's volunteer workers, Elizabeth Casson, went on to become a physician. After a few years in practice, she founded the first school of occupational therapy in the United Kingdom, at Dorset House in Bristol in 1930.

William Morris (1834–1896)

Some fifteen years younger than Ruskin, William Morris was influenced by Ruskin's works on art criticism while a student at Oxford in the 1850s.[22] Morris was initially interested in a career in theology. He also considered art and architecture, but he soon settled to craftwork, which he thought could bring great joy and beauty to his life.[23]

Morris taught himself many crafts: from stained glass window making, to ceramics, and metalwork, through tile-making, weaving, woodworking, bookbinding, and wallpaper design. In addition to being a highly skilled craftsman, he was associated with the group of painters known as the Pre-Raphaelite Brotherhood and shared much of their philosophy.

Like Ruskin, Morris was deeply concerned about the lives of factory workers. The industrial revolution had resulted not only in cheap and unattractive products, but it had become dehumanizing to workers. Many of those who had once used their craftsmen's skills, and were fulfilled by their work, were now without work. Those who had work in the new factories suffered the alienation that resulted from mechanized production methods.[24] For Morris, who had turned away from religion, salvation could now be found only in "art labour," work that involved the hand, the heart, and the mind.

The environment in which people lived and worked was an important source of spiritual well-being for Morris. He exhorted people to furnish their homes in a way that would ensure that their living space supported this notion, making the now well-known remark: "Have nothing in your houses which you do not know to be useful or believe to be beautiful."[25] Along with like-minded colleagues, he established Morris and Company to produce handmade furnishings for the home. However, Morris and Company was only a partial success; while it was able to set standards of beauty and integrity with its handmade goods, its high prices made these goods unavailable to the common man.

Finding the process of creating – and the beautiful objects created – spiritually uplifting, Morris stressed the importance of crafts for their health-giving properties. He also valued the sense of tradition that crafts brought and celebrated the variety of crafts found in different cultures and in rural communities.[26]

Morris honoured nature both in life and in his designs, which were replete with intricate patterns of flowers, plants, and leaves. He believed in the healing power of nature and saw it as a means of connecting people with the world, of enhancing their sense of belonging, and thus of meet-

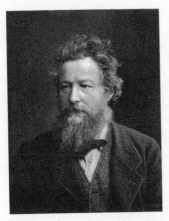 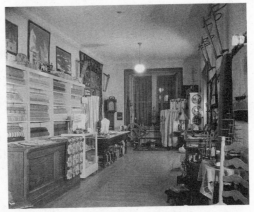

LEFT William Morris, craftsman, social reformer, writer and poet, and founder of the arts and crafts movement; RIGHT Interior of Canadian Guild of Handicrafts Shop in Montreal, c. 1930. Courtesy Canadian Guild of Crafts, Montreal.

ing a need expressed by many who felt alienated and longed for spiritual meaning. His art, with its simple, light, and utilitarian aesthetic and natural lines, celebrated the natural environment and stood in contrast to art of the Victorian era, which tended to be ornate and formal.[27]

To create social change through art, Morris proposed a return to earlier ways, when people with various skills and trades worked together within a community setting. He thought that in such a setting, an "organic society" would develop that would foster mutual aid rather than competition. Morris thought that there was something about artists' inherent nature that made them key workers for a better society.[28]

While Morris wanted to make the world an "earthly paradise" through art, he gradually realized that a better world would have to be created before his ideas could be accepted. This discovery led him to join the Socialist League, and he wrote and spoke of his political views widely in the United Kingdom. As a founder of the socialist journal *Commonweal* in 1885, he was a frequent contributor to its pages, decrying a system that resulted in a society of rich and poor. He remarked, for example, on the dearth of shelter for the poor while those with private property could state, "This is mine, and whether I can use it or not, nobody else shall."[29] In 1889, seven years before his death, he wrote about the role of art within a socialist milieu, convinced that art could not be made without there being a better life.[30]

Morris championed ways of life that valued collegiality, camaraderie, and interdependence. Like those involved in the settlement house movement, which was just being established, he wanted to build or rebuild social networks in the community. While his underlying reasons for changing society were as much about decreasing the benefits of the rich as increasing the benefits of the poor, he believed that the way forward for both goals was similar: building a sense of community, improving the environment, and enriching the day-to-day lives of workers.[31]

Sharing Ruskin's views about art as a means of educating and elevating the human spirit, Morris believed that art was important for everyone. He thought that crafts were essential to the well-being of all people and should be considered a right: "I do not want art for a few, any more than education for a few, or freedom for a few."[32] This idea, that all people could be artists in some way at some time in their lives, was revolutionary and was never fully accepted. Nonetheless, through Morris (and Ruskin), craftwork gained greater respectability as art while also becoming more popular in everyday life. It was considered appropriate for men and women (albeit in different roles)[33] to learn a craft that could be used as a means to earn a wage or as a leisure-time pursuit.

THE ARTS AND CRAFTS MOVEMENT IN NORTH AMERICA

Many North Americans visited and studied with Morris to learn a craft and/or to imbibe his socialist views.[34] However, when the arts and crafts movement came to North America, it lost much of its socialist leanings. Rather than fighting industrialization, the movement sought peace with the industrial world and tried to find ways of taking more control over the means of production.[35] Rather than focusing on how it could improve the health of society, the movement focused on improving the health of the individual.[36] Now the link between art and health was promoted for those who, stressed by working "for pay not for joy," could find refuge in art.[37] Craftwork was offered to adults, partly as therapy and partly in response to yearnings for a "real" life, where people could live, work, and create together.[38] For those suffering from stress (generally labelled as neurasthenia at the time), a popular form of treatment was a period of time at an arts and crafts retreat where one could work communally, make art, and be close to nature.[39] Handicraft workshops provided a cooperative environment in which people could enjoy the work they were doing; they felt a spiritual connection to life that had been missing, and as a result their health and well-being were thought to improve.

Oscar Wilde was also promoting the virtues of the decorative arts at this time, but his approach was focused on art for art's sake.[40] During his North American lecture tour, which included Toronto, Wilde shared his views on the appreciation of beauty above wealth. He pointed out that possession of the *right* objects was taken to be a sign of moral and spiritual superiority.[41] Advocating for the marriage of beauty and functionality, Wilde stated that the beauty of an object was in direct correlation to the amount of skill and intellect that went into its production. He emphasized that doing and creating were essential and basic human rights, saying "that beauty which is meant by art is no mere accident of human life which people can take or leave, but a *positive necessity of life* if we are to live as nature meant us to, that is to say unless we are content to be less than men."[42] Thus, for Wilde, art was of such importance that it could redeem the mind and spirit.

The physician Herbert Hall used this approach at Devereux Mansion, a retreat he ran in Marblehead, Massachusetts, at the turn of the century. Hall wrote about the importance of occupations in treating neurasthenia and stressed the idea of a "work-cure." He became very involved with the profession of occupational therapy in the early part of the century, serving as the president of the American Occupational Therapy Association (AOTA) from 1920 to 1921.

William Morris, the man and his philosophy, was a topic of great interest in academic and cultural circles in North America.[43] As Panayotidis-Stortz has noted, "Morris' spectre and the ethos of Arts and Crafts ideas were fundamental components of many cultural discussions in turn-of-the-century Toronto. Morris and the Arts and Crafts social-aesthetic philosophy, and especially its rhetoric of the centrality of art to daily life, pervaded many facets of Canadian life – especially art, social reform, and education in the late nineteenth and early twentieth century and was crucial in determining character and state-formation."[44]

A number of arts and crafts associations were formed in North America, each with similar principles: to celebrate the work of craftsmen in terms of design unity, joy in labour, individualism, and regionalism.[45] According to the magazine *Canadian Architect and Builder*, an arts and crafts association was founded in 1885 in Hamilton, Ontario, by fifty citizens "who felt an interest in matters artistic, and in the improvement of handicrafts on the part of mechanics and amateurs."[46] This group must not have been well known, as the first Arts and Crafts Society in North America is generally considered to have been founded in Boston in 1897 by Charles Eliot Norton, a close friend of Ruskin's and Morris's and a professor of art history at Harvard. Norton admired Morris's poetry as well as his designs and was largely responsible for his growing popularity in the United States.

The Boston Arts and Crafts Society came into being following the successful First Exhibition of Arts and Crafts held earlier that year, which had presented objects of everyday use as works of art. A process whereby societies were formed after successful craft exhibitions was followed in other cities, including Hamilton, Vancouver, and Chicago. Meanwhile, designs by Morris entered into everyday life.[47] Across Canada, furniture, tiles, fabrics, jewellery, tapestry, wallpaper, and stained glass in the arts and crafts style became popular and could be found in homes and churches built to arts and crafts architectural ideals.[48]

Some public buildings were also constructed on arts and crafts principles. Hart House, an athletic and social centre at the University of Toronto (U of T),[49] was inspired by William Morris and his arts and crafts fellow "art-workers" and designed by Canadian architects Henry Sproatt and Ernest Rolph.[50] The Founders' Prayer, which adorns the walls of its Great Hall, expresses Morris's social ideal of a guild of like-minded people inspired by the arts, working together for a better society.

Many who became involved with arts and crafts movements in North America had some connection with Morris. George Barton, an architect who had studied with Morris, was the Boston society's first secretary. He brought ideas about arts and crafts with him when, in 1917, he became a founder of the National Society for the Promotion of Occupational Therapy (NSPOT).[51] The Chicago Arts and Crafts Society was founded in 1897 by Ellen Gates Starr, who had studied bookbinding with Cobden-Sanderson, a colleague of Morris's. Professor James Mavor, chair of economics at the University of Toronto, was a friend and former colleague of William Morris in the Socialist League in the United Kingdom. He was also a friend of Octavia Hill (the social housing worker; see chapter 4) prior to immigrating to Canada. Mavor was a member of the Society of Arts and Crafts of Canada and the University Settlement House. These relationships and experiences likely influenced his academic work, including his study of compensation for workmen's injuries in 1899.[52] Seeing the value of occupations for the injured, Mavor helped raise funds for programs to aid in the functional re-education of injured soldiers toward the end of World War I.[53]

In 1903, George Reid, an artist, educator, and community leader, co-founded the Arts and Crafts Society of Canada with Mabel Cawthra

Adamson. The preamble to the constitution described the movement's artistic aspirations and noted that "[a] small band of workers, headed by William Morris, led the revival, which spread from England to the Continent and finally to our own country."[54] Like others, Reid had reverently recalled the worker of the nineteenth century "busy making with the aid of his hand and foot power machines and tools, a complete article" and compared his effort to the "typical workman of today keeping time to the beats of a machine as a minute piece of a complete article gets advanced a step." Restating Morris's ideology, he referred to the first worker as an "artist artisan" and to the second as a "mechanical drudge whose work debases him and saps his life by its monotony and lack of interest for him."[55] Reid was a highly respected artist, and in 1912 he became the first principal of what is now the Ontario College of Art and Design. Mabel Cawthra Adamson was an accomplished artist, craftswoman, and art collector. Her considerable inheritance, added to the profits of her own interior design company, allowed her to be a fervent supporter of the arts.[56]

The crafts of Canada's Native and immigrant populations were also being promoted. William Carless, a professor of architecture at McGill, described the vast array of crafts to be found across the country at the time: woven blankets, beaded moccasins, ivory carvings, intricate basketry, hooked and braided rugs, metalwork, pottery, needlework and lacemaking, quilting, sweet hay and raffia work, woodcarving, porcupine-quill work, glass beadwork, wampum belts, *étoffe du pays* (homespun of the habitant French Canadian), and the very complicated *ceintûre flechée* or sash. Echoing Morris's sentiments, Carless summed up the value of such work: "The desire to find artistic expression in the making of useful and beautiful things, particularly in those related to the home and our personal needs, is an instinct which should be encouraged."[57]

WOMEN, CRAFTS, AND OCCUPATIONAL THERAPY

In the nineteenth century, art, architecture, and many crafts were practised primarily by men. However, by the turn of the twentieth century, two groups of Canadian women had organized themselves into what would become very important art associations: the Women's Art Association of Canada (WAAC), founded in 1896 in Toronto by artist Mary Dingham, and the Canadian Handicrafts Guild (CHG), founded in 1905, in Montreal, by craftswomen Alice Peck and May Phillips. Both groups were inspired by the arts and crafts movement, seeing it as a means of uniting the world of the home with the world of social reform.[58] Both groups were dedicated to supporting women artists and craftworkers, preserving the arts and crafts of immigrant and Native Canadians, and promoting home industries as a means of helping women to contribute to household earnings. Many women learned crafts as part of a wider training as artists. Crafts gave women some profile in the world of art, where otherwise they were expected to take the roles of fundraisers or purchasers of art.[59]

Members of the Women's Art Association in Montreal supported the home arts and handicrafts of rural Quebec in the mid-1890s, echoing the arts and crafts ideals espoused by Morris. They sold handicrafts from their headquarters on Stanley Street in Montreal and held exhibits of Canadian handicrafts that included the craftwork of Native groups and immigrants. In her description of the early work of the CHG, Peck discussed the significance of crafts to well-being in rural areas: "Where the crafts flourish there will be found a happy and contented people who have interests outside their daily labour, and a chance to increase the income that the annual crops fail to give them."[60]

The first exhibition of Canadian craftwork, held by the WAAC in Montreal in 1902, was very successful and demonstrated that there were skilled craftworkers across the country.[61] Building on the success of the exhibition, the association started an educational program to promote good workmanship and design, using vegetable dyes and quality materials. In 1905, the Montreal Branch of WAAC split off from the parent organization and two members, Alice Peck and May Phillips, founded the Canadian Handicrafts Guild. The guild held annual exhibitions and competitions, opened and operated a shop to sell their workers' crafts, and collected examples of crafts for study purposes.[62]

The CHG was a resourceful group whose work met various needs. By supporting the craftwork of immigrant and Native women, both because of its quality and because of the disadvantaged conditions in which the women lived, the CHG was applying the principles first articulated by Ruskin and Morris in regard to community development.[63] When injured soldiers returned from the front in World War I and needed something to occupy them during lengthy periods of convalescence, the CHG was able to meet that demand as well. They supplied craft teachers to the hospitals and also displayed and sold the articles made by the men.[64]

It was from the membership of the CHG that many of the first occupational therapists emerged. During the war, they worked directly with the soldiers and were responsible for teaching other women to do the same.

Their contribution seemed a natural extension of the work they had been doing with immigrant and Native groups.

CHG co-founder May Phillips was concerned that when the injured soldiers returned to their homes, many would still need to work at their crafts. In homes where craftwork was already practised, the men could carry on with the work on their own. But in other homes, there was a need to monitor the work to ensure it met appropriate standards. Phillips very confidently noted that while other women could also provide this service, they, the women of the CHG, "undoubtedly can offer the best means of sale, and, exercise a restraining influence upon the production of useless, meretricious and inartistic work."[65]

One of the interesting activities promoted by the CHG was toy making. Before the war, most of the toys sold in Canadian stores had been imported from Germany. However, with the outbreak of war, German-made toys soon became unacceptable. The CHG set up a competition and provided prizes for the best toys made by soldiers in Canada. With this event, the term "Made in Canada" is said to have been coined.[66]

CONTRIBUTION TO OCCUPATIONAL THERAPY

Ruskin and Morris both started out writing art criticism, and both revered the decorative arts. Both men then moved on to social criticism and from there to political action. Ruskin supported individual causes (e.g., the Working Men's College, Octavia Hill's social housing projects) often to promote political change, while Morris promoted political change at the societal level through his socialist party involvement. Both men were involved in social reform during the latter half of the nineteenth century.

Ruskin's ideas were well known in political, intellectual, and art circles. His writings appeared in the popular press as well as in scholarly publications. Although some of his political writings met with negative reactions when first published, they gradually came to be accepted. As he wrote in the last half of the nineteenth century, a period that coincided with the decline of the moral treatment era in mental health, it is likely that his ideas about the importance of using one's hands would have been known to hospital superintendants and members of the all-important hospital boards. The notion that art might somehow "liberate the spirit" would have seemed attractive to those dealing with depressed patients.[67] At a time when mental hospitals needed to use occupations that would not directly support the institutions financially (e.g., agricultural work on the grounds or cleaning the buildings), craftwork would have been seen as an attractive option. Morris was very much in the public eye, and the example he set would have greatly broadened the choice of crafts available for patients (e.g., ceramics, bookbinding, weaving, metalwork, etc.).

The emerging world of occupational therapy was sensitive to the philosophy and sentiment of the arts and crafts movement. Many individuals who later became occupational therapists were connected to the movement through their early training as artists at, for example, the art department at Mount Allison University, the Ontario College of Art, or the Pratt Institute in New York. By the early 1900s, some of these craftswomen were working – either voluntarily or for pay – with patients in mental hospitals or other settings, such as so-called homes for incurables. The socialist philosophy of the arts and crafts movement would have suited their desire to help those disadvantaged by poverty, illness, and disease. Teaching crafts to these people would have echoed Ruskin's philosophy of helping those who were disabled so that they might become less dependent on others and Morris's ideas about the health-giving properties of creativity and joyful work.

4

The Settlement House Movement

Behold, this was the sin of Sodom, your sister: She and her daughters
had pride, surfeit of bread and peaceful serenity, but she did not
strengthen the hand of the poor and the needy.

Dead Sea Scrolls, Ezekiel 16:49

If occupational therapy is linked with mental health because of a basic
need for humans to engage in work or other activities, and if the arts and
crafts movement brought a spiritual, soul-saving dimension to occupations, then the settlement house movement might seem almost unrelated
to the notion of occupations being important to well-being. The occupations used in the settlement house movement served a larger goal: they
were planned for the well-being of the community within which individuals lived, and they were designed to help community members survive
and belong.

The activities of daily living constitute one of the cornerstones of occupational therapy practice. Being capable of carrying out the activities
of daily living helps people to imagine moving forward in their lives. All
sorts of people need help in managing their lives: the poor who were first
targeted by the settlement house movement; those who are ill; people
with disabilities; and those who must adapt to major life changes, like immigration. When people can manage their activities of daily living, they
decrease their dependency on the state and on their families and they
have hope for the future.

The advocacy of people's right to move forward is rooted in a belief
in social justice. People who believed in the ideology of the settlement

house movement broadened the basis for societal interventions. Many of those who were to become occupational therapists were involved in social reform, advocating for – and working with – communities as well as individuals.

HISTORY OF THE SETTLEMENT HOUSE MOVEMENT

Settlement houses were physical structures located within the impoverished communities they intended to serve. They reached out to the community and offered people a place to congregate and participate in educational activities. The activities were designed to enhance people's skills and generally included language classes (for immigrant groups primarily from eastern Europe), cooking, sewing and other handicrafts, and art and music. Some settlement house workers were paid, but most were volunteers. Volunteers tended to come from the middle and upper classes and were well educated. There was an expectation (not always met) that workers would live in residence at the settlement house for a period of time because doing so would give them a better understanding of the community they were serving.[1]

The settlement house movement began in the late 1800s with the goal of improving the living conditions of poor and immigrant populations in urban centres in the United Kingdom. The mechanism for effecting social reform revolved around two central ideas: one, that people could learn skills that would help them better manage their lives; and two, that those who wanted to help the poor should engage with them fully. Both ideas were in sharp contrast to the idea that one should give alms to the poor, as well as to the belief held by much of the middle class that the poor were to blame for the situation they found themselves in. The settlement movement challenged that notion and instead strove to preserve the dignity of those receiving help. According to Cathy James's study of Toronto's settlement house movement (1900–20), the movement helped "to reform Canadian social reform."[2]

Working in a settlement house brought different experiences according to the gender of the worker. For women, settlement house work provided an opportunity to be out in the world and to use their education and the benefits of their station in life to help others. The work, in most cases, was an end in itself, but some women used the experience to go on to become professional social workers. For men, the work was often considered more pragmatically; it was a means of gaining a broader experience of life, one that could be useful to them as they moved forward with their careers in business and politics.[3]

OCTAVIA HILL

A very early example of settlement house practices – and of their later connection with occupational therapy – is provided by the work of Octavia Hill (1838–1912) in England. Hill was raised in a family where social action was almost commonplace. Her father had died early, leaving his wife to raise their eight daughters and earn a living. Hill's mother, Caroline Southwood Hill, was a social activist and educator.[4] She followed the progressive ideas of the educator Johann Pestalozzi, who favoured the use of crafts, and established a Pestalozzian infant school.[5] In 1852, she managed a cooperative crafts workshop in central London, and Octavia – then fourteen years old – assisted with the work. Octavia also visited the children at their homes and remembers feeling horrified to see the families' very difficult and crowded living conditions.[6]

Hill's maternal grandfather, Dr Southwood Smith, was a well-known physician and health reformer. He fought for the abolition of child labour and for the improvement of housing conditions. Seeing the good works of both her mother and her grandfather and being deeply religious herself likely influenced her decision to do what she could to improve the lot of her fellow man. She chose to address the need for housing reform and community development by managing social housing projects in poor areas of London.[7]

Octavia Hill knew John Ruskin and interacted with him on two fronts. Initially, she benefited from studying with Ruskin the artist during a time when she considered becoming a serious painter. However, her work with the poor soon took precedence, and it was then that she benefited from her interactions with Ruskin the social reformer. Ruskin's wealth and generosity resulted in his buying houses for the poor that Hill could manage. Hill wrote to her sister Miranda in 1864 describing Ruskin's affirmative response to her housing plan and its costs. She quoted him saying that he thought "the homes of the poor *the* one question of the time."[8]

Although Hill's main role was to prepare the houses for residents and then collect the rents, she used her position to develop relationships with the immigrants and other poor families who were her tenants. She then worked with them, teaching them how to manage their finances and helping them find work. She encouraged the practice of traditional crafts

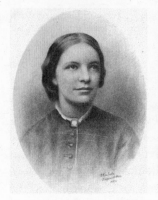

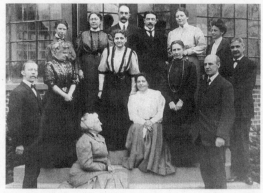

LEFT Octavia Hill, social housing reformer and early prototype for occupational therapy, c. 1870. Courtesy Wellcome Library, London, L0000062; RIGHT First board of directors of the University Settlement House, Toronto, with their chair and founder, Sir Robert Falconer, president of the University of Toronto (*front row, far right*), 1910. Courtesy City of Toronto Archives, fonds 1024, item 6.

as a form of livelihood and a means of helping immigrants maintain links with their home countries. Recreational activities were organized with the goal of community building in mind. These educational and social interventions helped the people in her housing projects improve their station in life while also developing a sense of community.

Hill was a visionary in her attempt to bring self-respect to those who had long since lost hope. It is curious to note that while her approach to improving the lives of the poor was innovative, she herself was conservative in many of her views; for example, she was opposed to state or municipal welfare and argued against old-age pensions. While she supported women's involvement at the local level, she opposed parliamentary votes for women on the basis that women were not fit to decide broader issues that involved international policy, defence, or national budgets.[9]

Hill's exemplary work received the attention of many. In 1870, a fourteen-year-old Canadian girl, Alice (Skelton) Peck, while at boarding school in England, was taken on a school trip to see Hill's projects. She remembered being moved by the work Hill was doing and how it seemed to improve the tenants' living conditions and their outlook. She kept that idea in her mind and built on it years later in her social work activities at home in Montreal. Alice Peck ultimately became known as an artist, a skilled craftswoman, and a prodigious organizer. As a founding member of the Canadian Handicrafts Guild (CHG) in 1905,[10] she built an organization whose goals were aligned with those of Octavia Hill and the settlement house movement: to celebrate craftwork while promoting self-sufficiency. Indeed, the motto of the CHG was "Self help – not charity."[11]

A more direct connection between Octavia Hill and occupational therapy came by way of Elizabeth Casson (1881–1954), a woman from Bristol, England. Casson worked for Octavia Hill in Southwark, London, as an estate manager from 1908 to 1913. Observing the link between the residents' poverty and their ill health, she decided she could do more to help as a doctor and so enrolled in the University of Bristol. When she graduated in 1918, she became the first woman to gain the degree of doctor of medicine at the university. Casson had a special interest in treating psychotic and neurotic diseases and, in 1929, established her own clinic at Dorset House in Bristol.[12] Having seen the value of recreational and educational work with Hill, she used these interventions, along with crafts, and found them valuable not only as treatment but also for prevention and maintaining health.[13] In keeping with the settlement house ideal, Casson applied the idea of the importance of community to her clinic. She tried to break down barriers between patients and staff, having them work and often live together in a community where everyone felt valued.[14] She promoted the idea of a full-time planned day for all patients; occupational therapy occurred in the evenings as well as during each day of the week. In 1930, she set up Dorset House School at Bristol, the first school of occupational therapy in the United Kingdom.[15]

Hill's contribution, though not widely known, was significant and greatly affected the ideology and the implementation of social welfare in the United Kingdom and elsewhere. Her influence on the development of occupational therapy has been described by Wilcock as "the once missing link between nineteenth century social activists and the development of occupational therapy in England."[16] The same could be said for the missing link in Canada.

TOYNBEE HALL

Hill's early work preceded that of the settlement house movement, which had its formal start in the United Kingdom with Toynbee Hall in 1884. The movement owes its origins to T.H. Green, a philosopher at Oxford, who, like Ruskin and Morris, believed that industrialization had destroyed the natural ties of interdependence that traditionally had held society together. Concerned about poverty and crime and the growing disparities between rich and poor, Green thought that social reform could occur only with the re-establishment of local communities. In his ideal community, members of different classes would live side by side, and the poor would have access to, and be influenced by, their more educated neighbours. Green expected his university students (all of whom were male) to give their time voluntarily to work with the poor and to live among them.[17] Improving the lot of the poor was to happen not by charity but through personal example: that is, through the friendship between the working-class tenants of the housing projects and the Oxford (and Cambridge) student volunteers.

Toynbee Hall was located in Whitechapel in London's East End and was run by Canon Samuel Barnett and his wife, Henrietta. Though the Barnetts had strong religious beliefs, Toynbee Hall was nonsectarian; its goal was to bring people closer to one another, rather than to God.[18] Barnett writes, "A settlement of university men will do a little to remove the inequalities of life, as the settlers share their best with the poor and learn through feeling how they live."[19] Their stated goal was to help people help themselves. Toynbee Hall provided a place for the settlement house members to congregate and to learn. Education was provided through night courses at the Working Men's College, one of whose better-known teachers was Ruskin himself.

THE SETTLEMENT HOUSE MOVEMENT IN NORTH AMERICA: HULL HOUSE

With all the visitors to Toynbee Hall, it would not be long before the settlement house movement was brought to North America. In 1886, Stanton Coit, who had lived at Toynbee Hall for several months, opened the first American settlement, the Neighborhood Guild, in New York's Lower East Side. However, the most important of the four hundred settlement houses that would soon appear in the United States was Hull House in Chicago. And it is Hull House that provides the strongest link between the settlement house movement and the work of occupational therapists.

Hull House was founded by Jane Addams and Ellen Gates Starr in 1889 in a poor area of Chicago. They saw it as a means of creating social change through interaction, activities, and education. Starr, an artist, attempted to instil an appreciation of art and creativity among the immigrant and poor residents of the neighbourhood. Like many reformers of her generation, including Ruskin and Morris, Starr thought that working at an art or craft was spiritually uplifting and civilizing, and would serve as an antidote to the demoralizing repetitiveness of the factory work that most residents performed. She had met William Morris while visiting England and shared his socialist ideals. Starr helped found the Chicago Arts and Crafts Society and supported its fight for improved conditions for workers. However, by 1900, Starr had left Hull House and her association with Addams to become more militant on social issues, championing labour reform and joining the Socialist Party.[20]

Jane Addams was a pacifist,[21] a social and political activist, and the driving force behind Hull House. She had visited Toynbee Hall in 1888 with Starr and had been impressed with its work. Hull House soon developed a roster of programs to meet the needs of its immediate neighbours. Unlike settlement houses in the United Kingdom, which served everyone but focused on men, Hull House focused on women and children. It provided language courses to ease the transition for new immigrants; it offered cooking lessons to help poor women provide for their families; and it provided lessons in dressmaking and millinery to prepare them for better jobs. For the children, there were clubs and recreational classes as well as crafts. Hull House staff also pursued large-scale reforms – of the courts, of child labour laws, and of the treatment of people with mental illness.[22]

As with other settlement houses, workers at Hull House were expected to live in residence, at least for a time. The future prime minister of Canada William Lyon Mackenzie King lived in residence at Hull House for several months at the end of the nineteenth century while a student in political economy at the University of Chicago. The experience of living among people who were unemployed or had low-paying, unpleasant jobs likely influenced his thinking when he became Canada's first deputy minister of labour in 1900 and, later, the minister of labour in Wilfrid Laurier's cabinet in 1908. Mackenzie King remained in contact with Jane Addams over the years, and in 1930, while prime minister, he was invited to the fortieth anniversary celebration of the founding of Hull House. As he was unable to attend due to matters of Parliament and an impending general election, he sent a congratulatory telegram to Addams. It read: "I can never feel too grateful for the period of my residence both at Hull-House and at Passmore Edwards, London [another settlement house] and what they afforded in the way of a wider acquaintance with fuller understanding of industrial, civic and national problems and the contacts which they helped to further with men and women who had a special interest in the betterment of social and political conditions."[23]

Addams believed in the power of the community and in the mixing of the classes, but unlike Green at Toynbee Hall, who expected the poor to be influenced by their educated neighbours, she believed that the purpose of social mixing at Hull House was for the classes to learn from one another.[24] Indeed, she suggested that the settlement movement was of more benefit to educated and privileged young people, and especially to women, than to the poor. In the case of women, she was referring to the opportunities the movement gave women to learn social work skills and become employed.[25]

Hull House became world renowned, and many people came to visit, observe, or volunteer. Addams was a guest speaker at numerous conferences and events and was invited to visit Canada on several occasions. In 1897, she spoke at the National Conference of Charities and Corrections when it met in Toronto. She shared her views on how living in a neglected neighbourhood and constantly meeting people with different ideas and notions would modify one's own thinking. In this way, she explained, one would come to see the sense behind working-class attitudes on a number of issues.[26]

She was invited to address this same group at its meeting in 1914 but had to decline because of the pressure of other engagements.[27] In the fall of 1919, she was invited to the University of Toronto to speak to the Department of Social Service. By that time, however, she was well known for her pacifist beliefs and her criticism of the war. Patriotic sentiment ran high in a Canada still mourning the deaths and injuries of so many of its soldiers. As a result, there were strong protests against her visit and the lecture was cancelled. The Department of Social Work sent letters of apology, and the president of the university (Falconer) wrote to the editor of the student paper, the *Varsity*, decrying the behaviour that led to the cancellation.[28] Addams did make another visit to Toronto in 1924 to attend the Conference of Social Work, giving several speeches without incident.[29]

A friend to occupational therapy, Addams spoke on several occasions at the profession's annual conferences. In 1919, for example, she welcomed members of the National Society for the Promotion of Occupational Therapy (NSPOT) to Hull House, where the society's third annual meeting was held.

A large part of the success of Hull House was due to Addams's ability to obtain the help of outstanding figures of that time, people like the educator-philosopher John Dewey and the psychologist William James. Dewey, who occasionally lived and worked at Hull House, saw in Addams a personification of his educational idea that people learn by doing – a sentiment that would also be at the heart of occupational therapy.

Upon Addams's death in 1935, tributes came from around the world. Agnes Macphail, the first female member of Parliament in Canada, writes, "Hull House has been a Mecca for socially minded and peace-loving Canadians."[30] William Lyon Mackenzie King, who within six months would again be prime minister of Canada, sent a telegram of condolence. He concluded his message with this statement: "Miss Addams influence will endure and her memory will be cherished so long as the opinions of peoples and governments continue to be moulded by humanitarian ideals."[31]

SOON-TO-BE OCCUPATIONAL THERAPISTS AT HULL HOUSE

One of the workers at Hull House in those early years was an artist and craftswoman from Rhode Island named Jessie Luther (see chapter 6). From 1901 to 1903, Luther taught crafts at Hull House and ran its Labor Museum. The museum was established to help immigrants maintain a sense of continuity with their past, a connection that often was not only ruptured but also devalued at the point of immigration. The Labor Museum program acted as a bridge between the immigrants' European and American experiences and provided the older generation an opportunity to display their skills, which included handicrafts.[32] Craft classes such as pottery, cooking, spinning, and bookbinding were offered by the Labor Museum and were often taught by residents of the neighbourhood.[33] Luther went on from Hull House to develop her skills in occupational therapy at Marblehead, Massachusetts; in St Anthony, Newfoundland; at Walter Reed in Washington, DC; and as the director of occupations at the Butler Psychiatric Hospital in Providence, Rhode Island.

There were likely many would-be occupational therapists who came through Hull House at some point, but the best known was Eleanor Clarke Slagle. During her social work studies at Hull House in 1911, she took a summer course called "Occupations for Attendants in Institutions for the Insane."[34] The course had been organized in 1908 by the newly formed Chicago School of Civics and Philanthropy,[35] and its goal was to teach attendants to substitute educational activities for custodial methods, using games and handicrafts as stimuli, thereby easing the plight of the patients while making the work of the attendants more appealing.[36] These concepts were supported by Dr Adolf Meyer, who, in addition to his own work at the Phipps Psychiatric Clinic in Baltimore, was working with the social activists Julia Lathrop and Rabbi Hirsch to effect mental health reform more generally.[37] Slagle joined Meyer at the Phipps Clinic in 1913, providing occupations that addressed her newly developed method of habit training.

In 1915, the Illinois Society for Mental Hygiene established the Henry B. Favill School of Occupations at Hull House, purportedly as the first such school in the world.[38] Slagle, a founder of NSPOT and a major contributor to the profession throughout her life, directed the school's program from 1918 to 1922.[39] She visited Canada in 1917 to observe the work of the Military Hospitals Commission of Canada (MHC). She came as the guest of T.B. Kidner (see chapter 7), the commission's vocational secretary, and the visit marked the beginning of a long working relationship between the two. Slagle also visited the University of Toronto, having been asked to make recommendations regarding the ward aides program that was about to begin.[40] After visiting the Canadian hospitals, Slagle returned home ready to oversee the training of four thousand therapists, much needed with the entry of the Americans into World War I.[41]

CANADIAN SETTLEMENT HOUSES

A Canadian woman, Mary Lawson Bell, and an American settlement worker, Sara Libby Carson, founded the first settlement house in Canada. Evangelia House was established in Toronto in 1902 on Queen Street East, moving to larger quarters as its numbers grew. Its main benefactor, E.B. Osler (the brother of Sir William Osler the physician), purchased and equipped a large building with extensive grounds for the project. Evangelia House had close ties with the Young Women's Christian Association (YWCA) and initially dealt only with women and young girls. It later severed its ties both with the YWCA and with religion, broadening its approach in order to reach out to the larger neighbourhood. The goal of this settlement house, like that of its predecessors in England, was to influence the community by example. "Settlers" lived among the residents and shared their learning and their views.[42] Evangelia House gave its workers, who were primarily university-educated women, the opportunity to have experiences that would broaden their horizons and ultimately their employment and leadership options in the larger world.[43] It was something of a symbiotic relationship, with the helpers and those being helped each needing the other.

Settlement houses sprang up across Canada wherever there were major cities and the accompanying poverty. By 1917, there were thirteen settlement houses, six of which were in Toronto.[44] All had a mandate to decrease dependency in immigrant and poor populations, to develop skills and knowledge, to build communities, and to improve the quality of life. Unlike their British counterparts, settlement houses in North America were in neighbourhoods populated by recent immigrants, primarily from eastern Europe, few of whom spoke English. As a result, language lessons became a priority. Virtually all of the language programs had a practical orientation and were delivered to groups rather than individuals. The first outreach was to children and mothers, through daycare settings and kindergarten classes. Education groups for mothers and lessons in arts, crafts, music, and drama followed.

Canadian settlement houses were slower to start up than their American or British counterparts because the problems they had to deal with – and their target populations – were not as large. However, as non-English-speaking immigrants began arriving in greater numbers at the turn of the century, the needs increased. New immigrants had to compete for jobs. Lack of employment and low salaries meant that many had no housing and were forced to move in with other families. Overcrowded living conditions made people more vulnerable to disease and, some thought, to immorality. When the parents in a family succeeded in finding work, their children were often left on their own and neglected.[45]

There was no support for the idea that government – municipal or other – should provide relief to the poor. The prevailing ideology suggested that governments should provide only meagre relief lest the poor become dependent and habitually indigent and indolent. Conventional philanthropic organizations and the church were expected to provide whatever help was needed.[46]

THE UNIVERSITY SETTLEMENT HOUSE

When the University Settlement House was founded in Toronto in 1910, there was an expectation that the volunteer workers would be university students, men at the start and in later years women.[47] Among other purposes and objectives, the University Settlement House sought to "arouse social consciousness in both the University and the Settlement communities by cultivating among the youth of both communities common interests in recreation, sports, arts, crafts, music, drama, debates and other activities."[48] In 1912, Mabel Newton was the first woman to be hired by the board. She worked in women's programs; visited homes; offered friendship, support, and advice; and organized sewing and needlework

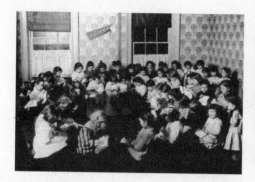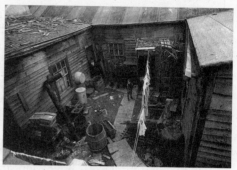

LEFT Sewing class provided to children at the University Settlement House, c. 1920. Courtesy City of Toronto Archives, fonds 1024, item 68; RIGHT Slum in an area near the University of Toronto, c. 1920. Courtesy City of Toronto Archives, series 372, sub-series 32, item 259.

classes. Newton was from England and had previous experience in nursing and social work.[49] Her background and the work she did could be seen as similar to that of early occupational therapists.

Sir Robert Falconer, the president of the University of Toronto at the time, was a founder and strong supporter of the University Settlement House, finding it a means of expressing his religious values as a Presbyterian – without proselytizing.[50] Falconer thought that educated people were morally bound to share their expertise with others.[51] Furthermore, it seemed appropriate that members of the university should undertake the scientific study of, and learn to understand, the factors that created a slum.[52]

The issue of religion was a difficult matter for settlement houses in Canada. Given their neighbourhood locations, their religious affiliation or orientation was bound to offend at least some of their members.[53] When the University Settlement House hired Milton B. Hunt away from his position at Hull House in 1911, a new relationship with religion was heralded. According to a new mission statement, the settlement drew "no distinction as to creed, race, colour," while one of its aims was "to establish in the community a permanent socializing agency for bringing about civic betterment."[54] Settlement houses were open to community groups whose goals for social reform were directed towards relieving the burden of the poor. They welcomed meetings of trade unions, ethnic groups, and civic organizations that fostered traditions within their communities.

Some settlement houses established summer camps to give children a chance to be away from the city and to give their mothers a much needed break. A precedent had already been set by J.J. Kelso, a newspaper reporter at the Toronto *Globe* who was a social reformer with a particular interest in the rights of children. He, too, had spent time at Hull House and had returned to Canada with many ideas, establishing the Fresh Air Fund for summer holidays for poor children. In 1910, he became a member of the Board of Directors of the University Settlement.[55]

Despite their lofty goals and their considerable accomplishments, settlement houses did not escape criticism. Some argued that the movement was a way to deal with the threat to the middle and upper classes posed by the poverty, sickness, and what were perceived to be low moral standards in the areas where the settlement houses had been established. There was a certain irony in the fact that it was often wealthy single women who were advising poor wives and mothers on how to run their homes. Affluent women often taught skills (such as caring for a home) that, given that they had servants, they had never practised themselves.[56] There were also cynical questions about whether some of the programs were developed to meet the needs of the student volunteers rather than the residents. With the development of schools of social work, critics asked if settlement houses existed primarily to provide experience for student social workers or if they were indeed meant to provide the impetus for social reform.[57]

PUBLIC HEALTH

The physical health of the community was a primary concern for many of those in settlement work. Sanitation was a major issue, and poverty made the community vulnerable to a host of health problems. Dr Charles Hastings was Toronto's public health officer in 1910 and a founding member of the University Settlement House. His work in public health – directed primarily at the pasteurization of milk and the development of safe water for drinking and bathing – addressed important needs of settlement house populations. Hastings set up free clinics for new mothers and their babies; sent district health nurses on home visits to educate mothers on cooking for the sick and caring for children; promoted birth control; liaised with hospitals and social services; and instituted inspections and improvements of lodging houses.[58] The work of the public health department was very congruent with settlement house concerns and with the later focus in occupational therapy on teaching skills for daily living.

The poor working conditions that members of the settlement house community had to endure were another major concern. There was a great need for laws to regulate working hours and to deal with child labour. The issue of worker safety was not yet on the horizon, and assistance for injured workers was virtually non-existent, although Ruskin, among others, had recognized the need decades earlier. James Mavor, a professor at the University of Toronto who was involved in the University Settlement House (and also the arts and crafts movement), provided one of the first analyses of the situation in his 1899 report on compensation for workmen's injuries.[59] In 1907–08, he conducted a study on the living conditions and the budgets of the poor working class.[60]

Some settlement houses were established with special purposes in mind. For example, in London, England, Honnor Morten, a nurse, established Passmore Edwards Settlement specifically for handicapped children.[61] This model school included physical therapy along with regular course work and meals. Grace Kimmins opened the Heritage Craft School and Hospital for Cripples in Sussex in 1903 in an effort to send "young cripples away before they had been contaminated by their environment."[62]

SOCIAL WORK AND OCCUPATIONAL THERAPY

The settlement house movement is acknowledged as having been the progenitor of the profession of social work. A course in social service was established at the University of Toronto in 1914. As with the movement itself, it was initially thought that men would fill the places and take the leading roles in the profession. However, the low salaries perhaps acted as a deterrent, and with most young men preparing to go off to war in 1914, it soon became clear that the profession was attracting more women than men. The timing was right, as large numbers of university-educated women were looking for a profession. Although most of these women had worked previously as volunteers, they had practised their skills and gained experience in planning and implementing programs that had far-reaching effects. Armed with that experience, they were now ready for something more. Many women wanted to be of service to others and seemed suited to social work. While the men might theorize about what should be done about social issues, the women set out to prove what could be done.[63]

There was also something adventurous about the new profession of social work for women; it allowed them to be involved in the world outside their homes, to take on challenges, and to have some control over their work. The women in social work were similar in their outlook to those who were to enter occupational therapy, and in fact, the work of the two groups often overlapped. While the goals of community development and decreased dependency of individuals are more generally associated with the profession of social work than with occupational therapy, in the late 1890s, the roots of these two as-yet-unborn professions developed – in several areas – along very similar paths. Like social workers, early occupational therapists worked with people in communities, helping them develop skills to become self-sufficient. In the early 1900s, the two nascent professions were seen as complementary, and there were even times when it seemed that the two disciplines might be combined.[64] In the early years of their university programs, each discipline provided courses for the other.[65] Social workers relied on occupational therapists for the successful reintegration of patients discharged into the community, noting that they needed to be occupied in a satisfactory manner.

The philosophy of the settlement house movement attracted people with means who wanted to help the poor and needy. Settlement houses offered educated middle-class women the chance to become involved in the world outside their homes, albeit often as volunteers. The concern for social justice, apparent a century ago, still attracts occupational therapists today, but instead of it being those with means who are the only ones to help, it is now those with skills. The settlement house movement gave occupational therapy its social justice genes.

5

Educational Reform

MANUAL TRAINING AND TECHNICAL EDUCATION

The acquisition of dexterity and skill of hand; the training of the eye to a sense of form and beauty; the formation of habits of accuracy, order and neatness; the inculcation of a love of industry and of habits of patience, perseverance and self-reliance, are some of the results which may be claimed as peculiarly belonging to work with the hands as a means of education.

Thomas Bessell Kidner, 1910[1]

The widespread use of crafts as a treatment modality in early occupational therapy can be credited in part to the popularity of the role of crafts in education at the end of the 1800s. Craftwork, or manual training as it was more generally known, was a significant component of educational reform.

The pedagogical philosophy in support of manual training found application in the use of crafts in the treatment of soldiers with injuries and illness in World War I. Though not made explicit at the time, there was an underlying rationale that if children learned through "doing," then injured soldiers could learn that way as well; the process of learning new skills or practising old ones was preparatory to employment. That the craftwork could also build morale and begin to rebuild self-esteem was equally important for the injured soldier returning home after living in the very different world of war. Thus, the rationale for the use of crafts with injured soldiers was similar to that which informed their use with the mentally ill population. With the new knowledge about learning that educational reform was adding, crafts could now be viewed in a more sophisticated manner.

The career of Thomas Bessell Kidner (to be described in some detail later in this chapter) bridges the two worlds of craftwork, the first focusing on facilitating new learning in children through manual training, and the second concerned with preparing those who were ill or disabled for the real world of work.

EDUCATIONAL REFORM IN THE NINETEENTH CENTURY

Until the latter part of the nineteenth century, learning by rote had been the accepted method of learning. However, educational reformers in Europe were becoming increasingly dissatisfied with that approach and began to stress the importance of *learning by doing*. Some work had been carried out in support of this idea earlier in the century. In Switzerland, Johann Heinrich Pestalozzi (1746–1827) advocated seeking balance in educating the heart, the hand, and the head, thinking that children learned best through activities in which they could manipulate objects. Pestalozzi believed that these activities also served as preparation for employment in later life.[2]

In Germany, Friedrich Froebel (1782–1852) introduced kindergarten as the starting point of formal education and advocated manual activities. In 1883, a "Froebel kindergarten" was introduced into the public schools of Toronto (Toronto being the second city in the world to have one), and kindergartens soon appeared throughout the province of Ontario.[3] Froebel, who was a disciple of Pestalozzi, used the word "gifts" to describe the use (or manipulation) of objects that could be used to discover the world and the word "occupations" to describe activities that could promote self-expression. The gifts were the toys and materials used, and the occupations were the arts and crafts that could help children express their thoughts and feelings about the world.[4] Froebel viewed play as preparation for "future industry, diligence, and productive activity."[5] With pressure on educators to pay more attention to new approaches to help their countries become more competitive, Froebel's gifts and occupations were considered a good basis for later technical education.[6]

Building on the work of Pestalozzi and Froebel, Otto Salomon (1849–1907) introduced what was known as the *sloyd* method in Sweden. Sloyd used graded craft activities at a level of difficulty that would stimulate but not dishearten the child and would thus promote self-efficacy.[7] The approach had both formative and utilitarian aims: it helped instil good work habits, independence, and a love of labour as well as dexterity in the use of tools. The activities cultivated accuracy, carefulness, patience, perseverance, attention, and concentration. The sloyd method was child-centred, the value of the work being in the *child* who made the object and not in the object produced.

Sloyd was originally developed to prepare the children of working men for the physical labour of adulthood and give them the capacity to use the hands on which their living would depend.[8] However, Salomon's concern was with developing that capacity, and not with whether the activities were a preparation for work in later life. He thought the sloyd method belonged to general education and should be for everyone in elementary and secondary schools.[9] In keeping with principles then emerging from the arts and crafts movement, Salomon suggested that all models used in craft activities should be useful and made of wood in its most natural form.[10] Normal schools (i.e., teachers' colleges) in Canada incorporated sloyd and Froebel in their teacher training programs at the end of the 1800s.

Pestalozzi, Froebel, and Salomon influenced Sir Philip Magnus (1842–1933), a leading British educator and the director of the City and Guilds of London Institute. The institute was founded in 1878, in part "to promote technical education of people of both sexes engaged in the industries and manufacturers of this country."[11] The institute was seen as a concrete example of how Europe was responding to the growing demand for workers in the new industrial age. It was now accepted that rote learning and knowledge for its own sake were no longer appropriate and that practical education was what was needed for the modern new world. Magnus, who came to education after a career as a reform rabbi, was a gifted educator, and his contributions to the field won him the honour of being the first person to be knighted for providing educational service.[12] He successfully fought to have learning by doing incorporated throughout primary education in the form of manual training; for Magnus, the "3 Rs" were reading, writing, and "real" work. He admitted to having a "vocational bias" and expressed his belief that education should prepare the pupil for a future career, beginning in elementary school with manual training.[13] He later claimed that introducing manual training to the education system made "the greatest improvement in our elementary education since 1870."[14]

The American philosopher and educator John Dewey (1859–1952) was another influential reformer. Like his fellow reformers, he too promoted the idea of learning by doing as an antidote to the practice of training the mind only and rote learning. For Dewey, manual training was not a means of teaching children to use tools; rather, he saw it as a means of preparing children for daily life – a "mode of activity on the part of the child which reproduces, or runs parallel to, some form of work carried on in social life."[15]

Dewey's curriculum included manual, artistic, and domestic work, and emphasized *working to learn* (i.e., using hands-on activities) rather than learning as preparation for work.[16] Dewey thought that through meaningful experiences, which included the outside world of work, a person would be able to constantly connect to his or her environment.[17] He was particularly interested in knowledge arrived at through problem solving. "[Normal thinking] arises from the need of meeting some difficulty, in reflecting on the best way to overcome it, and thus leads to planning, to projecting mentally the result to be reached, and deciding upon the steps necessary and their serial order."[18]

Along with William James, Charles Peirce, and George Herbert Mead, Dewey was one of the originators of the philosophy of pragmatism, which sees knowledge develop apace with change and adaptation. Pragmatism was adopted as a model for learning by Dewey and as a model for enhancing health and social welfare by those working in mental hygiene. This philosophy stressed the integration of mind and body and the unity of time and space. It saw the individual proceed through life according to active experience and the feedback provided by that experience. Thus, active experience (or engagement in occupation) was the essential starting point.

It has been suggested that Dewey's philosophy of pragmatism underlies the theoretical basis of occupational therapy. Breines notes that while "active occupation as a modifier of learning and health, was a theme of great social relevance in the early part of the century, [it] received less emphasis as time went by."[19] The relevance of occupations would have been acknowledged in the early 1900s when Dewey, as a faculty member of the University of Chicago, was intimately involved with Hull House. His ideas influenced the educational programs the settlement house offered, and these programs, in turn, were often carried out by soon-to-be occupational therapists like Jessie Luther and Eleanor Clarke Slagle.

Like Ruskin and Morris, who had spoken of instilling the "art spirit" in children and providing "art for all," Dewey thought that art should be a part of everyone's creative life and not just the privilege of a select group of artists. Instructional classes at Hull House were carried out in an atmosphere that valued art and manual work, and by 1917, the Chicago Public School Art Society had begun placing industrial-arts display cabinets in schools that had manual-arts training classes. The cabinets, which were filled with needlework, weaving, block prints, and other textile work, were designed to dignify handiwork, cultivate appreciation of quality, and encourage self-expression.[20]

MANUAL TRAINING FOR LEARNING OR AS PREPARATION FOR WORK

Although there was certainly support for learning by doing as a better form of education, there was another, more practical reason for the popularity of this method. There was growing concern over the need to prepare students to become more competitive workers, and manual training was seen as a means of building better work skills. In Canada, ever since Confederation, pressure had been increasing for educators to take a more practical approach to preparing workers for the new economy. In addition, the recessions of the 1880s and 1890s had alerted Canada to the need for more skilled workers if it wished to compete in world markets.[21] Some thought that manual training provided a foundation for the vocational training and technical education programs that were needed. As in Europe, however, this idea was not accepted, and it was not the rationale provided by Canadian educators for introducing manual training into the schools.

James L. Hughes, a prominent North American educator and leading reformer at the elementary school level, supported manual training in the schools as early as 1886. However, he was clear about its role in education, saying, "Manual training is not to be understood as a system of trade schools or as something to be taught chiefly for its economic value, but as a system of definite self-expression with things; as formative, constructive self-expression."[22] Knowing that Hughes was a follower of Ruskin helps one understand the emotion behind his statement that manual training was "not to make articles, but to make men and women."[23] Indeed, Ruskin, Morris, and the arts and crafts movement had a strong influence on education while also dignifying and elevating the place of labour. There was opposition in many quarters to the notion that those values were to be replaced by practicalities.[24]

The debate over the role of manual training in job preparation was somewhat artificial, however, because if there was agreement that manual training was a good way to learn, then whether or not it supported the later acquisition of job skills was not altogether relevant; the important thing was to see that manual training programs were implemented. At the beginning of the twentieth century, Professor James W. Robertson (1857–1930), then commissioner of agriculture and dairying for Canada, assumed the responsibility of carrying out a plan to implement manual training in Canadian elementary schools.[25] While Robertson oversaw the plan, it was Sir William C. Macdonald who provided the funds to finance it.

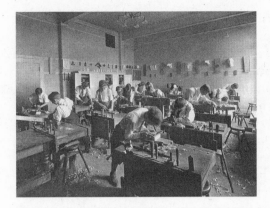 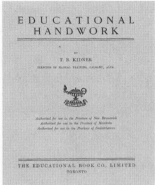

LEFT Manual training. Interior, Lower Canada College, Montreal, QC. Wm Notman & Son, 1910, 20th century, II-180773. McCord Museum, Montreal; RIGHT Cover of book for teachers of handicrafts, written by Kidner and published in 1910.

THE MACDONALD MANUAL TRAINING FUND

William C. Macdonald (1831–1917), a native of Glenaladale, Prince Edward Island, had become the very wealthy owner of the Montreal-based Macdonald Tobacco Company by the latter part of the 1800s. He was a great philanthropist, directing his efforts primarily toward supporting McGill University and improving rural education. Macdonald felt strongly that the young and expanding nation of Canada needed workers with the practical skills necessary for jobs in industry. He was also convinced of the importance of manual training in elementary school, seeing it as preparatory for the technical instruction at a later age that would lead to a vocation.[26] In 1900, he established the Macdonald Manual Training Fund (MMTF) with the express purpose of bringing manual training into the elementary school curriculum in Canada.

To promote his vision, Macdonald offered to provide salaries for three years for teachers of manual training in at least one town or city in every province in Canada. Payment was on the condition that local and provincial funding would support the program thereafter.[27] The funds also supported the instruction of teachers in training and provided the necessary equipment. The plan took hold, and by the end of the three-year period, more than seven thousand boys were taking the courses. Girls were soon enrolled as well, and by 1909, over twenty thousand boys and girls in Canadian schools had received the benefits of manual training as part of their regular school curriculum.[28] For Robertson, whose father had been a Church of Scotland evangelist, the work that the children did was important not only from an educational perspective, but from a religious one as well. He writes, "The happiness which springs from the consciousness of having begun and finished a piece of good, useful work by one's own labour, is more than a mental and physical tonic. In large measure, it allies the worker with the Power that maketh for righteousness. It gives power to overcome obstacles, and the power to overcome obstacles in the path of material mental, moral, and spiritual progress is perhaps the most desirable quality which can be acquired through education."[29]

There were no teachers of manual training in Canada at this time, and thus they had to be hired from abroad. Thomas Bessell Kidner, soon to be an important figure in occupational therapy (see also chapter 13), was one of twenty-seven teachers brought to Canada in 1900 through the MMTF.[30]

THOMAS BESSELL KIDNER (1866–1932)

Kidner was born in Bristol, England, and studied to become an architect. One of the courses he took was provided by the City and Guilds of London Institute, where Sir Philip Magnus (the educational reformer noted earlier) was in charge. Indeed, Kidner later identified Magnus as having been a particularly strong role model and mentor in his career.[31] With the offer from the MMTF, Kidner's career took a detour from architecture to manual training and technical education, and with the outbreak of World War I, this detour led to his involvement with the first systematic use of occupational therapy in Canada.

The MMTF sent Kidner to Truro, Nova Scotia, as an "organizer of technical work." He was well qualified for this new position, having already acquired carpentry and building skills, a certificate in technical education, and some teaching experience. Correspondence between Kidner and Robertson[32] suggests that Kidner spent much of his time in those early years organizing this new endeavour: ordering equipment, searching for household science teachers, consulting with schools, running training programs, and compiling instructional materials for teachers who could not attend his training programs.[33] When the three-year period sponsored by the MMTF ended, the province of New Brunswick hired Kidner to do the same type of work there. He moved with his family, which now included two children born in Truro and one born in Bristol, to Fredericton in 1904.[34]

That Kidner shared many modern ideas about educational reform was evident in his early writings. He was a regular contributor to the *Educational Review*, providing instructions for various crafts as well as philosophical articles.[35] While Kidner drew attention to the many intellectual skills that could be developed through active learning, he also noted another practical advantage of these classes: that both children and teachers would look forward to the manual training classes and that "the joy of 'doing' will appeal."[36] Kidner was concerned about the competence of the manual training teachers, noting the need for teachers who were "not only skilled in the use of tools but ... trained in the methods of pedagogy, the understanding of child life and the aims and ideals of educators of our future men and women."[37] This same concern would apply to those who were soon to teach crafts to injured soldiers.

Kidner believed that hand and eye training was a foundation for many other types of learning, and he wrote about the importance of acquiring these skills in his book *Educational Handwork*. In his introductory chapter, he remarks on "the value of the training of the hand in childhood as an aid to the development of the brain centres," and notes, "Wherever Handwork has been introduced into the schools, the literary and intellectual work has not suffered. On the contrary ... the ordinary work of the school has been much benefited by the introduction of 'Hand-and-Eye Training.'"[38]

Meanwhile, educational reform was continuing in Europe and gaining strength in the United States. The Italian physician and educator Maria Montessori (1870–1952) was promoting the need to educate the senses along with – and even before – the intellect. Like Salomon with his sloyd method, Montessori stressed using graded tasks, matching materials to a child's abilities and inner needs, and facilitating the development of the child's own initiative.[39] Her work caught the attention of the public and attracted many admirers, including Alexander Graham Bell and his wife, Mabel. In 1912, they founded Canada's first Montessori school, in Baddeck, Nova Scotia, where the Bell family spent their summers.

Mabel Bell, who had been deaf since the age of five, was actively engaged in various social reforms. She was interested in women's rights, advocated for women's suffrage, and used her considerable advocacy skills in Washington, DC, as well as in Baddeck. Like those women who would later be occupational therapists, she established a sewing cooperative in Baddeck, and when she found a market for the work in Montreal, the women were able to earn additional funds to support their families. Her concern for the health of the people in Baddeck led to the formation of a local branch of the newly established Victorian Order of Nurses. She also founded the Young Ladies Club of Baddeck in 1891 to help women acquire knowledge and social skills, and she purchased a building to be used for a public library.[40]

Alexander and Mabel supported one another's efforts at reform. Bell was particularly interested in educational reform, making it known that he valued experiential learning, whereby children would learn for themselves. "If their curiosity and interest can be aroused," he writes, "they will speculate for themselves as to the causes of the phenomena observed. This exercise of the mind is just what children need."[41] Arousing curiosity and interest was what the therapists were trying to do during the war as they attempted to engage the injured soldier in an occupation.

Canada was now coming to terms with the need to prepare young people for work in the industrial age. The Royal Commission on Industrial Training and Technical Education was established in 1910 to assess the readiness of the country to take on this task. By this time, Kidner was an expert in manual training and a proponent of the need for technical education. When the commissioners were travelling across Canada seeking views on the issue, Kidner was invited to appear before them. The commission was headed by J.W. Robertson, who had managed the MMTF and was the person to whom Kidner had been responsible when he had first arrived in Canada a decade earlier.

TECHNICAL EDUCATION AND INDUSTRIAL TRAINING

In 1911, Kidner was appointed as the director of technical education and technical adviser to the Commissioner of School Buildings in Calgary, Alberta. The city had a history of progressive education, having also been a recipient of an MMTF grant in the early 1900s, and so it was not surprising that it was ready to move forward with plans for technical education. Kidner's address to the Calgary School Board shortly after his arrival was significant enough to warrant coverage in the daily newspaper, the *Morning Albertan*. He announced that his new position meant that there would now be evening classes for building and machine work, architectural drawing, practical mathematics, shop arithmetic, and, in recognition of the large foreign population in the city, English-language classes. Household science courses would also be made available.[42] Kidner's annual reports to the board attest to the development of his programs and to increasing enrolments.[43] In 1913, a special anniversary edition of the *Morning Albertan* described the course offerings, which now included art classes and business courses. The domestic science program also expanded, with classes in cooking, laundry, and sewing in the elementary schools.[44]

While popular among politicians, technical education was a subject of controversy. The need to turn out enough workers for the increasingly industrialized country was not in dispute; however, it was clear that the student body for these courses was subject to class distinctions. In an effort to be more widely acceptable, some vocational high schools retained academic subjects such as mathematics, languages, and some science. In Ontario, for example, John Millar, the deputy minister of education, agreed that vocational training would be appropriate for a few high schools in Ontario and would provide some students with "ready access to the industries of a large manufacturing city."[45] However, his pedagogical preference was to have manual training in all levels of schooling. Like the educational reformers who had come before him, he believed that manual training was but a component of a holistic education. The reality was, however, that a dichotomy had begun to develop that was to "stream" students into vocational or academic programs, and the two approaches were rarely combined. It would not be long before it became apparent that the children of the working classes were being slotted into the vocational programs, effectively being precluded from joining the more academic stream with its concomitant opportunity for economic success.

Some have argued that the whole debate over the purpose of manual training was sparked by Morris (and Ruskin), whose ideology threatened the existing social, political, and economic order by attempting to elevate art and craftwork to the legitimacy of other curriculum offerings. The existing order much preferred the old order that had valued "the classical curriculum, and the life of the mind as the highest form of human achievement."[46]

With the outbreak of World War I, Kidner found himself volunteering to work with injured soldiers in Calgary, seeing that they were met on arrival and arranging for their future employment. He first interviewed the soldiers in order to understand their needs and work history. Then, knowing the resources for technical education well, he proceeded to find appropriate opportunities for their re-education.[47] However, his own life was about to change again.

CRAFTWORK AS TREATMENT FOR INJURED SOLDIERS

In December 1915, Senator James Lougheed, the newly appointed chairman of the Military Hospitals Commission, visited Calgary. He invited Kidner to take on a new position in Ottawa in connection with the re-education of injured soldiers, and Kidner accepted. When he informed the Calgary School Board of his imminent departure, the chairman of the board proudly responded that while they were sorry to see Kidner go, they were glad to know that they had had on their staff a man qualified to take on such work.[48] It was expected that Kidner would be away from Calgary for only two to three years, but when he eventually did leave Ottawa, it was to immigrate to the United States. In 1919, Kidner took a position with the National Tuberculosis Association and, at the same time, became fully involved with occupational therapy in the United States.

For Kidner, the transformation from educator and educational reformer to vocational rehabilitator occurred during World War I. At an early stage in his work in Ottawa, Kidner determined that just as manual training was a foundation for later work skills in children, so too would it be a way of preparing injured soldiers to return to their former work or enter a new field of endeavour.[49] Being able to make something with one's hands built morale and self-confidence and served as a preparatory step to returning to work. Now manual training would be provided to injured soldiers as bedside occupations and to those who were well enough, in workshops off the ward. The teachers of these occupations were known as ward, or occupational, aides. Within a few years, however, they would be known as occupational therapists.

6

Pioneering Women

LUTHER, PECK, AND SCOTT

It seems apparent that such normal and interesting occupations and the need
for continued effort in their accomplishment cannot fail to improve the
community 's social standards and have an influence on everyday life.

Jessie Luther's Diary, 1908[1]

In the decade or so leading up to World War I, women were taking on new roles, some of which would lead directly to occupational therapy. Roles for women in Canada at the turn of the century varied greatly and generally depended on social class, geographical location, and marital status. In these years, the pioneering women in occupational therapy differed in several ways from other women. Most were born to middle- and upper-class families, whether in major cities like Toronto, Montreal, or Winnipeg or in small towns. Many attended private schools and "finishing" schools, perhaps travelling abroad at some point to broaden their education. Most had artistic interests at some level, and virtually all had skills in handicrafts. They pursued art or handicrafts, if not as a vocation then as an avocation.[2]

These women managed to blend their artistic interests with doing good works, particularly in their encouragement of arts and crafts among poor, Native, and immigrant populations. They promoted self-sufficiency in these populations by selling the crafts that were produced. While many women pursued their interests for philanthropic reasons, others were gainfully employed teaching crafts and other skills for everyday living.

The work of three women – Jessie Luther, Alice Peck, and "Miss Scott" – represents early efforts in the use of occupations and presages the work of occupational therapists to come. Their stories shed light on the backgrounds, motivations, and contributions of the women who chose to undertake the work.

JESSIE LUTHER (1860–1952)

Jessie Luther's career as an occupational therapist exemplifies the relationship between the arts and crafts and settlement house movements (see chapters 3 and 4) and the profession of occupational therapy. Luther followed her profession in the United States and also in Newfoundland, the latter of which was then a British colony and still some forty years away from being part of Canada. Fortunately, Luther described her activities and feelings in a series of diary entries and letters and also published several articles about her work. These written records provide a means of understanding this early period of the profession and the people who helped to fashion it.[3]

Luther was born in Providence, Rhode Island, in 1860. She attended small private schools before studying for one year at the prestigious Rhode Island School of Design. She studied art at the Mary C. Wheeler Studio for four years, and during this time, she travelled with other students to Paris. She worked with various artists and taught art until 1899, and then she developed an interest in learning to do a variety of crafts, including woodcarving, metalwork, basketry, bookbinding, weaving, and pottery. As a member of the Boston Arts and Crafts Society and believing not only in the artistic but also in the social values of the movement, she willingly accepted an invitation from Jane Addams in 1901 to work at Hull House, in Chicago.[4] There she worked in the Labor Museum with immigrant and poor populations, teaching them new skills while nurturing their traditional crafts.[5] The Labor Museum served to ensure that art was a part of the daily life of the settlement community at Hull House.[6]

Luther's long hours of work, along with other personal issues, led to nervous exhaustion, and in 1903, she was admitted to a private clinic in Jaffrey, New Hampshire, for the "rest cure." The rest cure was a popular treatment in its day and expressly required the patient to remain in bed and avoid activity. During her recovery, however, Luther found comfort in doing craftwork, and she soon embraced the idea that involvement in crafts could benefit a person's recovery. This personal experience as well as the nervous illnesses of her mother and several friends led her to think that activities and work could bring on what she called "self-forgetfulness" and act as a cure for particular conditions. She explained her rationale,

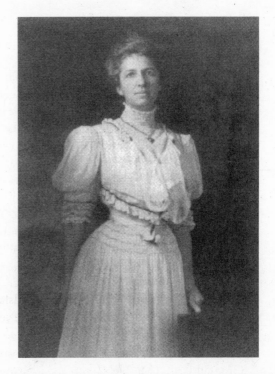

Jessie Luther at home in
Providence, Rhode Island,
c. 1890. Courtesy The
Rooms, Provincial Archives
Division, St John's, NL,
Martha Gendron Collection.

noting the importance of the timing of the intervention: "Nothing can
be more helpful than this cure if properly directed, while the will still has
the power to act."[7]

While at the private clinic, Luther met the physician Herbert Hall,
who was also a patient at the facility. He was an avid potter and painter
and, like her, advocated occupations as a means of treatment. In 1904,
Luther and Hall started a "handcraft shop" at Devereux Mansion at
Marblehead, Massachusetts, providing a practical application of the lessons they had learned from their own recoveries. Their program challenged beliefs about the rest cure for depression and nervous collapse and
opened the way for the therapeutic use of occupation.[8]

Hall described what he termed the "work-cure" in the *Journal of the
American Medical Association* in 1910. While many others had promoted
the idea of work as a treatment for mental health problems, Hall was the
first to interpret work more formally in terms of crafts. He approached
his patients with a variety of options, starting with weaving and gradually expanding the repertoire of crafts on offer to include woodcarving,
metalwork, and pottery. To build tolerance for activity during recovery,

he gradually increased the time spent on, and the complexity of, the craft. Hall noted that if a patient did not seem interested in the work, he would confront him or her with the statement, "Do this, and you will in the end benefit by it, although at present it may seem to make you worse."[9] In an early effort to provide evidence of the value of his new treatment approach, Hall reported some statistics regarding outcomes. He determined that of one hundred patients (nine males and ninety-one females), treated over a five-year period, fifty-nine had improved, twenty-seven were considered much improved, and fourteen had found no relief.[10]

The new approach to treatment carried out by Hall and Luther attracted many visitors, including the British physician Sir Wilfred Grenfell (1865–1940).[11] Grenfell worked for the Royal National Mission to Deep Sea Fisherman, providing medical and social services to fishing settlements along the coast of Newfoundland and Labrador. He worked from a hospital ship that stopped along the way as needed and also had a permanent mission in the town of St Anthony, located at the tip of the northern peninsula of Newfoundland.[12] Grenfell's interest in the link between economic well-being and health led him to found fishermen's cooperatives, home industries, farms and gardens, an orphanage, interdenominational schools, and a chain of hospitals and nursing stations.[13]

Grenfell visited Marblehead in 1905 during a fundraising tour. He saw Luther's work and was struck by the "non-medical application of … training [in crafts]."[14] He invited her to become part of the mission at St Anthony and she agreed. In the summer of 1906, after she had already been appointed as the full-time director of occupational therapy[15] at the Butler (Psychiatric) Hospital in Providence, Rhode Island, Luther arranged to take a leave of absence so that she could join Grenfell for the first of many working visits.

The voyage by sea from Providence to St Anthony was difficult, and when Luther arrived, there were few people and no resources to support her work. She assessed the situation, determined what she would need to begin the work, and gathered materials as best she could, meeting each challenge as it came. She eventually succeeded against great odds in establishing a variety of occupations.[16]

Luther set up a "loom-room," a pottery workshop, and a woodworking class for young boys, as well as mat-hooking and stone-carving classes for adults. In her spare time, she taught homemaking, social skills, and literacy, and established social clubs. She used the mission as a base from which to work with communities along the coast, directing her efforts toward the women in the hope of improving social conditions and build-

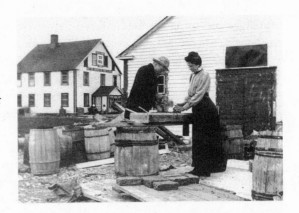

Jessie Luther at the Grenfell Mission in St Anthony, Newfoundland, supervising the construction of a kiln for pottery making, 1908. Courtesy The Rooms, Provincial Archives Division, St John's, NL, VA 118-93.4.

ing more self-sufficient communities. She visited both neighbouring and far-off communities to set up local workshops and would later return to them to arrange for the sale of the crafts they had produced.

Good entrepreneurial and interpersonal skills helped Luther develop these cottage industries. She made an arrangement with the Canadian Handicrafts Guild (CHG) in Montreal whereby the guild provided Luther with the raw materials needed for the crafts and Luther provided the guild with the finished products to sell. Sir Wilfred Grenfell was the popular intermediary who appeared periodically at the guild's meetings to make a personal plea to members to continue their support.[17]

Some years later, Dr Herbert Hall recalled their early work at Marblehead and Luther's departure for Newfoundland: "It began in a little cobbler's shop under the direction of Miss Jessie Luther, who is now the Occupational Director at the Butler Hospital in Providence, and was taken from me for his own occupational purposes by Dr Grenfel[l] who kept her in the Frozen North for a good many years."[18]

Although Luther worked with some people with disabilities, particularly those who were blind or had tuberculosis, her focus was on the well population. Her approach was that of a settlement house worker as she had experienced it during her years at Hull House. Her goal was to build a sense of community and to enhance productivity, particularly among the fishers' wives, who were left with long hours to spend on their own while their husbands were at sea. She was interested in issues of social and occupational justice – "in what people were doing, in what they were eating, in the education of their children, and in the community's capacity to care for its elderly and poor."[19] Describing her work in Newfoundland, she writes, "It seems apparent that such normal and interesting occupations and the need for continued effort in their accomplishment cannot fail to improve the community's social standards and have an influence on everyday life."[20] Her work in developing skills and supports in Newfoundland and Labrador in the early 1900s was a model of health promotion that used intervention at the community level. It was also an example of how crafts could be used to enhance the productivity of people with and without disabilities.

In 1916 Luther ended her involvement with what had become the International Grenfell Association.[21] She continued to work as an occupational therapist in Rhode Island until her retirement in 1937, and she actively promoted the value of occupation in her writings in both professional and popular publications of the day. She tried to have her letters and diaries published but was unsuccessful.[22] It would be another fifty years before her writings were finally in print.

Jessie Luther's story helps affirm the profession's roots in the arts and crafts and settlement house movements and is an endorsement of the profession's early values.

MARY ALICE (SKELTON) PECK (1855-1943)

Peck was born into a privileged upper middle-class family in Toronto in 1855. She contracted whooping cough at a young age and, following the suggestion that a change would speed her recovery, spent time with one aunt in Montreal and another in Saint John. By 1861, her parents, brothers, and sister had moved to Montreal and the family was reunited. Peck's father, James W. Skelton, was a businessman who shared his love of literature, music, and the stage with Alice. Her mother, Marianne Gault Skelton, originally from Montreal, was a member of the wealthy and influential Gault family.[23]

Alice's teenaged years were filled with travel abroad and visits to art galleries and museums. She enjoyed these activities, many of which appear to have influenced her future actions. For example, at age fourteen, while attending boarding school in England, she visited Octavia Hill's housing project in the poor area of South London. The memory of that visit stayed with her long after her return home. She later recalled being inspired by the social reform work that Hill was doing and impressed with Hill's patience in carrying it out.[24]

One experience that would influence her future came during a stop in England when she was fifteen and travelling with her older brother. She was impressed by "the joyous expression on the face of a young crippled

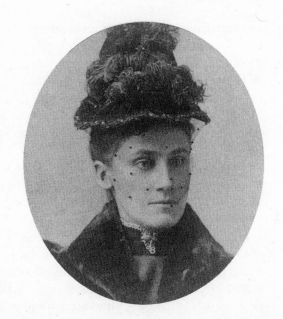

Alice Peck, c. 1890, co-founder of the Canadian Handicrafts Guild in 1905 and organizer of bedside occupations in military hospitals in Montreal 1917. Courtesy Barbara Carter Collection.

girl who was weaving the replica of a famous painting onto a loom."[25] They also visited Les Invalides, the seventeenth-century home for old and unwell soldiers in Paris. Alice later remembered their sad state – "poor men, legs, arms, eyes, gone, and many with years before them."[26]

Though clearly a sensitive young woman, Peck was also lively and had her share of fun and adventure.[27] She returned to Montreal and to her home at 28 McGill College Avenue for her debutante year in 1872. She married James Henry Peck in 1878 and thereafter was more commonly known as Mrs James Peck. They lived at "Undermount" a property of fifty thousand square feet in a well-established upper-class neighbourhood in Montreal. Mr Peck died in 1903, leaving Alice with seven children aged ten to twenty-three. Soon afterwards, she invited Patsy Andrews, an American with a background in fine arts whom she had met on one of her travels to the West, to stay with her at Undermount.[28] They became lifelong companions.

Although busy caring for her children, Peck's situation was sufficiently privileged that she still had the time and energy to pursue philanthropic work. She had founded the Montreal Branch of the Women's Art Association of Canada in 1894 and was its first president.[29] However, a decade or so later, it was decided that Montreal did not need the association, as it already had its own Women's Art Society. What Montreal did need was an organization to represent and preserve handicrafts, and thus in 1905 Peck founded the Canadian Handicrafts Guild with May Phillips. The guild's mandate was to "revive, preserve, and stimulate handicraft work and Home Art industries throughout Canada; and to encourage new and old settlers in the Dominion, to continue using their skill and knowledge in handicraft work."[30] In an address made in 1904 to the Conference on Art organized by the Women's Art Association, Peck spoke of the potential of craftwork to augment family income (particularly that of farmers and fishers), to preserve the arts as an asset for the country, and simply to make people happy. Echoing the view of Ruskin and Morris that making art was good for the soul, she said, "The practice of art in any form whatsoever tends to make men and women happy."[31]

In an entry in the 1904 yearbook of the National Council of Women of Canada, Peck spoke of the differing roles played by men and women in the promotion of Canadian handicrafts. She noted a straight-forward, almost mechanical role for men, saying, "It lies in the power of men to provide such a scheme [for handicrafts] with financial aid," and then went on to describe a more compassionate role for women: "To reach its utmost limit of good, it [the promotion of handicrafts] must ever be administrated by women, for in its personal element lies one of its greatest benefits. It is when heart touches heart that melody is struck."[32]

As a supporter of social justice and eager to comment on if not change practices she thought wrong, Peck noted the demise of the arts of the "red man." She attributed the phenomenon to the fact that "the white man is not willing to pay his red brother liberally, seeking a bargain and forcing the craftsman to accept the price to afford the necessities."[33] Throughout her life, she worked to celebrate and appropriately reward these arts.

The Canadian Handicrafts Guild organized displays and exhibitions to keep craftwork in the public eye. The guild also put a major effort into the sale of the handicrafts, the proceeds of which supported the many indigent craftworkers the CHG represented as well as those in a better financial position with high-quality work to offer. The business values of the CHG members came into conflict with their philanthropic ideas when they determined that they should teach and supervise their workers as necessary to ensure a quality of work that would result in sales. If the guild could train workers and "cultivate in them a natural and artistic sense in the use of colour design, then the likelihood of sales would increase."[34] Thus, while the CHG members celebrated the crafts produced, they also conveyed an air of superiority and maternalism in their notion that the craftworkers required their oversight.

In keeping with settlement house ideals, the motto of the CHG was, as noted earlier, "Self help – not charity."[35] When holding sales of craftwork, the guild was careful to appeal to a market that could afford to buy the work and would also want to lend support to the workers. With this demographic in mind, the guild chose to hold sales at the upscale retailer Holt Renfrew in Montreal, just down the street from the guild's location on St Catherine Street West. The CHG knew that the work would appeal to people in that class of society on philanthropic terms and that this population could afford the high cost of handmade articles.[36]

By the time of World War I, Peck had become an authority on handicrafts. She herself was an expert weaver, dye maker, and bookbinder, and she was an exceptional teacher. She had also had an interaction with the physician Alexander Mackenzie Forbes (1874–1929) that was to revive her interest in helping people with disabilities. Forbes was an old family friend who was to become an influential figure during and after the war.[37] The Peck and Forbes families summered in Métis, Quebec, and during one of these holidays, Forbes discussed a patient (Michel Massé) who had been a train coupler until he became paralyzed as a result of a railway accident. Unable to carry on his former work, he stayed at home and became a burden on his family. Forbes asked Peck to teach Massé to "do something with his hands" so as to keep his mind off his crippled body and perhaps, eventually, to earn a little money for himself. Peck taught Massé to make baskets, and he soon sold enough of them to support his entire family.[38]

With the outbreak of war, Peck, like many Canadian women of her class, went to England to volunteer. There she worked in a home for injured soldiers, teaching crafts at the bedside, and she saw the positive impact the work could have. On her return to Montreal in 1916, she set up craftwork in several military hospitals, determined to help relieve the monotony of convalescence for the newly returned injured soldiers. Peck had brought a small reed loom with her from England and used it as a model for special looms for patients who were confined to bed.[39] She was put in charge of the work done by ward aides (soon to be known as occupational therapists) in Montreal's military hospitals. Indeed, some credit Alice Peck with the official start of occupational therapy in Canada.[40]

Many of the women of the CHG became involved in the war effort. It seemed obvious that war work was just an extension of their regular work; that injured soldiers would benefit from handicrafts, which would help heal their bodies and their souls; and that the use of crafts would suit wartime every bit as much as it suited work with Native, poor, and im-

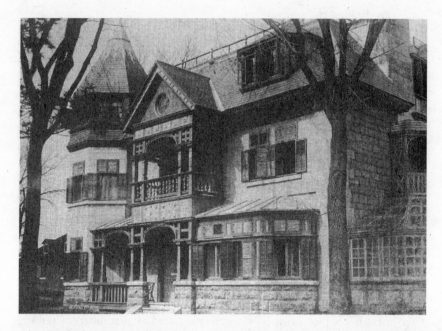

Alice Peck's home – "Undermount" – at 167 Durocher Street, Montreal. Peck started a workshop for veterans here, called "Undermount Industries," in 1919. Courtesy Canadian Guild of Crafts, Montreal.

migrant populations in peacetime. By volunteering themselves as handicraft teachers, these women could promote artistic standards that would make the work more likely to sell.

Peck also knew that for many veterans, their time in the hospital or convalescent home was only the start of a long journey toward a new way of life. With that concern in mind, she established a workshop for veterans in the basement of her own home. The workshop was known as "Undermount Industries," and at one point, Peck and her friend Patsy Andrews were providing instruction in handicrafts to twenty-five war veterans. Peck then sold the handicrafts produced by the soldiers, and the men not only gained a profit but also a level of confidence that enabled them become more self-sufficient.[41]

A strong advocate for her cause and a well-known figure before the war, Peck was asked to address the Royal Society of Canada in 1905. There she spoke about the Canadian Handicrafts Guild's exhibitions, its financial situation, its outreach to Aboriginal peoples, and its efforts to help workers throughout the country become more self-sufficient through the sale of their crafts.[41] Another noteworthy occasion came in 1910, when Jane Addams, the founder and director of Hull House in Chicago, invited Peck to a special lunch. There were forty guests, all specialists in some philanthropic work, Peck's being the preservation of the cottage industries in Canada. In addition to her philanthropic work, Peck was also a prolific writer. She wrote poetry, she wrote about her life and her extensive travels, and she wrote about the CHG. She interacted with many important people, including John McCrae, the Canadian army doctor who wrote *In Flanders Fields*, and T.E. Lawrence, famous for his activities in Arabia during World War I.

At her death in 1943, Peck was lauded by many for her good works. Her contributions to the preservation and promotion of crafts in Canada, to occupational therapy, and to posterity went beyond all that seemed likely.

Good historical records exist for Alice Peck as for Jessie Luther, and so their stories are easily recovered and told. But for the majority of pioneering women in occupational therapy little is known beyond some administrative information, such as a listing of their names at the institutions where they were employed or perhaps a fleeting mention in some official correspondence or report. While it is possible in these cases to recreate their stories in some measure, using knowledge of the times, those stories are but an approximation and await further information. One such story concerns "Miss Scott." Her work reflects the influence of the earlier moral treatment era on the development of occupational therapy in Canada.

"MISS SCOTT"

In 1883, the Homewood Asylum in Guelph was established as the first private asylum in Ontario. In 1912, "Miss Scott" was appointed director of the asylum's newly opened handicrafts department. The medical superintendent, Dr Hobbs, had been asking his board to approve such a program for some five years. Hobbs had reported that friends and relatives of patients often inquired about the possibility of some work being given to patients while under treatment or while convalescing. Hobbs, who had seen the value of occupations in his previous position under Dr Bucke at the London Asylum, had become increasingly concerned about the lack of activities for his private patients at Homewood. In 1912, following recently completed renovations to the building, the board of directors finally put forward and approved the following motion:

The question of providing some useful employment for patients has been under consideration for some considerable time, but owing to lack of room for carrying on such industrial work nothing was ever done. Now that we have ample space to enable this work to be done, it is recommended that ... we should establish certain branches of industrial work, such as the making of leather articles in various forms, brass work, knitting, etc., to be given effect under the supervision of a proper instructress.

To that end it is recommended that the services of Miss Scott, a Canadian girl who formerly resided in Windsor but who has been under instruction [at the Pratt Institute in Brooklyn, NY] in Arts and Crafts in the US for some considerable time, be engaged at a salary of $60 a month, together with board and lodging.[44]

When Dr Hobbs decided to provide activities for his patients, he would have been thinking not only of their welfare but also of Homewood's ability to compete with nearby private mental institutions in the United States. In 1913, Hobbs proudly described the rooms in the asylum devoted to arts and crafts: "The Homewood Sanitarium now compares favourably with the McLean Hospital at Waverley, Boston, the Butler at Providence, RI,[45] Bloomingdale at White Plains, NY, and the Sheppard-Pratt at Towson, Maryland. These are the leading institutions now in the United States for the treatment of nervous and mental diseases."[46]

Hobbs notes the great success of the occupational work in the arts and crafts room: "It fills in the spare time of patients, keeps them busy, at the same time turning their energies into useful work. This is all free, and a gift of the institution to the patients. The only expense involved is the cost of the raw material on which they work."[47] While the space and the materials were essential, the success of the program that Hobbs describes had to have been due in large measure to the role played by Miss Scott, the instructor in handicrafts.

Little is known about Miss Scott, as there are few records to be found. She was likely Jessie Scott, born in Windsor in 1893 and educated at the Pratt Institute. Her education at an art school such as the Pratt was not uncommon for would-be occupational therapists. Nor was it uncommon for Canadian women to attend art schools in the United States. Courses offered around the turn of the century at the Pratt provided useful knowledge and skills for women with artistic interests and abilities. Along with classes in drawing, painting, design, and colour, there were also courses in manual training and domestic science.

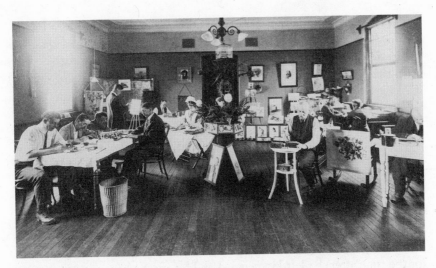

Patients doing artwork at the Homewood Retreat in Guelph, Ontario, where, in 1912, "Miss Scott" became the first instructor in handicrafts. University of Toronto Archives, Farrar Collection, B1999-0011/007P.

It was also not unusual for American women to attend art schools in Canada, especially in the East.[48] The register for the early years of the American Occupational Therapy Association shows that American occupational therapists attended the Mount Allison University Art School in New Brunswick, as well the Ontario College of Art. Such cross-border exchanges were also common for work. For example, an American woman, Kathryn Root, taught weaving and pottery in the School for the Blind in Halifax, Nova Scotia.[49] She too had attended the Pratt Institute and held a diploma from the normal art course, which included classes on teaching clay-modelling and woodcarving. She also attended the domestic science program offered at the Pratt, which included subjects such as emergencies, home nursing, hygiene, biology, chemistry, psychology, physics, and dietetics. Root's personnel file indicates that she had taken a short course in manual training in which she studied the sloyd method, a popular approach in education at the time (see chapter 5), and that she had worked at Devereux Mansion with Dr Hall.[50]

There are no details of Jessie Scott's training at the Pratt; however, it is likely to have been similar to that of Miss Root. Neither is there any information about her personal characteristics. Judging from comments made at the time, it is likely that her personality enabled her to get along with various groups and that she was enthusiastic about her work.[51]

The ideal instructor of handicrafts was described at the time as a multi-talented and somewhat unique person, "able to teach, and participate in the games, drills, and various sports that would interest the patients; in brief, the director should be brimming over with enthusiasm and energy, and able to impart the same spirit to his or her pupils."[52]

There was a Jessie Scott who taught in the ward aides course in 1918 and 1919 and was said to be from Windsor. She was likely the same woman who had taught at Homewood in 1912.[53] Her boyfriend went overseas in 1915 and returned in 1919. It is possible that he was seriously injured because although they married in 1920, he had died by 1924 when he was but thirty. Jessie remarried in 1927.[54]

Jessie Scott made a much-needed contribution to Homewood's treatment options and was an important figure in the training of ward aides. It is unfortunate that no information exists to describe her activities for the time after she left Homewood and before she began instructing at the University of Toronto. However, by 1915, a Miss Bathgate is listed in the Homewood brochure as the handicrafts instructor.[55] Scott is but one of many pioneering women in occupational therapy whose history remains to be recovered.

PART TWO

World War I

World War I

OCCUPATIONS AS TREATMENT DURING THE WAR

Except for Belgium ... Canada is the only one of the belligerents who from the first recognized the national responsibility to her disabled soldiers. This should be recorded to the great credit of our neighbor to the north. From the first year of the war, no Canadian soldier has had need to depend on charity for his convalescent care or industrial training.

D.C. McMurtrie, 1917[1]

By the start of World War I, several ideas about the use of occupations as a means of treatment were already in place. In mental institutions, occupations for patients reduced the need for physical and chemical restraints and lifted morale. In some segments of society, occupations, mainly in the form of crafts, were used to relieve stress, restore the soul, and develop a sense of community. In settlement houses, occupations helped immigrants preserve their sense of identity and self-image and learn new skills for work and daily living. In schools, occupations – in the form of manual training – were used to enhance children's learning and prepare adolescents for work. The pioneering women in the field before the war – women like Luther, Peck, and Scott – worked in a relatively isolated fashion, each using occupations in her own way to help others. These varying purposes for occupations would have seemed disparate at the time and might not have taken hold in a cohesive manner had it not been for World War I. The war was a major turning point in the development of occupational therapy, as it helped it coalesce as a profession.

Injured soldiers created a demand for a new kind of care. Their injuries were different from anything seen during peacetime. Where people with disabilities had been ignored in the past or sheltered and hidden away, the sheer numbers of injured soldiers meant that the need for a vigorous response was obvious. It was difficult for nations unaccustomed to actively caring for their disabled to suddenly have to come to terms with

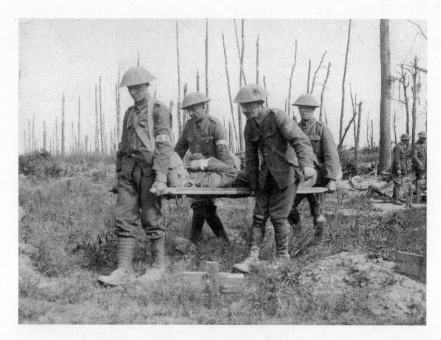

Soldiers of the Fifth Battalion of the Canadian Expeditionary Force carrying a wounded soldier away from the battlefield for treatment. "To the Railway," CWM 19920044-509, George Metcalf Archival Collection, © Canadian War Museum.

the new situation. The injured soldiers were thought to have been at the height of their masculinity when they enlisted, but were now dependent in a way that was then considered appropriate only for women or children. Work with so-called crippled children had shed some light on the needs of the injured soldier, but there were no clear guidelines as to what should be done. There were also no directives as to "the state's obligations to assist those who, through no failing of their own, could not provide for themselves."[2]

The psychological and physical aspects of war injuries prompted considerable concern and compassion from society. Determining treatment for injuries never seen before presented a huge challenge to the medical profession. However, it was the economic consequences of the war that quickly focused society's attention on the need to lessen the impact that the wounded soldiers' dependency would create. As before, occupations would have a role to play – to boost morale, to increase self-confidence, and to build skills – only this time, the population and the context were new.

TREATING SOLDIERS BACK HOME

Canada had no choice but to enter World War I at Britain's side in 1914. Initially it was thought that the war would be over quickly and that any injured Canadian soldiers would be treated overseas.[3] Not only would the soldiers be treated abroad but they would be treated as quickly as possible in field hospitals so that they could return to the front lines. If the field hospital could not manage the injuries, soldiers were sent to stationary hospitals further away from the battlefield or, if necessary, to hospitals in England.[4] In fact, soldiers often spoke of wanting a "Blighty" – that is, a wound that was sufficiently severe or complicated to require treatment in England and hence an opportunity to be away from the front lines.[5] Complete "hospitals" were organized and equipped by various organizations and universities across Canada and shipped overseas. In all, there were some twenty-six "Canadian" hospitals abroad – sixteen general and ten stationery.[6]

As the war dragged on and the numbers of injured mounted, it became clear that many wounded soldiers would not be able to return to the front lines. Instead they would be sent home for further treatment or to convalesce, even though Canada was unprepared for their arrival, having few hospitals and fewer ideas about how to deal with this new and complex situation. The soldiers' convalescence would be lengthy, and many would be at risk for later psychological problems as they attempted to return to normal living. In addition, it was soon apparent that growing numbers of injured soldiers would be unable to return to their former jobs. If these men were to work at all, they would need to be retrained.

Some 600,000 young men and women served in the Canadian Expeditionary Force. Of these, 66,000 were killed and a further 173,000 were injured by the end of the war. How could such a young country continue to grow and prosper with so many men cut down in their prime? And how could the country afford the cost of caring for those men who had become disabled? It was quickly becoming clear that economic issues would overwhelm the country unless the injured soldiers could find employment and be re-established as productive citizens.

The scheme that Canada devised for enabling injured soldiers to enter or re-enter the workforce was lauded as the first comprehensive plan in the world.[7] The Military Hospitals Commission (MHC) was established on 30 June 1915 to "deal with the provision of hospital accommodation and convalescent homes in Canada," and Sir James Lougheed (then a senator from Alberta) was appointed its president.[8] By October 1916, the commission had provided 2,193 beds in forty-seven institutions. However,

with the Battle of the Somme the following year, the MHC gained a more
realistic picture of the work to come. Shiploads of wounded men began
arriving home from Great Britain, and the injured soldier population in
Canada grew to 11,981 by early 1917.[9]

The need for rehabilitation and job retraining was clearly greater than
anticipated. A report published in the *Canadian Medical Association Journal* in 1916 described the plans to accommodate to the new situation:

> The [Military Hospitals] Commission is devoting serious attention
> to the functional and vocational reeducation of returned soldiers
> who are unable to carry on their former occupations. Mr T.B.
> Kidner, who has had much experience in such work, both in Eng-
> land and Canada, has been appointed Vocational Secretary. It has
> been realized that both physical and mental training must be given
> concurrently in order to obtain the best results and the value of
> occupation has been duly considered. Schools have therefore been
> established at the convalescent homes where instruction is given
> to the men in general education and in such manual work as will
> prove recreative.[10]

Even as the war was drawing to a close, the problems associated with
injured soldiers continued to grow and a reorganization of the Military
Hospitals Commission was needed. In 1918, soldiers not yet discharged
and requiring medical treatment would be cared for within the Department of Militia and Defence, while those who had been honourably
discharged, or were suffering from incurable diseases or diseases of long
duration (including tuberculosis, insanity, and mental deficiency), would
remain within the care of the commission.[11] A new department, the Department of Soldiers' Civil Re-establishment (DSCR) – whose name described its role and function – was formed. The mandate of the DSCR
was to prepare injured soldiers for return to their former work or, in cases
where they could no longer perform that work, to train them for work
that they could do.[12]

ORIGINS OF THE PLAN TO RE-ESTABLISH SOLDIERS

There are several very similar accounts of how the retraining program
itself was first devised. According to the records of the MHC, F.H. Sexton,
the director of technical education for Nova Scotia, and a woman named
Ina Matthews, who had been working with convalescing soldiers in

Sydney at the Ross Convalescent Home, developed the idea.[13] (See chapter 8, for Ina Matthews.) They presented their plan to E.M. McDonald, member of Parliament for Pictou County, and also consulted the premier of Nova Scotia, George Murray.[14] Their preliminary plan was sent to Ernest Scammell, the executive officer of the MHC. A series of meetings followed that included Miss Matthews and others. Scammell presented the final plan at the Conference of Provincial Ministers held in Ottawa in October 1915.[15]

The plan for re-education, Sessional Paper 35a, was comprehensive, taking the injured soldier from the bedside to the workplace. It included a special disablement fund to support soldiers and their dependents while the soldiers were retraining for suitable work, as well as funds to support those deemed totally incapacitated by their injuries. The paper expressed a certain urgency, as its authors thought it important to provide the re-education program as soon as possible lest the invalided men "degenerate into unemployables."[16] The report (which was in the form of a letter to President Lougheed) also stressed the need for a vocational adviser who would know more about the whole issue of employment than the soldier would and could suggest work that would remain economically viable. The report cautioned, "There must be a minimum of sentiment and a maximum of sound hard business sense concerning the future of the returned soldier to civil life."[17]

An appendix to Sessional Paper 35a set forth a principle very familiar to occupational therapists: that an injury that might appear minor might nonetheless render someone unable to earn a living in his former profession. Hand injuries, for example, would affect a musician, but a leg amputation would not affect an accountant. As Bourillon notes, "The relation between infirmity and profession is therefore the essential factor to consider from the point of view of the invalid's future."[18]

IMPLEMENTING THE RETRAINING PLAN

The three-part program to be delivered by the Military Hospitals Commission included bedside occupations for those still convalescing, workshop occupations for those well enough to leave the ward, and job training for those ready to pursue a vocation. While job training was considered the major purpose of the plan, the sequence of steps was generally acknowledged as important and necessary. Bedside occupations were needed to help restore the man's spirit and prepare him for the more strenuous activities in the workshops, where he would start building work

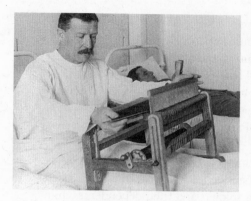 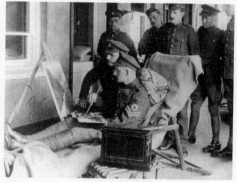

LEFT Injured soldier working on a loom specially constructed for use in bed. Courtesy CAOT Publications ACE; RIGHT Convalescing soldier painting on the grounds of College Street Hospital, Toronto, c. 1919. Courtesy CAOT Publications ACE.

skills. Ward aides provided the bedside occupations and some of the off-ward activities at the start of the recovery process, and vocational officers prepared the soldier for a specific position. The local citizenry provided apprenticeships and job placements for the soldiers at the end.[19]

Bedside occupations generally involved the use of crafts. They were designed to be diversional at the outset in order to influence the soldier's mental attitude; a positive mental attitude would contribute to a successful recovery, while idleness led to despair, which would have a negative influence on recovery.[20] Occupations that raised morale had been important in mental health settings for some time and were now of interest in recovery from war injuries and illnesses.

The importance of diversional activity in maintaining morale was widely subscribed to by physicians and others connected with the treatment of injured soldiers of World War I. The issue of whether diversional activity was a preliminary step in recovery, or whether that first step should be directly related to stimulating vocational interests and a return to work, was a matter of debate in both the United States and Canada. Occupations that could both divert *and* prepare the patient for return to work were considered the ideal.[21]

Motivating some of the injured to get well would be no easy feat. They had been witness to the horrors of war and seen their comrades fall and die. In their own cases, their injuries meant that their day-to-day lives would drastically change. Yet, while it would be difficult for them to think in a positive way about the future, many commentators of the day considered it essential that the soldier be invested in his own recovery. Galsworthy, the celebrated British author and philanthropist involved with the war effort, saw the options open to the soldier and the consequences: "If a man's mind, courage and interest be enlisted in the cause of his own salvation, healing goes on apace, the sufferer is remade. If not, no medical surgeon, no careful nursing will avail to make a man of him again."[22] It now fell to the ward aide to enlist the man's mind, courage, and interest.

EXPECTATION FOR SOLDIERS

The re-establishment of injured soldiers into society was fraught with moral issues for society and for the soldiers themselves. The war brought with it a deep respect and concern for the sacrifices the soldiers had made for Canada. All citizens of the dominion, and particularly those who did not go overseas, felt – or were exhorted to feel – a great sense of duty toward the men. This duty translated into fundraising activities and volunteer efforts aimed at restoring soldiers' physical and mental well-being. Businesses were expected to help the men return to work by providing jobs, and citizens were asked to buy savings bonds to help finance the rehabilitation programs. The work of the MHC – and later the Department of Soldiers' Civil Re-establishment – was widely publicized through posters and films, thus keeping the soldiers' needs at the forefront of people's minds.

While the aim of the MHC was to "do its best for the physical and economic well-being of the man [i.e., the soldier]," there was also an expectation that the soldier would continue to do his duty. The MHC urged the injured soldier to "perform for his country a service not less important than those on the firing line, namely, that, instead of being an idle ward of the State, he becomes a shining example to the young, of self-dependence, of courage and perseverance in overcoming disabilities."[23]

Just as it was morally right that society should help these men, so was it now morally wrong that the men be idle. In describing Canada's work for its wounded soldiers, Major J.L. Todd stated this *quid pro quo* in the *Canadian Medical Association Journal*: "There must be a general appreciation among Canadians, not only of that which Canada owes her disabled soldiers, but of that which a disabled soldier, still a citizen, continues to owe to his country."[24] This seemingly tough approach could legitimately be taken because injured soldiers remained militarily obligated to do their duty. Thus, discipline was to be upheld during rehabilitation; indeed,

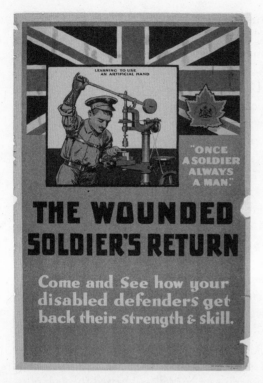

One of many posters issued by
the federal government urging
Canadians – and injured
soldiers – to do their part
in returning the country to
economic stability.

exercises designed to remediate an injury were often presented in the
same manner as army drills.[25]

Propaganda materials painted a promising picture of the road ahead
and were intended to reassure the injured soldier that all would be well.
The film *Canada's Work for Wounded Soldiers* (which was silent but had
subtitles) was shown in hospitals in England,[26] on troop ships bringing
soldiers home, and in theatres across Canada in 1918. The film was widely
publicized and included a segment on occupational therapy (considered
the most interesting part of the film, according to one Toronto newspaper).[27] However, the film also made it clear that those who did not in-
tegrate and thrive had only themselves to blame and that it was only the
soldier who refused to try to overcome his wounds who was destined for
hardship. Soldiers with psychological damage were shown little compassion and were instead simply urged to face their fears.[28]

A similar approach was followed in the United States after it entered
the war in 1917. Harris expressed his government's stance: "There will be
no more pensioned men in semi-charitable jobs; the redeemed disabled

will be given regular pay for regular and efficient work. There will be no more burdens on the communities; for these men will pay their taxes and bear their share of whatever other burdens the community may have to shoulder."[29]

MEETING THE GOALS OF THE RE-EDUCATION PROGRAM

With the employment of soldiers returning from the front as its major task, the MHC required staff knowledgable in work-related matters. The director of vocational training for the commission was Walter Segsworth, a former mining engineer from Toronto. The vocational secretary was Thomas Kidner, recently the organizer of manual training and technical education in Calgary and previously the organizer of manual training in Nova Scotia and New Brunswick (see chapter 5).[30] Vocational officers were appointed in each province and were responsible to the MHC.[31]

By the time of his appointment in 1915, Kidner was an authority on manual training and technical education and had had some experience as a volunteer in finding work for injured soldiers returning home.[32] Now, as vocational secretary, he would implement and oversee a program of vocational training for all soldiers undergoing treatment in hospitals and convalescent homes across Canada. It was from this vantage point that Kidner developed the knowledge and interest that led him to become a major contributor to occupational therapy within a few short years.

Kidner described the benefits of vocational training (as the whole process of rehabilitation was known) while speaking at the College Street Convalescent Home in Toronto in 1916,[33] soon after his appointment: "First it will prevent the 'lazy bug'; second, it will have a therapeutic value; third, it will tend towards better discipline in the home; and fourth, it will improve the men's positions in life."[34] Improving the soldier's position in life was an important issue, as many – if not most – infantry soldiers in World War I (as in later wars) had been poorly educated or unemployed when they enlisted. Thus, a vocational program could provide an opportunity for advanced education and retraining.[35]

When asked to share his views on the need for occupations, Kidner reflected on the evils of idleness. "In many cases," he said, "they [the soldiers] were being spoiled by over-indulgence, in most luxurious surroundings with nothing to do but sit around and smoke cigarettes. In consequence, many of them, following out the old adage of idle hands finding mischief to do, got drunk and there were various disciplinary troubles, due largely, it was considered, to the lack of occupation."[36]

Although the control of the soldiers was of concern, there was also an understanding that the men needed to be involved in their own futures. They could not be regimented in their handling of major life changes, such as those brought about by a disability or the need to train for a new type of work. In fact, Kidner thought that the soldier should be "demilitarized" at a certain point and treated as a civilian, because only then would he see himself as an individual and be motivated to improve.[37] This idea was stressed by the ward aide Mary Trent, who reflected on her own interactions with soldiers at the Inter-Allied Rehabilitation Conference in 1919. Noting how army men had to lose their initiative and become slaves of discipline, she pointed out how the ward aide needed to be not only gentle, patient, and kind but also a student of character to determine how to awaken each soldier's individual interests.[38]

Simply finding out what jobs were available was a major task and required careful and comprehensive labour surveys. Determining which job would be appropriate for each man also required great care, as taking on a job that would later disappear or could be done by someone less qualified would only bring trouble further on. American architect George Barton, who was soon to suggest the founding of the National Society for the Promotion of Occupational Therapy, commented on the gender and disability stereotypes then very common: "If we can train the public, or persuade the uninjured man, that it is hardly respectable to do work that can be done by a cripple, in short time the well man would feel much as the small boy feels about something that girls can do; that is, he respects the work itself, but taking pride in the fact that he is a boy, he cannot be induced to do it himself."[39]

In Britain, John Galsworthy voiced the concern that young soldiers might not properly recognize the need for retraining. He warned that a soldier might take a job appropriate for someone young without realizing the long-range implications – that is, whether the job would be good enough for the next thirty or forty years of his life. In a few years, when jobs might be harder to get and public sympathy for veterans might have subsided, that man would not have the needed skills, having missed the opportunity for retraining.[40] Galsworthy's concern was prophetic. The majority of soldiers deemed eligible for retraining rejected that option in the United Kingdom, and great numbers were indeed unemployed within a decade. His prediction regarding the waning of public sympathy also proved true; people tried to forget the war and thus their concern for the veterans dissipated in the ensuing years.[41]

The option to allow retraining to be voluntary created much debate. France had encountered difficulty with this approach, reporting that in order to get 350 soldiers to retrain, they had to interview 2,000 men. It was thought the problem lay in "alcoholism and a certain ingrained idea that, as the men had been wounded in defence of the State, the State should support them for the rest of their lives."[42] Thus, a delicate balance had to be struck between setting the men in what the state considered the right direction and supporting their right to determine their own future.[43]

Perhaps the most salient issue that needed to be addressed prior to the start of the retraining process was the injured soldier's pension. Until that matter was settled, invalided soldiers took little interest in any plans for their return to civilian life. It was decided, therefore, that the pension issue had to be resolved as quickly as possible. There was also a need to assure the soldier that if his earning power increased following retraining, his pension would not decrease. The pension was based on the disability and not on earning power. It would always remain the same.[44]

VISITORS TO THE PROGRAM

While Kidner was the vocational secretary at the MHC, he and his program received many American visitors. For example, Jane Addams, the founder and leader of Hull House in Chicago, came to visit, as did the soon-to-be prominent American occupational therapist Eleanor Clarke Slagle.[45] Representatives of the US government also visited, wanting to learn how to set up their own programs. One visitor, writing in the (American) Red Cross Magazine, stated "the MHC is attacking this problem [of soldiers disabled by war] ... in a way that might well be imitated by the United States."[46] Under the auspices of the American Red Cross, thirty vocational educators came to Canada to observe the industrial re-education work during a four-week tour of Ottawa, Toronto, Montreal, Winnipeg, Calgary, and Saskatoon. With the United States not entering the war until April 1917, these visitors had the opportunity to benefit from the Canadian experience. By the time the injured American soldiers started coming home, their reconstruction aides were ready to follow the Canadian initiative.

Kidner's re-education program was seen as the one to emulate. Indeed, it seemed as if his program could achieve what everyone had been striving for: the program helped the men move from the role of invalid to one of productivity, it kept them from dwelling on their traumatic experiences, and it gave them some hope for the future. It provided a beginning step toward the restoration – of body and spirit – of each soldier. In a speech to a conference on the after-care of disabled men, Kidner cited Galsworthy's opinion: "A niche of usefulness and self-respect exists for every man, however handicapped; but that niche must be found for him. To carry the process of restoration to a point short of this is to leave the cathedral without a spire."[47]

Kidner had staked out an interest in the value of occupations as treatment. His reputation in the field preceded him and was such that in March 1917 he was invited to Clifton Springs, New York, to meet with a group of six other like-minded individuals to discuss the work. In joining this group, Kidner, the Canadian, became a founding member of the (American) National Society for the Promotion of Occupational Therapy, later to become the American Occupational Therapy Association.[48] In 1918, Kidner was invited to appear before the Federal Board for Vocational Education to share his views on soldiers' re-establishment. Soon thereafter, he agreed to assist that board in organizing the work in the United States.[49]

The injured soldiers of World War I were a new population to benefit from engaging in occupations. While the mentally ill, immigrants, the poor, and those who struggled with the stresses of everyday life had been the primary recipients of this unique form of treatment previously, now the work would be extended more broadly to people with physical injuries and illnesses in the civilian as well as the military population. One good example of how the use of occupations had already been extended to the physically ill lay in the treatment of those with tuberculosis. For this population, the long-established regime of rest, fresh air, and a good diet had been augmented by "exercise," which was generally in the form of work for the institution – either in the fields or within the sanatorium walls. However, just as in the asylums, work for the sanatorium became a source of conflict and other forms of occupation were needed. With the disease being so prevalent, the use of graded occupations, not only to raise morale but also to build physical tolerance, took on an important role. The idea of grading occupations – whether to maintain interest or for physical strengthening – soon became a basic principle in occupational therapy.[50]

Speaking at the annual meeting of the American Orthopedic Association in 1918, US Army Major Henry Hayes stressed the importance of occupations for all patients with an illness lasting over three weeks. He saw the work as an essential adjunct to medical treatment that should be extended to all military hospitals whether overseas, at home, or on the seas. Furthermore, there should be no interruption of the work, as that would have a depressing influence: "Once having been given the stimulation of work, with the attendant joy of accomplishment and of thinking of something else than himself, he will become dejected only too soon." Hayes notes that "within a very few days after work was started in the orthopedic wards at the Walter Reed Hospital, the improvement in the aspect of the ward was marked and the gleam in the men's faces was really inspiring."[51]

THE WARD AIDES

Two cohorts of women became ward aides in Canada. The first were the women who took on the job early in the war, often as volunteers with no specialized training for the work but with an aptitude in crafts and a comfort in teaching (see chapter 8). In this pre-professional stage, these women performed activities of a similar nature and developed methods that they passed on to new workers. However, the rapidly increasing number of casualties meant there was a need for more ward aides. It was decided not only to recruit more ward aides but also to provide a formal training program designed especially for them. Thus, the second cohort of ward aides were those women who trained in special classes in 1918 and 1919 (see chapter 9) at the University of Toronto and McGill University.

The training courses served to develop common methods for occupational therapy. They also helped to organize the women into what sociologist Eliot Freidson would call, in his discussion of the characteristics of a profession, an "occupational group."[52] By the 1920s women who were now calling themselves occupational therapists were lobbying for positions in civilian hospitals, establishing professional societies, and planning educational programs. The war had confirmed the need for their work and provided them with the impetus to move forward.

8

Women at Work during the War

MATTHEWS, LIGHTHALL, AND GOODMAN AS
UNTRAINED WARD AIDES

Most of all, the occupational therapeutist assists the man himself,
and by giving him encouragement, new power, and increased determination,
helps him to fight his way back again to the normal civilian life.

Hilda B. Goodman, Strathcona Military Hospital,
Edmonton, Alberta, 1918[1]

WOMEN AND THEIR GOOD WORKS PRIOR TO WORLD WAR I

Many middle- and upper-class women were already involved in philanthropic work before the war. They were generally well educated and
had the means to work as volunteers; indeed, there was an expectation
that they would do such work. They worked primarily with the poor,
but also with immigrants, children, and those who were disabled. They
raised funds, served on organizing committees, and sometimes performed
hands-on tasks in caring for the sick or teaching skills in the home. Their
work made a much-needed contribution to society at a time when there
were no formal supports.

Philanthropic work often led to political activity. Denied a formal role
in politics – which was seen as a somewhat immoral arena and inappropriate for women – they became activists and lobbied for special causes,
including prohibition, suffrage, sanitation, the pasteurization of milk,
minimum wage, and control over child labour. Having come from what
were considered "good" families, they had connections with those in
power, which meant they could bring pressure to bear on politicians and
their issues had a chance of being brought to the government's attention.

Many women also engaged in cultural endeavours, supporting music,
drama, literature, and especially art. Some had studied painting formally,
but few practised as artists, as their works were not welcomed in what

was still primarily a male enterprise. Women with interests or skills in craftwork had more opportunities to pursue their work and to join organizations, such as the Canadian Handicrafts Guild or the Arts and Crafts Society of Canada.

All of this involvement on the part of women helped improve society while, at the same time, allowing women to develop their administrative abilities and leadership skills. While their activities gave them an acceptable role in public life, many women of the day still felt unfulfilled. They were frustrated at their inability to be more fully involved in public life, to be employed, and to have careers of their own. By the time of the war, they were more than ready to take on new roles as new options for work came open for them.

WOMEN'S WORK DURING THE WAR

Women were soon taking up civilian positions left vacant when men joined the army.[2] The Department of Public Information encouraged women to take on work that had previously been done by men – or indeed work that had been done by women who were now doing men's work. The department's leaflets told women to "Substitute! Support! Carry on!" Women started to work the land (as "farmerettes"), took on higher-level clerical work, assembled munitions, and even drove streetcars.[3]

Other women supported the war effort directly through volunteer work. They assembled food parcels to send to the soldiers, sewed bandages, and knitted scarves and socks for them. The socks were in great demand because of trench foot, an infection that resulted from the soldiers' feet being wet and cold for lengthy periods (while they were in the trenches) and from which gangrene could follow. The condition could be prevented with better foot care and enough socks to allow for frequent changes.[4] Women also organized entertainments for returned soldiers and raised funds for their rehabilitation and for the support of their families. The Red Cross, the Khaki Club, the Soldiers' Comfort Club, the Imperial Order of the Daughters of the Empire (IODE), and the YWCA took on these special tasks, and many women found an outlet for their aspirations within these organizations. The mayor of Toronto reported that the women's organizations were the backbone of the war effort "in keeping the home fires burning," in encouraging their men to enlist, and in working on patriotic campaigns.[5]

Still other women wanted to be more closely involved. Lacking the training to serve as nurses overseas, they looked for other ways to work directly with injured soldiers. Many women joined the Voluntary Aid Detachment (VAD) to serve as support for nursing staff in Canada or over-seas. The VAD, formed in the United Kingdom in 1909 when the British Red Cross Society joined forces with the Order of St John of Jerusalem, attracted educated, middle-class women to its ranks.[6] Women who were craftworkers – either because they had developed such skills as a part of their expected role as women or because they were in fact artistic and creative – had special skills to offer. Educated at art schools or trained as teachers, they now saw an outlet for their talents that could also help the war effort. They knew of the need to help soldiers during their lengthy convalescence – to lift their spirits and take their minds off the horrors of war and the fears of the life that lay ahead. Thus, it was not surprising that when the position of ward occupations aide was established by the Military Hospitals Commission (MHC), many women were eager to offer their services.

Applications for the job of "ward occupations aide" were made to the Vocational Branch of the MHC in Ottawa. Information on educa-tion, special training, and experience was required, as well as references. While everyone knew people at the front, women whose close relatives or boyfriends had died or were seriously injured formed a special group of ap-plicants. These women had pride of place when selections for posts were being made. The Red Cross, St John's Ambulance, and the VAD were major sources for recruiting ward aides, as women in these organizations were already familiar with hospital care and routine.

While the ward aides were employed by the Vocational Branch of the MHC, it was the Army Medical Corps (under the Department of Militia and Defence) that directed their work. This dual oversight placed the ward aides in a difficult position, especially in the hospitals, and they found themselves having to use all their social skills to keep relation-ships harmonious.[7] Professor Herbert Haultain, the vocational officer for Ontario, recalled their situation in a letter to Dr Alexander Primrose, then dean of the Faculty of Medicine at the University of Toronto: "The situation that the girls had to face in the hospitals was an extremely dif-ficult one. By specific orders from Ottawa, they were placed in the hospi-tals by the Vocational Branch and they remained in the hospitals under the jurisdiction of the Vocational Branch, and on their entry into the hospitals, neither the doctors nor the nurses were their friends. They had to make their own way and they did it."[8] Looking back on the difficulty faced by the ward aides in winning over the patients, the doctors, and the nurses, and stressing their role in motivating their patients, Hault-ain notes their assets: "bravery, unselfishness and self-repression, and that something which defies analysis – the 'eternal womanhood.' They concerned themselves heart and soul and hand with the deeper, the intangible phases of man's being. Handicrafts were incidental."[9]

WARD AIDES ON THE JOB

The stories of three women, Ina Matthews MacKinnon, Hilda Goodman, and Cybel Wilkes Lighthall, exemplify the different experiences of the women who took on the role of ward aide. They brought their ideas and skills to their work with injured soldiers and made their own way with little direction. They carved out a path for those who were to follow.

Ina Matthews MacKinnon (1886–1952)

Ina Matthews (MacKinnon) is something of an enigma in the early history of occupational therapy in Canada – albeit a very important one (see the earlier reference to her role in chapter 7). She was born in Toronto in 1886 to a very wealthy and influential family. Her father, Wilmot Deloui Matthews, was the co-founder of the Canada Malting Company and known as "The Barley King of Canada." At the time of his death in 1919, he was considered the second most influential business figure in the Dominion of Canada.[10] Ina's mother, Annie Jane Love, was interested in the arts and took an active role in the Women's Art Association of Canada, serving as co-convener of the Exhibition Committee and, in subsequent years, as a vice-president of the association. In a pamphlet on the curative workshop, Mrs W.D. Matthews (as she was known) is listed as an honorary member of the Toronto Association of Occupational Therapists.[11]

Ina's siblings all married well and expanded the influential position held by her father. Her brother Wilmot married Sir William Osler's niece Annabel, while her brother Arnold married Constance Greening, a wealthy socialite from New York. Ina's sister Ethel married J.K.L. Ross, the son of James Ross of Montreal, a founder of the Canadian Pacific Railway. Ross (senior) had a home, known as "Dumbrow,"[12] in Sydney, Nova Scotia, where his business (the Dominion Coal Company and the Dominion Iron and Steel Company) was located. By 1901, J.K.L. had become the assistant manager of the company and was spending time in Sydney for business as well as for pleasure, as he was an ardent yachtsman.[13] Ethel and J.K.L. kept a permanent home in Montreal and in 1905 built a summer home beside Dumbrow in Sydney.

As injured soldiers began returning home to Canada and it became clear that there were few places to house convalescing soldiers, many wealthy families offered their summer homes to the Military Hospitals

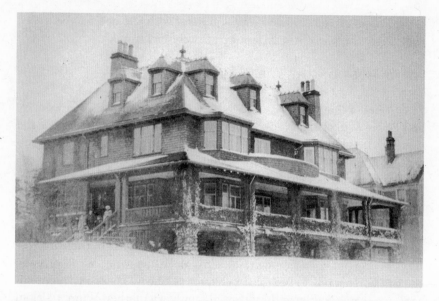

Ross House (Convalescent Home), *c.* 1930, 116 King's Road, Sydney, Nova Scotia, given by Mrs J.K.L. Ross (née Ethel Matthews) for convalescing soldiers in 1915. Photographer unknown (copy), 81-246-5316, Beaton Institute, Cape Breton University, NS.

Commission. James Ross had died in 1913, and in 1915 J.K.L. and Ethel offered what had been his large, three-storey home in Sydney to the MHC, renovating it to create bed space for some forty-five patients. A covered squash court was converted into a workroom and classrooms for courses in carpentry, mechanical drawing, English-language classes, and furniture making. Ethel Ross fitted up and maintained the home at her own expense. She also hired and paid the medical and nursing staff.[14]

Ina Matthews was twenty-nine years of age and unmarried when she joined her sister Ethel in Sydney in the summer of 1915. Wanting to help the convalescing soldiers and being an able craftswoman herself, she taught crafts to the injured soldiers.[15] Little is known of Ina's (or of Ethel's) early life other than that it was one of substantial wealth and privilege. Their home at 89 St George Street in Toronto was built for the family in 1890,[16] and a ballroom was added specially for Ethel's wedding in 1902. There was a tower in the turret, and the story is told that Ina was supposed to read her Bible there on Sundays but always had a novel handy to hide inside the Bible's cover. Ina and her family were great travellers, and as would be common with their class, they were often cruising at sea.[17] There is no record of Ina's or Ethel's education, and it is likely that private

Ina Matthews, c. 1920.
Ina worked with her
sister Ethel at the
Ross Convalescent
Home, using crafts at
the bedside. Based on
this experience, she
worked with others
to devise the plan for
re-educating injured
soldiers. Courtesy
Matthews family.

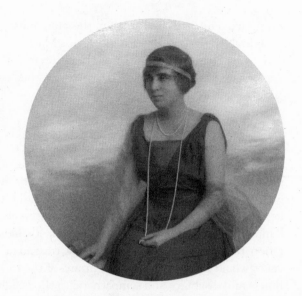

governesses taught them at home. Fluent in several languages, including German, Ina has been described as "quite a force"; she was known as an energetic and hard-working trailblazer "who would get an idea and then go and do it."[18]

It seems that the work Ina was doing with the soldiers during her visit in Sydney was worthy of notice. On 8 October 1915, Frederick Sexton, the director of technical education for Nova Scotia, wrote to J.W. Robertson of the Canadian Red Cross: "The question of training disabled or partially disabled Canadian soldiers who are returning home from the front has arisen here in Sydney where two Ontario women, Miss Ina Matthews and her sister, Mrs J.K.L. Ross, are conducting a convalescent hospital for soldiers."[19] Just a few weeks later, the Halifax *Morning Chronicle* featured an article on the need for rehabilitating injured soldiers, for "getting our gallant sons back into our industrial and agricultural life and making them again respected and self-respecting members of the community."[20] The article went on to describe the movement to train disabled soldiers for useful work that had originated in Nova Scotia:

> To Miss Matthews, who has taken a keen interest in the Convalescent Home established by Mrs J.K.L. Ross [i.e., Ina Matthews's sister Ethel] at Sydney, is due the credit of directing this important matter to our consideration. From her experience in Sydney, Miss Matthews speedily discovered that while the Convalescent Home

fulfilled a most useful function, the State must go further in its care of disabled soldiers. Accordingly Miss Matthews took the matter up with Premier Murray, whose keen interest in all humanitarian problems is so well known to us all, with the result that Professor Sexton, Principal of the Nova Scotia Technical College, was asked to make a report.

The newspaper report recognized the role of Premier Murray, who aside from his usual sympathy for humanitarian causes, may well have had a personal interest in the issue. He had two sons fighting in the war, and he himself had suffered bouts of depression and had had an above-knee leg amputation. Treatment for his nervous breakdown took him to the United States and away from Parliament for most of 1902. The amputation resulted in a lengthy period of treatment in 1910. Both experiences would have made him cognizant of the difficulties of adjusting to illness and disability and sympathetic to the need for occupations during a lengthy convalescence.[21]

By 4 April 1916, Nova Scotia could proudly claim to have established the first curative workshop classes in the dominion at the Ross Convalescent Home.[22] Convalescing soldiers remained there through 1919, under the jurisdiction of the Military Hospitals Commission. At that point, the home was no longer needed, and any remaining veterans were sent elsewhere for treatment.

Ethel moved back to Montreal, divorced Ross in 1930, and then remarried and resided in Montreal. Whether she worked alongside her sister Ina at the Ross Convalescent Home in Sydney or whether either sister had any further connection with the emerging profession of occupational therapy is not known. Of interest is the fact that the list of students in the ward aides course in Toronto in 1919 (see chapter 9) includes the name "E. Ross"; however, there are no further details, and the surname "Ross" was very common at the time. Ina was among some thirty thousand Canadian women who travelled to Britain during the war. Many women of means went overseas to help out and to be with their loved ones when they were on leave. Ina's brother Arnold Matthews, who was an officer in the 3rd Tunnelling Company of the Canadian Engineers, mentions her in a letter home in March 1916: "Have seen Ina several times in London and she seems to be enjoying herself also doing a certain amount of work in canteens, etc."[23] Whether she stayed on in London or visited only briefly and then returned to Nova Scotia to continue her work at the Ross home is not known.

It appears that Ina did not continue with the work after the war. She met Bruce MacKinnon, a tea merchant from Scotland, while on a cruise ship with her parents in the Far East. They married in 1918 in the Philippines and lived there for a number of years. After the birth of their two children, they maintained a flat in Montreux, Switzerland, where the children attended school. Ina's husband died just after the end of World War II, and Ina died in 1952 after suffering from a heart condition for several years.[24] It is unfortunate that nothing further is known about Ina and what may have motivated her to instigate the retraining scheme – a scheme that was to influence both the re-education of injured soldiers and the development of occupational therapy.[25]

The ideas and the work of Ina Matthews were clearly known to at least seven individuals of influence during the war – Sexton, Scammell, McDonald, Smeaton White, Kidner, Robertson, and Murray – as well as to the readers of the Halifax *Morning Chronicle*. In 1919, Ernest Scammell, then the executive officer of the Military Hospitals Commission, recalled the beginnings of the re-education program, noting that while an initial "short and valuable suggestive report" had been provided, "the writer's name was not given, but it was afterwards found that it was written by Miss Ina Matthews, sister-in-law of Mr J.K.L. Ross."[26] Even though Matthews was a signatory to Sessional Paper 35a, which set out the plan for soldiers' re-establishment, her role was not known among her family or recognized in any official manner. Her contribution has certainly never been acknowledged in the literature of occupational therapy. That the name of Ina Matthews is at least now recorded in this early history of the profession is of some consolation, and additional information may yet come to light.

Hilda Goodman (1884–1967)

Growing up in London, England, Hilda Goodman remembered working with what she called "crippled children," teaching them simple crafts, serving them refreshments, and singing hymns along with them in her church hall. She later qualified as a teacher and came to Canada in 1912 to teach school "on the Prairie." In 1914, she held a teaching position in Lethbridge, Alberta, and from 1915 to 1918, she taught at the Donald Ross Public School in Edmonton. At the request of the district vocational officer, Goodman was given an extended leave of absence from the Edmonton School Board so that she could provide "fingercraft instruction" to bedridden injured soldiers at the Strathcona Military Hospital.[27]

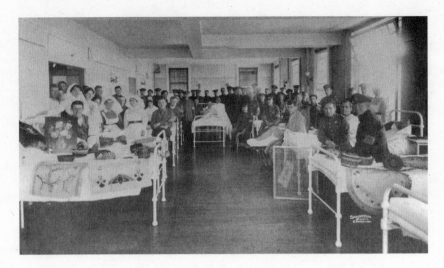

Hilda Goodman (*just visible on left without a cap*) at Strathcona Military Hospital, Edmonton, where she was a teacher of handicrafts in 1918. Archives Department, University of Wisconsin-Milwaukee Libraries.

Goodman began her leave from the Edmonton School Board in May 1918.[28] At Strathcona Military Hospital, she was given a small office and storeroom and five dollars to buy supplies, including some paints and reed for basket making. In a letter written to colleagues in 1954, she recalled starting that work: "Most of the men were lying on their beds in their uniforms with nothing to do – one boy broke the ice, [saying,] 'I'll paint.' Soon most of the boys were working." Goodman tells the story of a soldier who had been ordered to stay in bed for eight weeks to allow his leg to heal but had great difficulty following those orders. She convinced him to make a basket and said he could get out of bed when it was finished. Then she saw to it that it took the soldier eight weeks to complete the basket.[29]

In September 1918, Goodman was asked to take charge of the craftwork for all the military hospitals in Alberta, from "Frank to Edmonton."[30] However, by this time she had also been offered a position at a new school for occupational therapy about to open in Milwaukee, Wisconsin. She asked the board for an extended leave to pursue that work, intending to gain new skills and likely return.

Elizabeth Upham, then the director of the art department at Milwaukee-Downer College (MDC; now part of the University of Wisconsin), was one of the many Americans who toured Canadian military hospitals during the war to learn more about treating injured soldiers. She met Hilda Goodman during her visit to Strathcona Military Hospital in

1918 and decided that Goodman would be perfect for the occupational therapy program she had been asked to establish at MDC.

With its entry into the war, the United States had recognized the need for what it called "reconstruction aides." The Surgeon General's Office established training centres for teachers of "invalid" occupations, one of which was to be at MDC. There would be three months of practice teaching under supervision in a hospital (this would be called fieldwork today) in addition to six months of courses at the college. Goodman was being asked to organize and supervise the practice teaching.[31]

Upham was faced with a dilemma: she had to raise funds for the new program at the same time as she was trying to set it up. In a note to Ellen Sabin, the president of the college, she described one aspect of the problem: "I cannot see what we can do without her [referring to Goodman] nor what we could do with her if we do not give the course!" Upham and Sabin decided to proceed on faith, believing that if they showed the college trustees the importance of this form of war work and the need for fieldwork to accompany the classroom learning, the trustees would support them. Ultimately, their faith was rewarded and the trustees gave their support.[32]

In her president's report of 22 November 1918, Sabin noted that the opening of the occupational therapy department was the result of an appeal from the national government for nurses and reconstruction aides. MDC considered itself equipped to carry on the work because its art department included work in applied arts. The new department opened on 6 November 1918 with a faculty of four, including Hilda Goodman, and seven students. Sabin went on to note that the college, in offering this work, supported its extension to civilians and its importance as a profession for women: "Its place in our College came as a war measure, but we think it likely to continue as furnishing a permanent civilian service, and as giving to women an opportunity to apply academic training to practical sociological needs."[33]

Goodman remembered her journey to Milwaukee via Winnipeg as filled with anxiety. The influenza outbreak was a great worry: "Everyone in Winnipeg was wearing masks; trains were locked going through the town so I thought I should probably get the flu." She also had difficulty trying to cross the border between Canada and the United States because the US officials did not understand the nature of the work she was going to do: "I was stopped at the border for a week for no custom official had ever heard of such a job [as occupational therapy]."[34] As it was wartime, there was greater surveillance at the border and Goodman was warned that she would be watched to see if she tried to cross the border at another point. Finally, after a series of letters involving the American consul general, the president of MDC, and contacts in Washington, Goodman's intended work was presumably considered legitimate and she was allowed to cross into the United States.[35]

Goodman had initially hesitated over accepting the offer from MDC. Although she wanted to work in Milwaukee, her position in Edmonton was very attractive. In a letter to Upham dated 2 September 1918, she wrote that the Military Hospitals Commission of Canada wanted to send her "to the east for 2 or 3 months to see the work in other hospitals and the training courses being given. They would pay all my expenses and salary during the time I was making the trip. Then I was to return to Alberta and look after this work in all the Military Hospitals in the province." Her arrangement in Edmonton also meant that at the end of the war she could return to her permanent teaching job. She did not want to "throw these [opportunities] over unless I am certain I am the right person for the other position." She went on to say, "It seems such a big thing, and I would be sorry for you to get me there and then be a failure." Then she added what was to be a prophetic phrase: "so far though I have made a success of everything I have undertaken."[36]

Indeed, Hilda Goodman made a great success of her time in Milwaukee. She developed the first fieldwork placement program, opened additional programs at new sites as needed, and saw to it that the directors at each site felt that their program's success was their own doing. Hospitals soon became concerned when the training of students ended at their site, and this concern became the impetus for their hiring occupational therapy staff.[37]

A student recruitment advertisement in the *Milwaukee Journal* in 1918 described the occupational therapy program at the MDC and traded on Goodman's reputation. The course was described as an opportunity for people "to learn how to serve their country and mankind by teaching wounded soldiers handicrafts and other manual work to occupy their hands and minds while convalescing." The ad referred to the work as "the science of curing by work known as occupational therapy" and went on to state that "Miss Hilda B. Goodman, of Strathcona Military Hospital, Edmonton, Canada, will supervise the practice teaching in Milwaukee hospitals."[38]

During her time in Milwaukee, Goodman was involved in the work of the National Society for the Promotion of Occupational Therapy (NSPOT), becoming a member in 1919.[39] She continued her professional involvement nationally and also with the Minnesota Society of Occu-

Hilda Goodman
leading a class for
children at the Cura-
tive Workshop, Mil-
waukee, Wisconsin.
Wisconsin Historical
Society.

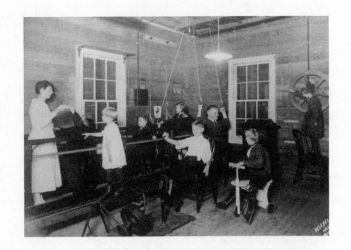

pational Therapists. She published a number of articles and was seen as
an expert in several areas, including the work in TB sanatoriums, industrial rehab, muscle strengthening, and the occupational therapy role in
general hospitals.[40] By 1921, Goodman was the director of the curative
workshop and occupational therapy department of Columbia Hospital,
Milwaukee, and in 1927 she was appointed director of the Junior League
Curative Workshop in Milwaukee.[41]

Goodman was something of a citizen of the world with her early life
in England, her adventures in Canada, her work in Milwaukee, and her
periodic travels in Europe to study art and architecture. When Kidner
was president of the American Occupational Therapy Association, he
was entertained by the Wisconsin Occupational Therapy Association;
he would likely have met with Goodman and perhaps recalled some earlier interactions in Canada when she had been employed by the Military
Hospitals Commission.

By 1932, Hilda Goodman had left Milwaukee to return to England.
She later set up a large private practice on England's east coast and remained there until the outbreak of World War II. In her retirement, she
continued her work of helping others and reflected that it seemed she had
been "doing OT in one way and another most of [her] life."[42]

Cybel Wilkes Lighthall (1869–1958)

Cybel Lighthall represents a class of women whose formal education and
life experience gave them specialized knowledge and skills. After marry-

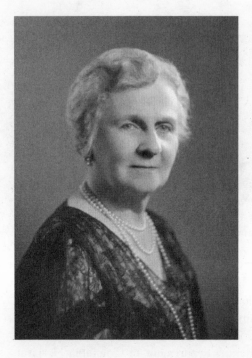

Cybel Wilkes Lighthall, c. 1930.
Cybel was a member of several
cultural and philanthropic
groups, including the Canadian
Handicrafts Guild. She helped
form the Quebec Society of
Occupational Therapists in
1928. W.D. Lighthall Family
Papers, Rare Books and Special
Collections, McGill University
Library.

ing and particularly after having children, however, these women seemed
to all but abandon that preparation. In Lighthall's case, World War I was
the catalyst that put her specialized knowledge and skills back into action.

Cybel Wilkes Lighthall was born in Montreal in 1869 to a family of
fairly modest means. Her maternal grandfather (Reverend Henry Wilkes)
had been a prominent Congregationalist minister in Montreal. All of her
siblings went on to some form of higher education, and Cybel chose to
become a teacher, leaving home to attend normal school in Ottawa from
1888 to 1890. Cybel had planned to work as a kindergarten teacher, a
position that was well accepted for women at the time. However, she soon
met W.D. Lighthall, who was originally from Hamilton, Ontario, but had
studied law at McGill University in Montreal. Their courtship, described
in a series of letters, ended with marriage in 1890 just after Cybel graduated from normal school. Their first child was born the following year,
and two more children were born soon thereafter.[43]

Cybel's education in Ottawa is chronicled through a number of her
essays and copies of her exams that have been preserved. Of particular
interest is the fact that her teacher training followed the model set out by
the educational reformer Freidrich Froebel, described in chapter 5. Oc-

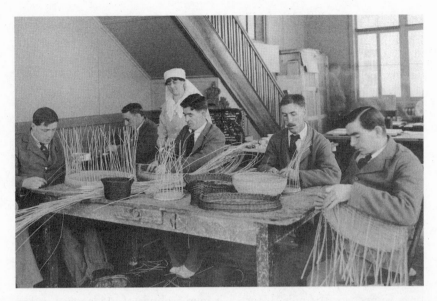

Cybel Wilkes Lighthall working as a ward aide with soldiers at the military hospital at Ste Anne de Bellevue, Quebec, in January 1919. W.D. Lighthall Family Papers, Rare Books and Special Collections, McGill University Library.

cupational therapy mirrored Froebel's philosophy in many ways. Froebel expected children to use their hands and would present them with what he called "gifts" and "occupations." Craftwork started at a point where the materials (which were the gifts) dictated the structure of the activities (which were the occupations). Gradually, structure decreased and the opportunity for greater freedom of expression increased.[44]

During the early years of her marriage, Cybel would have been engaged in raising her family and helping her husband, who was becoming a major public figure as a lawyer, writer, historian, and poet, and as mayor of Westmount from 1900 to 1903. In addition to her roles as a wife and mother, Cybel also became involved with artistic organizations and engaged in philanthropic work. She was a founding member of the Canadian Handicrafts Guild, the Women's Art Society of Montreal, and the Antiquarian and Numismatic Society.

With the outbreak of war, Cybel knitted "mufflers" and rolled bandages to be sent overseas. She also took first aid and home nursing courses through the St John's Ambulance program and worked for the Canadian Patriotic Fund, which supported the families of the soldiers of the Canadian Expeditionary Force. However, by 1917, with her own son serving in

Cairo and her daughter a VAD in France, she wanted to be more directly involved and thus became a "ward occupation aide." She was soon in charge of the other aides at the Drummond Military Home in Montreal despite feeling unqualified for the role. In 1919, at age fifty, she became the "Lady in Charge of Ward Occupations" at Ste Anne de Bellevue Military Hospital, then a new facility for injured soldiers.[45]

Cybel Lighthall's abilities and experiences were soon recognized, and she was asked to instruct new ward aides, now being trained in the Divinity Building at McGill University. She agreed to address the class on the topic of "Hospital Etiquette and Deportment," and her rough notes for the lecture suggest her understanding of hospital etiquette – and hierarchy. "Chief Medical Officer is King," she writes. "Matron has absolute control and is to be treated with absolute respect and deference; for example, always stand when she enters the room and continue to stand unless she requests you to be seated." Her explanation for this protocol was that if the patient sees that the aide has respect for the nurse, he will have respect for the aide.[46] With her own feelings of inadequacy in her role at Ste Anne's and the stress of worrying about her son at the front, it is not surprising that she should have felt somewhat overwhelmed. When asked to take on the additional duty of taking students in training as ward aides at her hospital, she declined, stating, "I could not undertake to do one thing more and certainly could not add instruction."[47]

After the war was over, Lighthall went back to her various charitable works. She was one of nine directors of the newly formed Association of Junior Leagues and its only Canadian. She remained a member of the Canadian Handicrafts Guild, and although nominally the vice-president, she took on the role of president from 1924 to 1925. In 1923, she was, rather surprisingly, listed as a member of the advisory council of the Toronto Curative Workshop. Whether she travelled to Toronto from Montreal for meetings or was simply a good name to have on the council's letterhead is not known.

Cybel Lighthall supported the formation of the Quebec Society of Occupational Therapy in 1928 and continued her involvement with the profession for several decades. In 1953, just five years before her death, she served as the honorary president of the Quebec Society of Occupational Therapy. She was a highly accomplished woman who proved to be a major contributor to a number of organizations, despite her own feelings of inadequacy and lack of self-promotion. Her formal education and her work during the war had led her to occupational therapy. She may have seen a role in the profession that fitted her own vision of what women "should" do. It is curious that her own daughter, Alice Light-hall (1891–1991), who attended the arts program at McGill and was an excellent student, was not allowed to complete her degree, her mother having stated that she did not want a "bluestocking" in the family.[48] Still, Alice followed her mother's example of giving service to the community. In 1991, she became the first person to receive a posthumous honorary degree from McGill University.[49]

℘

The stories of Ina Matthews MacKinnon, Hilda Goodman, and Cybel Wilkes Lighthall each describe a different facet of the work of the ward aide during the war. Ina's story describes the organization of the work in its early days when it was seen as a small but significant part of the larger scheme for re-establishing injured soldiers in society; Hilda's story tells of a woman's journey from the practice of teaching to the profession of occupational therapy; and Cybel's story shows the contributions made through philanthropic efforts by those with special skills. Not surpris-ingly, Hilda, as the only one of the three who did not marry, was the only one to continue to work in the profession.

Of interest in this discussion of "a new women's profession" is the fact that a few men were also hired as ward aides during the war. They were usually involved at the vocational end of the training programs, teach-ing specific trades. One example was George Wiltshire, a returned soldier skilled in cabinetmaking and fretwork and a resident in the Manitoba Military Convalescent Hospital in Winnipeg. After some negotiation, his appointment was approved by Kidner in March 1918. He was to be paid $100 per month, while the women hired as ward aides received $80 per month. In reviewing the issue, Kidner expressed the hope that there would soon be enough properly trained instructors of ward occupations, but he expected they would be young women "who would work for a scale of pay similar to that of the masseuses in the commission's employ."[50]

Thus, no sooner were women gaining a place in a profession, than issues of equity were again on the horizon. It was soon evident that women, having finally achieved paid work, were not receiving the same pay as men who were doing work of equal value. Furthermore, women who were working at higher levels were not being paid their due.[51] Whether it was because of the apparent need for higher salaries for men or other fac-tors, it appears that no men enrolled in occupational therapy anywhere in Canada until sometime after 1945.[52]

9

More Ward Aides Needed

COURSES AT THE UNIVERSITY OF TORONTO
AND MCGILL UNIVERSITY

Mrs Alice Bailey, Public school education, Leeds, England, and special training
in nursing, with five years' experience as a nurse. Mrs Bailey has done a certain
amount of fancy work and is quick at picking up information. A war widow,
with two boys at the front.

– *description of applicant to Bedside and Ward Occupation Course, 1918*[1]

On 21 February 1918, the newly formed Department of Soldiers' Civil Re-
establishment (DSCR), took on the task of overseeing the training course
for ward aides previously organized by the Military Hospitals Commission.[2] The end of the war was still not in sight and the number of injured
soldiers returning to Canada was increasing daily. More ward aides were
needed to help these men begin their long road to recovery. Even if the
war was to end soon, the soldiers' re-establishment would be ongoing and
ward aides would be needed for some time to come. It was recognized
that the women who worked as ward aides differed greatly in their pre-
paredness, and it was decided that a formal training program was now
necessary.

The courses for the ward aides, offered at the University of Toronto
in 1918 and 1919 and at McGill University in Montreal in 1919, were
popular for several reasons. Most importantly, they would provide a way
for women to contribute directly to the war effort. The courses were also
popular because while the work was perceived to be a feminine occupation like nursing, it did not involve cleaning up or caring for people's
bodily needs. It was seen as an appropriate role for women of "good families," women who might otherwise be doing charity work and could now
be engaged in "real" work.

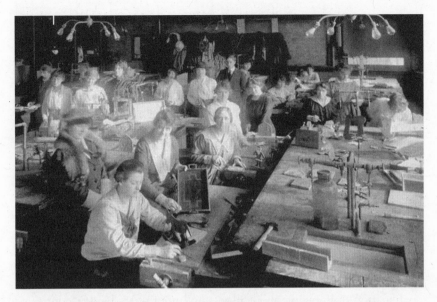

Students in the first ward aides course at the University of Toronto taking carpentry lessons in the Mining Building, Faculty of Applied Science and Engineering. Courtesy CAOT Publications ACE.

THE WARD AIDES COURSES AT THE UNIVERSITY OF TORONTO

It is unclear how the course first came about. However, by 22 February 1918, a department had been established by the Council of the Faculty of Applied Science and Engineering "for the purpose of training instructors in Bedside Vocational Training, Occupational Therapy, Diversional Occupation or what ever else it may be called."[3] Haultain, a mining engineer in the Faculty of Applied Science and Engineering, had gone to President Robert Falconer with a request to establish the course, and Falconer had readily agreed.[4] Falconer was a firm supporter of the war; his previous training as a Methodist minister had left him with the strong view that all people were meant to do their part to make the world a better place, and for him, the war came into that category.[5]

Born in 1869 and thus too old to go to war, Haultain was among the many who nonetheless wanted to play an active role.[6] As the vocational officer for Ontario, Haultain was charged with organizing the industrial retraining programs in his province. He had already proven himself a leader within the Faculty of Applied Science and Engineering and had been helping out with mining students who had returned from the war.

Haultain's primary task was to organize vocational classes that would teach soldiers new skills and then to place the men in a work setting that would give them practical experience. However, the national plan for re-establishing injured soldiers in the workplace had also included the important steps that preceded skills training. While the soldier was still confined to his bed, ward aides were to provide bedside occupations to help him regain his self-confidence and self-esteem and motivate him to start on the path back to work.

Up to this time, ward aides had been taken on as needed and came to the job with a variety of background experiences and varying abilities to do the work. The actual work also varied widely, depending on the physical setting, the ward aide herself, and the medical personnel in charge. Most ward aides had previous training as teachers, nurses, social workers, or handicraft workers, but only the nurses had the additional qualification of knowing about illness and injury. As the war continued and casualties mounted, it soon became clear that not only were there not enough ward aides to provide occupations at the bedside, but that these women could do a better job if they had better training, including some medical knowledge.

Haultain organized the courses to train new ward aides at the University of Toronto. He arranged for classroom space in the Mining Building, which belonged to the Faculty of Applied Science and Engineering, and he played a role in hiring the staff. C.H.C. Wright, professor of architecture, was the chairman of the Committee of Management that ran the course. Signifying the commitment of the faculty, the ward aide's certificate that graduates were given bore the crest of the university and the signature of its dean (Professor W.H. Ellis).

Proud of his role in the development of occupational therapy, Haultain was quick to clarify any misunderstandings about it. In a letter to Dr Alexander Primrose, then dean of the Faculty of Medicine, he pointed out that it was he – and not the psychologist Dr E.A. Bott – who, as Primrose had claimed, had started and run the program.[7] The confusion about Bott's role was understandable. While Haultain had clearly started the ward aides course in 1918 and had referred to it as "occupational therapy," Bott had been running a voluntary – and unofficial – program to treat injured soldiers since sometime in 1916. In an article in the *University of Toronto Monthly*, Bott made a distinction between his re-educational

Soldier with amputated
limb bowling as part
of his functional re-
education program at
Hart House, c. 1918.
University of Toronto
Archives, Hart House,
A 1980-0030/002(22).

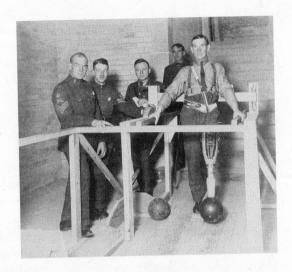

efforts, which were to lead to improved function, and the vocational programs led by others that were directed toward employment.

Bott's "functional re-education" program used a variety of approaches
to achieve restoration of function. In addition to using exercise, massage,
and electrical stimulation, Bott's staff had devised mechanical appliances
(these would be called "adaptive devices" today) to facilitate the patient's
own efforts. The appliances would enable the patient to perform activities or play games designed to provide movement for the muscles that
needed to be strengthened. As Bott put it, "the co-ordination of a partially paralysed arm, for instance, improves more rapidly by driving a nail,
catching a ball, whittling a stick, or threading a needle, than simply by
having the lame joints flexed."[8] His program, which he called "mechanotherapy," could easily be considered similar to the occupational therapy
given in a workshop at the start of a return to work program.[9] Bott notes,
however, that whereas treatment in the curative workshop was designed
to help the patient forget his injury, his approach brought the patient
"face to face with his incapacity and encouraged him to use his whole
power to overcome it."[10]

Bott had started his program at the College Street Military Hospital
in Toronto and had then moved it to a university building.[11] By 1917, the
work had moved into Hart House, where it became part of the training course in massage and electrotherapy for people who would soon be
known as physical therapists.[12]

Haultain's concern about who was to take credit for the beginning of occupational therapy was such that Dean Primrose made a formal statement in the university senate to acknowledge his error in attributing the start of the occupational therapy course to Bott (and Wilson).[13] In retrospect, it seems that Haultain was only partly right in correcting Primrose. The more reductionist approach to occupational therapy – where activities are designed for the purpose of improving physical strength and mobility and not for the psychological value of engaging in occupations – does have its origins in Canada with Bott.[14] Indeed, since the late 1800s, a similar premise had been used in occupations for people with tuberculosis; for example, graded activities (particularly "graduated walking" on hills) were used to improve strength and endurance. By the early 1900s, other occupations simulated hill walking in facilities where there were no nearby hills.[15] As the medical model grew, the use of graded activity for physical outcomes became more common within occupational therapy.

Haultain noted that he had studied Dr Bott's work at Hart House, but claimed that his ward aides course was developed on a very different psychological basis. He was likely referring to the treatment approach to be used with the many soldiers suffering from what was then called neurasthenia (also known as shell shock or battle neurosis). Many mental health issues needed to be addressed along with, and even before, the soldiers' physical disabilities could be considered. Here the ward aides were able to intervene most effectively, helping to rebuild confidence and self-esteem, just as their predecessors had been doing in mental hospitals and other treatment centres over the years.[16]

When Haultain retired in 1919, five hundred members of his vocational staff presented him with a McLaughlin touring car. Note was taken of his long service and the fact that the male vocational staff in Ontario (92 per cent of whom were returned officers and men) had come to see him as a personal friend. It was also noted that Haultain apparently accepted no remuneration for his work.[17] A renowned engineer and academic, Haultain took special pride in his work with occupational therapy, saying, "[T]he origin and early growth of this work is a thing of which I am more proud than of anything else I have done."[18] Years later Haultain recalled how occupational therapy "flourished in Ontario as it had done in no other part of the world."[19]

The first ward aides course began on 20 February 1918 at the University of Toronto with just four students: Misses Stupart, Trent, Bruce, and Challis. By 21 March 1918, twenty-four "girls" had enrolled. The initial course was just six weeks long, but there was an expectation that the

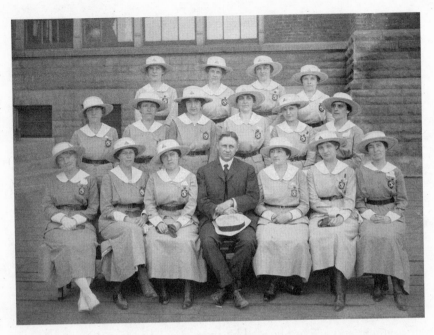

Professor H.E.T. Haultain, vocational officer for Ontario, and graduating class of ward aides, 1918. University of Toronto Archives, H.E.T Haultain, B1972-0005/001P.

students would return later on for additional instruction when the course had been further developed. By the time of the second class of ward aides, the course had been extended to three months. The students spent the first half of the course in the university and the second half partly in classes and partly in the military hospitals doing practical work. Enrolment varied from fifty to eighty students at any one time.

Winifred Brainerd, an American handicraft teacher, was brought from the United States to assist in the running of the first course. Thomas Kidner, the vocational secretary, had met Brainerd when he attended the founding meeting of the National Society for the Promotion of Occupational Therapy (NSPOT) in 1917 at Clifton Springs, New York. The founding members were invited to visit the Clifton Springs Sanitarium, where Brainerd worked. Anticipating the start of the ward aides course, Kidner had told her then that he would soon send for her to come to Toronto.[20]

As both a teacher and a handicrafts expert, Brainerd was well qualified for the position. She had taught handwork in the normal school in

Indianapolis, Indiana, and elementary handwork at the University of Virginia teachers' session prior to joining the staff at the Clifton Springs Sanitarium in 1911. There, in her first experience with patients, she worked alongside nurses who helped her with bedside and recreational activities and also in the Industrial Workshop.[21]

Upon arriving in Toronto to begin her job, Brainerd was faced with teaching a new course with no curriculum. She decided what to do as she went along and realized early on that her primary role was to "tie up" what the expert craftworkers were teaching the students to the actual work being done in the hospitals. She recalled that "the 'tieing up' process was not popular at all times for it interfered horribly with what would have been otherwise delightful occupations [for the students]."[22]

Wanting to ensure that her course content was relevant, Brainerd consulted business people in the choice of handcrafts to use with the soldiers. She sought the advice of department stores on the types of toys that would sell and the kinds of baskets that were appropriate for different seasons. She encouraged the ward aides to consider how some work might have commercial value, knowing that the official organizer of the course, an engineer and a "hard-headed business man," thought that everything should have a commercial value.[23]

Despite her ingenuity and other qualities, it appears that Brainerd had difficulties in her role and needed to be replaced. According to Segsworth, while Brainerd had been brought from the United States "as a woman fit to undertake the training of all our teachers of ward occupations for the Dominion," she apparently "developed certain weaknesses when she was given the training of other teachers, and it was found she could not occupy the position, it was so large."[24] However, they did not want to discharge her altogether and suggested transferring her to Winnipeg at a salary commensurate with her recent experience (i.e., at $125 per month). While discussion was going on about her salary level – which was considered too high and to be setting a bad precedent – she apparently did several things that led to her resignation being accepted.[25] There is no further information as to what these "things" were.

This situation caused concern across the border as well. The psychiatrist W.R. Dunton, then president of NSPOT, was supportive, noting the importance of Brainerd's work and asking her to contribute articles to the *Maryland Psychiatric Quarterly Journal*, for which he edited a section on occupational therapy.[26] When she left the University of Toronto after four months, she had helped to train thirty students, all of whom had been sent out to work in various hospitals in Ontario and Quebec.

Brainerd's replacement was Norman Burnette (1884–1962), a man with a broad background and several careers. Born in England and educated at Cambridge and the Royal School of Science in London, Burnette trained as a survey engineer. When he came to Canada, he initially worked as a surveyor in the Arctic Circle.[27] However, by 1917, Burnette was working at the Whitby Military Convalescent Hospital in Ontario,[28] where he was listed as doing "elementary and civil service teaching."[29] How or why he went from surveying in the Arctic Circle to working with injured soldiers in Whitby is not known. However, Segsworth's account of the development of ward occupations has Burnette taking on a pioneering role at Whitby in 1917 and, more widely, promoting occupations (along with Alice Peck) to the Vocational Branch of the Military Hospitals Commission.[30]

Burnette spent a comparatively short time working in the area of occupational therapy (from about 1917 to 1923) before moving on to a position in health and welfare with the Metropolitan Life Insurance Company in Ottawa.[31] Yet he appears to have been deeply invested in the work and a strong advocate. At an early stage, he went to Chicago to meet with Eleanor Clarke Slagle and to visit the Henry B. Favill School of Occupational Therapy.[32] He also toured hospitals with occupational therapy departments, including Bloomingdale (psychiatric) Hospital in New York and the Elgin State Hospital in Illinois.[33] And, as did a number of other Canadians, he became a member of the American Occupational Therapy Association (AOTA).

During his time overseeing the ward aides course at the University of Toronto, Burnette set out a curriculum that was co-authored by Ms Aletha Wathen, an instructor in the course.[34] He also wrote a training manual, entitled *Invalid Occupations in War Hospitals*, for students and graduate ward aides. It recorded many of his own experiences at Whitby and observations from his hospital visits in the United States. He included chapters on the history of occupational therapy and set out the various fields of work, always stressing the psychological aspects underlying the work with injured soldiers.[35]

Burnette thought it important to provide "manly" occupations for the men, describing the wounded soldier as having his manhood sapped by hardship and nervous strain, the latter considered a typically female ailment in the Victorian era. The contrast between the highly masculine soldier going off to war and the returned soldier now injured and dependent was an issue of general public concern.[36] Burnette was also concerned with the need to develop a certain resolve in patients. He encouraged the ward aides to help their patients select an occupation they would enjoy, but he also noted that "strengthening of the will is developed through sticking at work we don't like."[37] Didactic in nature, his training manual included statements such as "curative work is social because all sick people are anti-social. They are unable to do their own share of the world's work, and they take up the time of others."[38]

In 1919, Burnette wrote an article for the *Canadian Journal of Mental Hygiene* entitled "Invalid Occupation as a Guide to the Vocational Fitness of the Handicapped." The article stressed many of the same points made in his manual, but here he reached a larger audience and was perhaps more eloquent. Fascinated with the use of the hand in daily life and with what it symbolized, he writes, "Primitive man was a creature of the hand; through it he expressed his thoughts, his hopes, his fears, his strivings for communion with God. Machinery has tyrannized our lives, but it has not conquered us. We are the manipulators. The hand of man is still the master."[39]

Burnette saw occupations as an *in vivo* experience that could be used to assess the patient's mind and body and to aid in decisions about work placement and discharge.[40] Presaging occupational therapy's later interest in the environment and how it could support or impede occupations, he recognized the importance of "placing the man in an environment where he can function."[41] At a time when the focus of occupational therapy was starting to address physical dysfunction directly by remediating the patient, this broader perspective was unusual. Burnette also advocated for the creation of aftercare branches in social service departments – rather like contemporary mental health aftercare programs – citing the need for occupational therapists who could carry the work into the home.[42]

Adding to the debate in occupational therapy regarding "process versus product" and to discussions of the economic value of occupational therapy to an institution, Burnette argued that the emphasis be changed from *what* the patient did to *how* he did it. Underscoring the psychological aspects of engagement in occupations, Burnette noted that despite being "diagnosed as unable to function in ordinary surroundings, [people] could produce useful and beautiful things and evince joy in their work." "This," he said, "was a matter fraught with deep psychological significance."[43]

Burnette joined the Canadian National Committee for Mental Hygiene soon after it was established in 1918 and was a member of the subcommittee on educational and industrial psychology. Demonstrating his belief in the value of occupational therapy, he wrote an entire issue on the topic for the *Mental Hygiene Bulletin* in 1921.[44] The publication was divided into six sections designed to educate readers and advocate for a wider use of occupational therapy. Using a dramatic turn, he included photos of patients in two different situations with captions that read: "Which shall it be? This?" (over the picture of patients sitting and staring idly into space), "Or this?" (with patients actively engaged in occupational therapy).[45] Burnette reiterated the commonly held view that engaging the mind of the patient could chase away morbid thoughts and at the same time lighten the workload for nurses. He also commented on the need for more occupational therapy positions and bemoaned the fact that many of Canada's well-trained occupational therapists were leaving the country for work elsewhere.

Like many others, Burnette was concerned about where occupational therapy fit in relation to vocational training. He noted that the idea of providing occupations to fit "the needs of the invalid was an offshoot, not of medicine, but of the vocational training scheme."[46] However, Burnette was probably conflicted when it came to the relationship with medicine, noting elsewhere that occupational therapy was one of the handmaidens of medicine and should not be confused with vocational training.[47]

After the courses at the University of Toronto ended in 1919, Burnette continued his involvement with the Vocational Branch of the DSCR, often filling in for Haultain and his successor, George Drew, taking on some of the duties of the vocational officer for Ontario. One of these tasks involved overseeing work at the Vetcraft Shops in Toronto, which were now under the jurisdiction of the Vocational Branch of the DSCR. Burnette apparently overstepped his authority at some point and became the subject of a series of complaints. He was accused of calling himself "Chief Psychologist, Vocational Branch, D Unit," diagnosing patients on his own without consultation, and making decisions about their referrals.[48]

There is no information on why, after some five or so years with occupational therapy, Burnette changed his line of work and joined the Metropolitan Life Insurance Company in Ottawa as its director of welfare services – although it is possible that the above unpleasant episode contributed. He remained a member of the Canadian National Committee for Mental Hygiene and in that capacity continued to promote the development of occupational therapy. In particular, he voiced his concern that there were not enough trained occupational therapists available in civilian mental hospitals in Canada.[49]

WARD AIDES' UNIFORMS AND THE NAME FOR THE WORK

Captain Stanley Fryer (an architect on the Vocational Branch staff of the DSCR) designed the ward aides' uniforms. These were two-piece

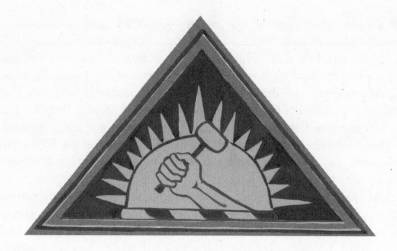

Insignia designed by S.T.J. Fryer and N.L. Burnette. The clenched fist holding a hammer and resting on a bar signifies the nobility of work, while the rising sun suggests that the nobility of work could light up mind, body, and spirit, which are represented in the insignia's triangular shape. Author's collection.

outfits made of dark-green linen, with a brown leather belt. The letters "SCR" (standing for "Soldiers' Civil Re-establishment") and a shield were embroidered on the top-left pocket. A white veil was worn, except in summer, when it could be replaced by a white panama hat with a broad green ribbon. A small badge, designed by Fryer and Burnette, was attached to the hat.[50] The badge was triangular in shape and showed a clenched fist holding a hammer and resting on a bar, with a rising sun in the background. The symbols related to the nobility of work and how it could light up the mind, body, and spirit.[51] These three components were seen as "the essentials necessary to be built up (after having in all probability been shattered through some unfortunate illness) in a manner that will bring back nature to its original happiness and prosperity."[52] The design of this badge was a reminder of the importance attributed to "restoring the spirit." It was also a reminder of how closely tied occupational therapy was to work in those early days. According to the DSCR, the vocational idea applied not only to the work of the ward aides but also to all of the DSCR's work.[53]

Haultain remembered the uniform: "It was bright. It had military cut. It attracted the sick man. It was not hospital, and it was not discipline. It worked. It suited those days."[54] The uniforms were certainly distinctive; even the Prince of Wales commented on them during his visit to Canada in 1919: "You have the most attractive uniform that I have seen."[55] The ward aides were often referred to as "the girls in green" and on occasion as "the green goddesses."[56] Ward aides who had not yet qualified and were still on probation were apparently dressed all in white.[57]

That there was as yet no agreed-upon name for the work of the ward aides is evidenced by an exchange of letters between Haultain and Kidner in 1918. Haultain writes that the Faculty of Applied Science and Engineering "has established a department for the purpose of training instructors in Bedside Vocational Training, Occupational Therapy, Diversional Occupation or whatever else it may be called." In reply, Kidner says that he wants a term wider than bedside occupations because some occupations will be carried out elsewhere on the ward. He suggests the term "ward occupations." Haultain's response is that while occupational therapy is a better title from the doctor's point of view, he feels that they must emphasize the vocational side. He writes, "[T]hough it is not specifically or entirely vocational work, it leads up to the vocational idea."[58] Ultimately, the women doing this work were known as ward aides in Canada[59] and as reconstruction aides in the United States.[60]

The early confusion over the name of the ward aides' work continued for some time, and it mirrored the uncertainty over where occupational therapy ended and vocational training began. For example, Burnette writes that when attempting to restore function the activity should "include motions which are normally used by the worker in his trade. In many cases tools could be altered to fit deformities of the hands, or injuries to the arm."[61]

THE WARD AIDES COURSE AT MCGILL UNIVERSITY

Alice Peck, founder of the Canadian Handicrafts Guild (see chapters 3 and 6), was instrumental in developing the ward aides course in Montreal. Peck was likely asked to organize the course because of her long history with the guild, her own expertise as a craftworker, and her experience using crafts to help others improve their productivity. An early account of the work with soldiers states that Major R.T. MacKeen, the district vocational officer for the province of Quebec, asked Peck to organize craftwork for the soldiers who were confined to the wards of the hospitals in Montreal.[62] The Hospital Committee of the CHG organized voluntary teachers of handicrafts for the injured soldiers and arranged for

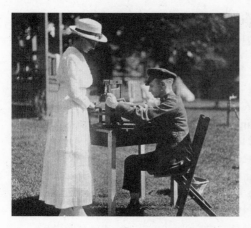
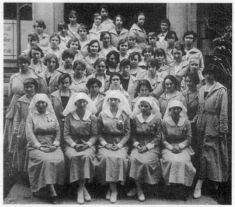

LEFT Doris Stupart, a student in the first ward aides class at the University of Toronto, dressed in the white uniform of the probationer, working with a soldier on the grounds of College Street Hospital, spring 1918. Courtesy CAOT Publications ACE; RIGHT Students in the ward aides course in Montreal on the steps of Divinity Hall at McGill University, summer 1919. Courtesy CAOT Publications ACE.

the soldiers' metalwork and woodwork to be shown and sold on a regular basis.[63]

In addition to leading the program, Peck was herself teaching crafts such as weaving and bookbinding at the bedside. For weaving, she used the small reed looms that she had seen in England, which had been specially made for use in bed. Her expertise became well known and was sought after as others started programs elsewhere.[64] Peck's work for the war effort was also a result of her very strong belief in the positive power of art and creativity, as well as in the need for humanitarian efforts in life.[65]

The course in Montreal was held in Divinity Hall at 740 University Street adjacent to the Montreal Diocesan College (at what was then 743 University). The building, also known as the Co-operating Theological Colleges of McGill University,[66] had been a gift from Sir Andrew Frederick Gault, the "Canadian Cotton King."[67] Gault was Alice Peck's adored uncle, and it is possible that the space for the Montreal ward aides course was made available because of this family connection. The course did not start until June 1919 and was offered only once, as the demand for ward aides was beginning to decrease by then.

The principal of the School of Occupational Therapy, as it was known, was C. Wenonah Brenan. Born in 1885 in Saint John, New Brunswick, she completed grade 11 at St John High School and then did two years of an arts course at Mount Allison University in New Brunswick. She also completed studies in the Graduate Department of Industrial Arts at the Pratt Institute in Brooklyn, New York. By 1918, she was working as an instructress at Camp Hill Hospital in Halifax.[68] Before she started that job, Kidner had recommended that she spend time in Montreal under Mrs Peck to learn more about occupations at the bedside. He wrote to Captain MacKeen, the district vocational officer for Montreal, saying, "As a part of the penalty for success, you will probably have some visitors from time to time, who are sent to you by us to look into this work."[69] The following year, Brenan attended the ward aides course in Toronto and was out of school just two months when she was appointed principal of the ward aides course in Montreal. After her teaching duties in Montreal ended, Brenan returned to the Atlantic coast, where she was appointed as the unit ward occupation aides supervisor in Sackville, Nova Scotia. In that position, she proved herself a strong and questioning leader: she tried to prevent undue staff stress by using rotations between work in TB sanatoriums and asylums; she lobbied for improved salaries; and she complained about her staff having to wear their winter uniforms in 85°F weather.[70]

The length of the course at McGill was meant to be up to three months,[71] but students could work at their own pace. It was understood that some students might finish the course sooner, depending on their abilities and previous training. The number attending that one course offering at McGill is uncertain. A class photo shows forty-one students, while other references suggest that twenty-eight were enrolled.

V.G. Rexford, then the acting director of vocational training for the DSCR, had organized vocational training classes in the old College of Pharmacy at the corner of Ontario and Jeanne-Mance Streets in 1918. Shoemaking and shoe repairing, art and metalwork, varnishing and painting baskets, and weaving were taught to soldiers and likely to the students from the school of occupational therapy as well. Artificial limbs, which were often made by injured soldiers, were also fabricated there.[72]

One important aspect of the curriculum at McGill University, as at the University of Toronto, was the provision of information on "hospital etiquette."[73] The emphasis on hospital etiquette was not surprising given the uncertain place of the ward aides within the hospital organization and their dual reporting lines (to the Vocational Branch of the DSCR and to the hospitals in which they worked). However, hospital etiquette was also important because of the need for the ward aides to work closely with the nurses.[74] Nurses were often expected to keep their patients occupied, especially in mental hospitals. Their own training generally included some classes in occupations, as well as massage, and exercise, areas that were considered as potential areas of specialization for nurses.

The idea that nurses should take on the work of occupational therapists, while a popular notion at the time, invited debate. The American physician Herbert Hall, who promoted occupational therapy, cautioned that nursing was already a full-time job and it would be better if nurses did not have to further expand their role. He suggested that the whole team would benefit from having what he called the "O.T. Aide."[75] The neurologist Goldwin Howland – a key individual in the growth of occupational therapy in Canada – recommended that all nurses receive some training in occupational therapy.[76]

One of the reasons that occupations were seen as part of the nursing role was that the parameters of the nursing role were not yet determined. Moreover, while the ability to teach and a knowledge of handicrafts were much needed for the work, it was also recognized that medical knowledge, together with the "nursing spirit," was an essential ingredient in this treatment option.[77] However, as occupational therapy and physical therapy became organized as separate entities and as nursing itself became more complex, nursing gradually gave up these extended roles.[78]

APPLICANTS TO THE WARD AIDES COURSES

A large number of women applied for the ward aides courses in Toronto and Montreal, and many were turned away. Some applicants made it known that they were war widows or had sons, or brothers, or sweethearts at the front, and it is likely that their applications were given precedence just as their applications for positions as ward aides had been. Recruitment materials and correspondence at the time make it clear that applicants were to be "girls of good education and suitable personality who had some training or showed aptitude in handicraft." All applicants were required to have previous education and experience.[79]

Applicants to the courses were expected to be between twenty-five and thirty-five years old, an age where women were thought to be compassionate, responsible, and able, if necessary, to tend to a soldier's broken spirit.[80] Middle-class women were thought to be ideal for the work, as they were considered the guardians of culture and morality, skilled at relationship building, and able to connect with the larger world around them.[81] The course attracted women from across Canada. Women living in neighbouring US states applied for the courses as well, eager to be ready to help now that their country was also at war.

Many applicants for the training courses made it known that they were from prominent families. Dorothy, the daughter of Sir James Lougheed (president of the Military Hospitals Commission of Canada and minister of the interior and soldiers' civil re-establishment) was accepted into a special course at the University of Toronto in 1918 that was designed for women from western Canada.[82] Doris, the daughter of Sir Frederick Stupart, national director of meteorology, was in the first course at U of T. The wives of important faculty members, such as Mrs Haultain, the wife of Professor Haultain,[83] and Miss Lash Miller, the daughter of Professor Lash Miller, were registered but not considered "official" students. C. Helen Mowat, the great niece of former Ontario premier Sir Oliver Mowat, was also enrolled in the course. Much like the recruitment process for the reconstruction aides courses in the United States, the attributes expected of applicants restricted the pool to a privileged and sophisticated group of women.[84]

There was no fee for the ward aides courses. In fact, students were paid to attend. After graduation, depending on the type of work required and the ward aides' abilities, they were paid between $60 and $75 per month. This amount was to cover their board, lodging, and clothes. Students undertook to stay with the Military Hospitals Commission for at least twelve months after completing the course.[85] It was expected that most graduates would return to their home area to work, but it was understood that they could be sent wherever they were needed.[86] Despite this agreement, there is correspondence to indicate that many of the graduates sought changes in their original placements and used their social connections to achieve them. Physicians, members of Parliament, and fathers wrote letters to their friends in high places, who then wrote to those responsible for assigning work locations.[87]

While many women had been working voluntarily as ward aides, it was decided that they and the trained graduates would now be paid.[88] There was a newly formed consensus that work with injured soldiers should explicitly not be charitable work; benevolence was perceived as particularly inappropriate in this instance, for if the ward aides were not self-sufficient, how could they promote economic independence among the men they were treating? However, a less philosophical and more practical reason for paying the ward aides was expressed by W.E. Segsworth, the director of vocational training, who found paid workers easier to manage. "[W]orkers who were not paid," he noted, "were hard to control and were inclined to give up their work on short notice when other things interfered." He went on to state that "continuity and a certain measure of uniformity and discipline are necessary, and these things it would seem can best be obtained by regular organization and paid workers."[89]

By the end of the war, some 350 newly trained ward aides had spread out across the country and were working with soldiers with a variety of conditions – war wounds, orthopaedic problems, tuberculosis, and mental illness. It was beginning to be recognized that if soldiers were benefiting from the work, then so too would civilians benefit. Requests for occupational therapists to work with civilians in general hospitals and other settings were starting to be made.

Many of the ward aides who had worked during the war retired at war's end, returned to their former lives, and were not heard of again in occupational therapy circles. A few went on to attend the diploma course offered at the University of Toronto in 1926. Ward aides who did not marry, were widowed, or married late tended to have more noteworthy careers and became familiar names in the profession as it grew.

Attending a training program, which was often away from home, would have been an interesting experience in and of itself. Working with soldiers across the country must have seemed an adventurous undertaking for many women, especially those who were previously sheltered and had lived with limited options for the future. It is no wonder that the ward aides courses were popular and the applicant rates high.

Graduates of the Ward Aides Courses

The actual work done is not really the chief thing, although that is very important, but it is the psychological factor, the changing of the mental attitude of the men towards themselves and towards the world which is the real work accomplished.

Doris Stupart, 1920[1]

The women who took the ward aides courses differed in several ways from the untrained ward aides who had gone before them. Application criteria meant that they were of a certain age and already had some advanced education or training. However, there were other, perhaps more subtle factors at play. Having some credentials already in hand, many of the women who took the courses were looking for a career and a proper working life. Approximately 12 per cent of the women in the ward aides courses were married when they began and many of those women were widowed.[2] The single women were already age twenty-five or over, and many would have thought their lives would not include marriage. Thus, an opportunity to earn a living would have been welcomed. The courses signalled a means of going beyond the world of handicrafts and into the fields of health care and social service.

Records for the ward aides courses are incomplete and somewhat inconsistent,[3] and records of the women who took the courses are few and far between. It is possible, however, to piece together the stories of several ward aides that, in turn, provide a picture of the women who practised occupational therapy in these early years.

(EMILY) DORIS STUPART

Doris Stupart was a graduate of the first ward aides course at the University of Toronto. Her privileged background was typical of many who took the course. Her father, Sir Frederick Stupart, was the director of the meteorological service of the Dominion of Canada and a faculty member at the university. Stupart attended Bishop Strachan private school for girls and the University of Toronto, from which she graduated in 1910 with an arts degree. Her activities from that date until she entered the ward aides course are not known other than that she did charitable work with the Junior League. Her brother was killed in action at the Somme in 1916,[4] and an uncle was also killed overseas. Soon thereafter Stupart became actively involved in the war effort. Her first step was to take a nursing course from the St John's Ambulance Corps and then to join the Voluntary Aid Detachment (VAD). As a VAD she was posted to the Spadina Military Hospital and worked there until she enrolled in the ward aides course in 1918 at age thirty. She worked for five years, married at thirty-five, started a family, and was not heard of professionally again.[5]

Although Stupart worked only for a brief period, she made significant contributions to the practice and the development of the profession. She started out working at the Christie Street Hospital, which, at the time, focused on orthopaedics, and then moved to the College Street Military Hospital, where she was made supervisor of ward aides. Stupart seems to have had a good sense of the wider world of occupations and to have understood how what was happening elsewhere might benefit her program. In October 1919, she requested permission to send two aides to the Roycroft Craft Shops in East Aurora, New York, to expand their knowledge. Roycroft, which was based on and followed the ideals of the arts and crafts movement, had become a highly successful retreat, teaching crafts to people suffering from neurasthenia and other stress-related disorders. Stupart's request was eventually granted, and two aides were selected on the basis of their qualifications in design and art. Their three-week stay at Roycroft was highly successful, and on their return, the aides began teaching several new crafts, including leather tooling and hammered metalwork.[6]

Stupart must have been held in high regard by her superiors. By 1920, when she was listed as the superintendent at the College Street Military Hospital, she was paid $115 per month, the highest wage of any ward aide at the time. She was responsible for the work in "Unit D," which included the more than sixty ward aides who worked in the convalescent facilities in central Ontario and the sanatoriums in Hamilton and Muskoka.[7]

As part of her responsibilities for Unit D, she was asked to undertake a review of the ward occupations being carried out in all of the Department of Soldiers Civil Re-establishment (DSCR) hospitals in central Ontario. Her ten-page report to the director of medical services was com-

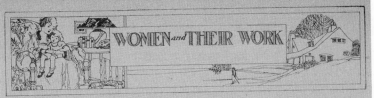

"God Bless the 'Girls In Green'!"

Story of a New Vocation for Women—Occupational Therapy —in Which Dominion of Canada Leads the World

By GERTRUDE E. S. PRINGLE

OUT of the strain and stress of the War there has sprung up in Canada a remarkable movement, which is now pointing the way to a new profession for educated women.

In 1917-8 our wounded were returning in numbers from the Front, and the military hospitals throughout Canada were rapidly filling up. Most of the cases were slow in recovering and, because the patients had nothing to do to while away the tedium of convalescence, they were becoming bored, listless, indifferent or despondent, mental states that retarded their progress and also made them less able to face the problems of civil life again. When pronounced physically and mentally well enough to leave the hospital they frequently were found industrially unfit. Long sheltering in an institution where everything was done for them had robbed them of initiative and ambition, and left them in a condition of mental apathy.

It was realized that something must be done to bridge the gap between hospital and civil life. The solution of the problem was some kind of bedside or ward occupation. And so the aid was sought of Occupational Therapy which been defined as an activity, mental or physical, especially prescribed and directed for the distinct purpose of contributing to and hastening recovery from disease or injury.

It was not a new idea. It had been used in various institutions even before it had been given the medical term of Occupational Therapy. Light, curative work for patients had been the rule for very many years in the Sisters' Hospital, Quebec, while Rockwood Asylum, Kingston, can show a beautiful bird fountain made as far back as 1900.

The work was first started in a small way by Mrs. Peck of Montreal, in the hospitals in that city. Then Toronto took it up, engaging two women trained in the United States, who commenced their labors in the College Street Military Hospital. It soon was seen that the situation called for a very special effort, for there was urgent need of many workers.

Accordingly, after some informal negotiations with the Government, the Engineering Faculty of the University of Toronto, acting entirely without precedent at a time when precedents were dead and buried, and when things were done with patriotic fervor and at white heat, formed a committee with Dean Ellis as chairman. This committee, acting upon the authority of the D.S.C.R., who supplied the funds, and backed by orders-in-council, started, in the Spring of 1918, special classes in Occupational Therapy. This action constituted a notable departure, and put Canada in the position of leading the world in such organized effort. The classes were held for eighteen months

and, in all, 375 girls passed through them. The first class numbered twenty, and before they had finished their eight weeks of instruction the second class was at their heels. A longer time of training could not

MISS E. DORIS STUPART,
Daughter of Sir Frederick Stupart, Dominion meteorologist. Miss Stupart is supervisor of Ward Aides of D. unit.

be given in view of the urgency of the situation.

How the Girls Were Chosen

APPLICANTS were chosen, not as might be thought for manual dexterity or knowledge of craftwork, but for personality and charm. The officials knew human nature. They chose the sort of girls that the soldiers would like,— nice girls who would be companionable, womanly and tactful, and who would meet every emergency in the right spirit. The fact that they would have to keep always in view the curative aim, and act in harmony with the medical and nursing staff, called for tact of a high order. Only girls endowed beyond the ordinary could meet these requirements and withstand the physical and emotional strain of the work. Practically every girl chosen made good, so well judged were the selections.

The committee was fortunate in procuring splendid teachers. One who rendered great assistance was Mr. Chester, of the Toronto Technical School. He was placed in charge of the classes when they grew large, sixty being the largest class handled. Dr. Graham of the D.S.C.R. who is now Chief Coroner for Ontario, was also closely identified with the work

from its inception, and was a member of the committee directing it.

Norman L. Burnette took a leading part in the training of the girls, giving them lectures on the psychology of their work. These talks were helpful in training them to get the viewpoint of the patients, and taught them not to view the work from a commercial standpoint but to keep the curative idea uppermost. Upon Professor H. E. T. Haultain, Vocational Officer for Ontario, fell the responsibility for the whole plan, and his enthusiasm, energy and boundless optimism piloted the scheme to success.

An Intensive Course

IN THE first course of two months eight handicrafts were explained to the students. After that they had to work out their own problems and teach themselves even while they instructed, keeping perhaps just a lap or two ahead of their soldier patients. But that practical training proved to be the finest possible. That is why the United States, even with the advantage of two-year College courses in Occupational Therapy, is engaging our girls trained in military hospitals as fast as they can secure them and at higher salaries than Canada pays.

The girls are given in Canada $65 a month while in training, and from $85 to $125 a month when they take up the active instructional work. With the official title of Ward Aide went a smart uniform of green linen, especially designed by S. T. J. Fryer, an architect of Hamilton. The Prince of Wales declared it was the prettiest uniform he had seen, and the pictures will bear out his verdict of approval.

When the first class was ready for its work among the invalid soldiers it appeared that the doctors, matrons and nurses did not want them. Since the hospital staffs were overworked, knew little of Occupational Therapy and feared that discipline, always difficult, would be rendered more difficult still, it is not to be wondered at that newcomers sent in by an outside organization were not given a very cordial welcome. However, the Aides were backed by the authority of an order-in-council, so the hospital doors had to open to them.

Aides Win Their Spurs

IT WAS a difficult situation for the girls, going daily to work where they were not wanted, and knowing that they were considered in the way with their raffia, their beads and their clay littering up the neat wards. Meantime Dr. Ellis, who was the friend of all the medical men, aided with his tact in clearing away many of the barriers of prejudice, and it began to get a little easier for the Ward Aides. But the girls themselves won a complete prehensive, and her comments provide a good picture of what the work must have been like and what the issues were at the time. For example, she emphasizes the quality of the articles produced by patients and expresses concern for their saleability. The commercial side of the work is also noted in reference to acquiring contracts for the workshops to produce baskets for florists and to linking up with merchandisers such as the T. Eaton Company that would sell the toys.[8] Stupart comments on the negative consequences for patients when equipment and workspace were inadequate and is not afraid to point out organizational issues, including poor performance where she saw it. She found that a wide range of occupations were offered to patients, such as basketry, clay modelling, toy making, weaving, reed furniture making, knitting, and beadwork. Stupart also reports on the occupational work of the social service department, noting the growth of that new work and describing how much the men welcomed the home visits.[9]

Stupart saw a future in occupational therapy and took an active role in helping to move the profession forward. She was a member of the organizing committee for the founding of the Ontario Society for Occupational Therapy (OSOT) and was the society's first president. She helped establish the first curative workshop in Toronto and was one of the leaders in a campaign to establish a permanent program in occupational therapy at the University of Toronto.[10] Her standing was such that she was chosen by OSOT to represent Canada at the American Occupational Therapy Association's convention in Baltimore in 1921.

When Stupart was awarded an honorary life membership by OSOT in 1923, the society noted that she "had the heaviest burden and responsibilities of this society during its formation, and with untiring efforts and unlimited patience did establish it on a firm foundation."[11]

M. LEONA HUDSON EDWARDS

Leona Hudson Edwards was also a member of the first ward aides course at the University of Toronto, having entered a few weeks after the course had officially begun. Her experiences differed considerably from Stupart's in that she left Toronto for Saskatchewan immediately after graduation. She described her work in the West in a series of letters written in 1970 to Helen LeVesconte, then director of occupational therapy at the University of Toronto, who was collecting material for the history she was writing.[12] Hudson painted another picture of what the work was like in those early days and also told something of the character of the ward aides.

Hudson had been chosen by Professor Haultain as the first graduate to go to Saskatchewan, seemingly on the basis of her ability and character. She was joined in her adventure by her classmate Kathleen de Courcy O'Grady. They were welcomed at the railway station in Regina by Mr F.M. Riches, the district vocational officer for the province. Riches, after being injured in the war, had been hospitalized in England and in France and had had ample opportunity to see men who had nothing to do unless "kind old ladies" visited and brought knitting and crocheting materials. On his return to Canada, Riches joined the chorus of those who believed that rehabilitation should start as soon as possible after hospitalization, and he wrote Ottawa to that effect. Riches was particularly concerned about the large proportion of soldiers from Saskatchewan who had worked on the land before going off to war but would now be unable to do so. He wanted to help them make the best use of their time in hospital to prepare for other work and that meant establishing occupational therapy programs. According to Hudson, Riches did so much for occupational therapy in Canada that he could be considered the father of the profession.[13] Riches also became a member of the National Society for the Promotion of Occupational Therapy (NSPOT) in the United States.

Hudson first worked at the Saskatchewan Military Hospital in Moose Jaw. The building was a converted public school with two large sixty-bed wards added on. A large vocational school was built on the ground floor, and the occupational therapy department was initially located on the upper floor. However, it was soon realized that the department would have to be moved, as there were no elevators and many of the men could not use the stairs. After a short time, de Courcy O'Grady, who had been placed at the Earl Gray Sanatorium in Regina, moved back to Toronto to take over the curative workshop. Hudson remained in Saskatchewan working in a variety of settings: at a TB sanatorium in Fort Qu'Appelle, at the asylum in North Battleford, and at St Chad's Military Convalescent Hospital in Regina.[14]

One issue that stood out among Hudson's memories was the problem caused by civilian patients (who were mainly women) wanting to join in the work they saw her doing with the soldiers. While they begged to be included in the handicraft classes, the aides were only allowed to teach civilians when all of the ex-soldiers had been cared for. But this criterion presented a problem: if the ward aides acknowledged that they had time to spare after completing their work with the soldiers, then the number of ward aides on staff might be cut back. There was apparently some confusion on this matter, and Hudson and other aides were reprimanded for allowing civilians into their classes.[15] Once the matter was settled and the need for expanding the work to civilians was accepted, the demand for ward aides increased; for example, where one aide had been sufficient for the soldiers at Fort Qu'Appelle Sanatorium, three more were needed to work with civilians.[16]

Hudson was able to see the broader implications of illness for a patient's family and was a good problem solver. In one instance, when told that she could do anything that might aid in the well-being of a hospitalized soldier, she arranged for a housekeeper to care for the children in his family, thus freeing his wife to visit and relieving him of his worries. She was also adventurous and eager to take on new challenges. Asked to make a home visit to a soldier who had been blinded in the war, she travelled by train to the town of Biggar, on the prairies, "near to nothing." She was met late at night by someone with a lantern who took her to a mud house where she was warmly welcomed. The blind soldier had been taught to make fishing nets during his rehabilitation at the special training centre for blind soldiers at St Dunston's in England, but he found that the method was not right for him on his return home. Hudson stayed with the family long enough to help the man develop a new method of netting. She later summed up her reminiscences about her work out west: "The story of our work in Saskatchewan is one of which we may be proud. The men were a noble lot, and one can accomplish things in the clean, bracing air of the West which would seem to me to have been impossible anywhere else."[17] Her feelings about working with the soldiers in Saskatchewan were reciprocated; when she left after just over two years, she received presentations from the injured soldiers with whom she had worked. One said, "As long as this generation lives, Saskatchewan belongs to you."[18]

When Hudson returned to Toronto in 1920, she found herself troubled by what seemed to her to be a "highly localized viewpoint" that did not value experiences elsewhere.[19] She felt she would not fit into the work there and chose instead to take a position in the United States. Hudson was in touch with members of the American Occupational Therapy Association (AOTA), corresponding with individuals such as Eleanor Clarke Slagle, to whom she turned for advice. Slagle invited Hudson to attend the third annual NSPOT convention, which was held at Hull House in Chicago in 1919. Hudson reported that Slagle had stated in her speech that "the best thing the American OT society could do was to 'follow the Canadians.'"[20] Another proud moment for Hudson occurred when she attended a summer course at an artists' summer colony in Woodstock, New York, which provided "a splendid selection of medical and arts and crafts lecturers." Hudson was the only Canadian in attendance, and when she was elected president of the class, she considered it a tribute "to our Canadian War work."[21]

Hudson met the man she would marry during one of her visits to Toronto. After her marriage, she settled in Brantford, Ontario, and appears to have stopped working soon thereafter. Commenting on why she became involved in occupational therapy in the first instance, she stressed her own experiences with what she saw as the healing powers of creativity: "My physical experience has put me in close creative contact with countless lonely people. I know that everyone can become creative in some way."[22]

EDITH A. GRIFFIN

Edith Griffin was among the early graduates of the course at the University of Toronto.[23] Her story highlights a number of interesting issues of the day, including early attempts to organize the profession, the issue of "the West" feeling slighted by "the East," and the potential for occupational therapy to align itself with social work.

There is as yet nothing known about Edith Griffin's early background, but it is likely that she had some training in art. By 1906, she was at Marblehead, Massachusetts, working with Dr Herbert Hall at Devereux Mansion, using her design expertise to develop the flower pots that Hall was then promoting. It was her idea to use cement for the flower pots and bird baths, as well as for the large "architectural" projects. She designed the moulds and cast them in cast iron. Hall loved this craft because supplies were cheap and plentiful and there was great interest in it.[24] Thus, by the time Griffin entered the ward aides course at the University of Toronto, she was well in her thirties and a skilled craftswoman.

Griffin worked at the Manitoba Military Convalescent Hospital in Winnipeg following her graduation from the course. She must have had good leadership skills because by 1920 she was helping to found the Canadian Society of Occupational Therapists of Manitoba (CSOTM) and was elected its first president. The establishment of the society, complete with a constitution, was an attempt to organize the work and the workers in occupational therapy across Canada. Griffin wrote George Drew, then the district vocational officer in Toronto, asking for help in promoting their efforts. Believing that occupational therapy was only in its infancy and that "study, experiment, and exchange of ideas would best assist its growth," she sought his support for the formation of a national association of provincial societies.[25] There is no record of Drew's response, and Griffin's plans were not realized for a further six years, when the national organization was eventually founded.

While working in Winnipeg, Griffin was asked to come back to Toronto as an instructor in a two-month ward aides course that was being run especially for western ward aides. News of the course was sent to vocational officers and other representatives in Regina, Vancouver, Winnipeg, and Calgary. Although there had been some uncertainty about the course since the fall of 1918, with periodic announcements that it had ceased, the session for the western aides did take place.[26] Griffin went to Toronto to assist as requested, but since final arrangements were not made for her as promised, she was left "hanging around Toronto for several months to no advantage." She expressed her annoyance at this treatment, and the organizers in Ottawa feared that she would go home feeling that the western work was being discriminated against.[27]

Griffin was not afraid to speak up for herself or her staff. She complained that her staff in Winnipeg had to wear uniforms that were worn and tattered and that her own winter coat and hat needed to be replaced. To her credit, her requests for replacements were met.[28] Griffin fought the same battle as Hudson had in Saskatchewan – to extend the work with injured soldiers to civilians. Aides in several facilities had been asked to help with civilian cases, and they worked after hours to do so. Rexford again responded that the ward aides should be doing work only for the military and that the DSCR should not be paying for work – and providing supplies – for civilian patients unless the ward aides had free time. However, this time he added that if they did the work, they should not report it and should donate whatever funds were collected.[29] Rexford took the same stance when told about work with civilians at the Queen Street Asylum in Toronto, but in that case, he ordered that the work be stopped immediately.[30] Although it was difficult at the time, dealing with this issue cleared the way for the growth of occupational therapy. It was this demand from civilians, their physicians, and their families that drove the expansion of the work after the end of the war.

Griffin must have also made her voice heard locally, as occupational therapy began to grow in the city. Reports from the director of the psychopathic department of the Winnipeg General Hospital showed an increasingly high regard for the service since it was inaugurated in 1920. In 1921, he noted that the psychopathic clinic regarded the occupational therapy department as one of the most important areas of its work. In 1922, the board authorized the extension of the occupational therapy work into the General Wards "as soon as finances will permit."[31] By 1920, Griffin

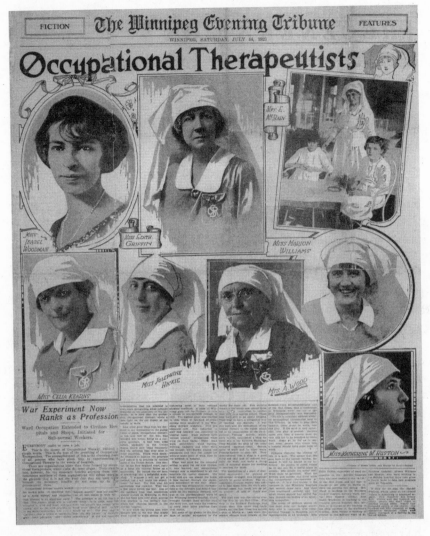

Story in the *Winnipeg Evening Tribune*, 1923, featuring eight occupational "therapeutists," including Edith Griffin (*centre top row*).

had become a member of the American NSPOT,[32] and like a number of other Canadian ward aides, she attended its meetings and conferences and presented her work. She served on the advisory board of the *Archives of Occupational Therapy*, the AOTA's first journal. Not having a national organization of their own until 1926, Canadians had a great need for support and information, and they seemed able to find it through the AOTA.

JEAN BLANCHARD CARTWRIGHT

Jean Blanchard Cartwright, a resident of Truro, Nova Scotia, applied for the ward aides course in Toronto when she was twenty-one. Not unlike others, Blanchard already had a university degree. She had earned a BA in English from Mount Allison University and planned to teach school. However, with the war still not over and her youngest brother a stretcher-bearer in France, she felt the need to contribute directly to the war effort. Although skilled in crafts and with the right educational background, she was told that she had applied too late. Determined to make a stronger application for the next available course, she – or more likely her father – arranged for a letter of reference from Mrs Jean Fielding, the owner of the *Windsor Tribune* in Nova Scotia. Fielding wrote to F.B. McCurdy, a member of Parliament for Nova Scotia and the parliamentary secretary in Ottawa. She asked that if another class was made up, whether he, "with his usual consideration for the 'Bluenose Province,' can see to it that one of her fairest daughters has a chance." Fielding added that Blanchard was "admirably fitted both by education and sterling character to qualify." McCurdy then wrote (on House of Commons letterhead) to the DSCR on Blanchard's behalf. By 14 September 1918, Blanchard was en route from Halifax to Toronto to enrol in the next course.[33]

It was a record-breaking cold and rainy fall in Toronto when Blanchard arrived. She found a room in a boarding house where she could sleep and a second boarding home where she could take her meals. She enjoyed the start of her courses at the Mining Building, but by 9 October, the Spanish influenza was declared an epidemic and a week later her classes at the University of Toronto were cancelled. The students were instructed to volunteer where they could.[34]

The citizens of Toronto, already exhausted from the war, soon became overwhelmed by the number of people suffering from the flu. Hospitals had no more room. Hotels were turned into hospitals, staffed by workers from City Hall.[35] Blanchard recalled the deserted streets and people collapsing unexpectedly; in one instance, she saw the driver of the streetcar on which she was riding slumped over the wheel. When a roommate at the boarding home where she lived took ill, Blanchard was the only one who could take care of her.

When the epidemic subsided, Blanchard returned to the ward aides classes. After graduating, she returned to the East Coast and worked briefly in Charlottetown, Prince Edward Island, at the military hospital. For Blanchard, being a ward aide was a means of contributing to the war

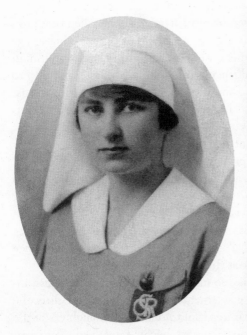 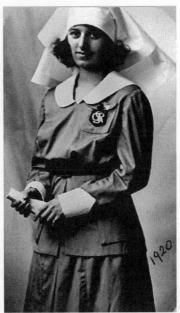

LEFT Jean Blanchard as a graduate of the ward aides course in Toronto. Her course began in September 1918 during the height of the Spanish influenza outbreak. Courtesy of Ann Kerr, daughter of Jean Blanchard; RIGHT Mary Black, c. 1920, was a graduate of the ward aides course in Montreal in 1919. She worked as an occupational therapist in both Canada and the United States and became widely known as an expert on weaving. Courtesy CAOT Publications ACE.

effort, and when she was no longer needed in that capacity, she decided to return to her original career choice of teaching. She then married and moved to Montreal, where she continued to teach until she became pregnant with her first child. As was customary at the time, she was required to leave her position. Blanchard's interest in crafts remained throughout her life.

MARY E. BLACK

Mary Black represents yet a different picture of an early ward aide. Never marrying, she had a lengthy career working in Nova Scotia and in the United States. Black was the daughter of a prominent family from Wolfville, Nova Scotia, although she was actually born in Nantucket, Massachusetts, where her maternal grandparents lived.[36] She recalled that from an early age she did things with her hands. She remembered that at age twelve, while at the family summer cottage, she saw a picture of an Indian weaving a grass mat. Black used the picture to help her figure out how to weave what she called "a coarse and crude mat" from a handful of grass gathered from the nearby marsh. This experience foreshadowed what was to be a lifelong interest in weaving. Looking back, she recalled that she "was always drawn to weaving, although I couldn't tell why."[37]

Black's early education was primarily in private schools in Wolfville. She was a bright young woman, and when she graduated from the Acadia Ladies' Seminary collegiate course, she was the youngest in her class. It is not known why she did not go on to university, but it is likely that post-secondary education was considered inappropriate for her as a young woman. Instead, she worked as a secretary in the Wolfville town office and from 1916 to 1919 as a clerk at the Royal Bank of Canada.[38]

During the war, Black was, like so many other women of her class, involved in charitable works. She was a member of the Camp Fire Girls, the Sir Robert Borden Branch of the Imperial Order of the Daughters of the Empire (IODE), and the Red Cross. She soon became involved in organizing war-related volunteer efforts. With this experience and with a brother already at the front for four years and her father in the Reserves, it was not surprising that she too decided to become more directly involved in the war effort. She had known of women using crafts to help injured soldiers and decided to apply for the course at the University of Toronto.[39] She was no doubt disappointed to receive a letter dated 23 January 1919 from F.H. Sexton, the vocational officer for eastern Canada and the Maritime provinces, informing her that the courses were ending.[40]

There is no information on what transpired over the next few months, but by 18 June 1919, Black and six other girls from Kentville and Wolfville had been accepted into the course at McGill that had started on 1 June. Her late start was made possible because of the flexible nature of the course; it was to be no less than eight weeks and no more than twelve, the time depending on the ability of the student as determined by the principal of the school, C. Wenonah Brenan (see chapter 8). Black travelled with the other girls to Montreal on 21 June 1919.[41]

Black must have progressed well, as she managed to graduate from the course in just over two months. She received a subsistence allowance of $55 per month, was "on probation" from week to week, and could be dismissed with a week's notice. As a graduate of the course, she was to be known as a "ward occupation aide" and could be sent at the discretion of the district vocational officer to any facility, "whether tubercular, insane, neurasthenic, medical or orthopaedic, in which soldier patients of the Allied Forces are receiving treatment, and whether these patients have been overseas or not."[42] Like the students in the course at the University of Toronto, she had to make the commitment to stay in service for at least one full year.

By September 1919, Black was back in Nova Scotia and working at the sanatorium in Kentville. After a few months, she transferred to the Nova Scotia (psychiatric) Hospital in Dartmouth. Just as Hudson had experienced in Saskatchewan and Griffin in Manitoba, there was recognition in Nova Scotia that the work needed to be extended beyond injured soldiers to the civilian population. In this instance, it was the medical superintendent of the Nova Scotia Hospital who took on the cause and Black who filled the first such position. "Recognizing the value of vocational work among those mentally ill, we decided to extend the work to our civil patients, and in September 1920, Miss Black was engaged to carry on the work." By then Black had completed the required year of service for the DSCR and was free to take on the task of organizing a program for civilian patients. When the work was fully underway, four "classes" were held each day to provide vocational – or occupational – work for fifty-five patients.[43]

By the summer of 1922, Black had decided that there was not much future for advancement for an occupational therapist in Nova Scotia. As she wanted more experience and knowledge, she looked for work in Boston, the nearest "big city" at the time.[44] Correspondence between Black and Harriet Robeson, the Director at the Boston State Hospital, and with Eleanor Clarke Slagle, then secretary of the AOTA, shows that Black was held in high regard. One of her letters of recommendation noted that "she lays the emphasis on the right thing, the treatment and the results, not on a beautiful product as many aides are prone to do."[45]

Black spent twenty-one years in the United States; she worked at the Boston State Hospital, at two state hospitals in Michigan (Traverse City and Ypsilanti), and at the Milwaukee Sanatorium.[46] Meanwhile, efforts were ongoing to bring Black back to Canada, especially as her experience in the United States had made her particularly valuable. One such request came from Verdun Protestant Hospital in 1926, and another from the Junior League in Winnipeg.[47] Interestingly, in 1930, the Winnipeg job offer for the position of director of occupational therapy came via the AOTA and not the Canadian Association of Occupational Therapists (CAOT), which by then was in place. While considering the Winnipeg position, Black wrote to Slagle, who was overseeing the hiring, stating that she had references from people who knew her family and background but would rather "obtain a position because of what I can do, rather than because of who I am."[48]

While in the United States, Black served on the executive of both the Michigan and Wisconsin Occupational Therapy Associations. She was the assistant editor of the *American Journal of Occupational Therapy* from 1938 to 1943 and wrote several professional and popular articles over the years. However, Black's major contribution came as she developed her knowledge of European handicrafts and began to focus on weaving. In 1945, she published *Key to Weaving*, which came to be known as "the handloom weavers' bible." It is considered essential reading for serious weavers and remains in use today.[49]

Black finally returned to Canada in 1943. From that time until 1955, she served as the director of the Handcrafts Division of Nova Scotia's Department of Industry and Publicity, later known as Trade and Industry.[50] She is especially remembered for starting weaving guilds locally in Halifax and provincially with the Atlantic Society of Handweavers. In 1948, she collaborated nationally to form the Guild of Canadian Weavers and served as its honorary president in 1949.[51] Over the years she was invited to help with various occupational therapy programs as well as with government handicraft programs. Black died in 1988. The Mary E. Black Gallery in Halifax – which specializes in crafts – is named for her.

Many other ward aides have left behind information that conveys their interesting experiences. Helen DeLaporte established her own clinic for children with learning disabilities in Toronto; the Eastmure sisters went west to work in Regina; Amy DesBrisay pioneered the work at Toronto General Hospital and then, along with another early graduate, Mabel McNeill McRae, helped to establish occupational therapy at the Astley Ainslie Hospital in Scotland; Kathleen de Courcy O'Grady ran the curative workshop; and Jean Hampson was the first occupational therapist to work in a public school.

Taken together, the stories of the graduates of the ward aides courses paint a picture of women who were intent on doing what they could for their country in its time of need. However, they are also seen as women who were ready to take on an important and completely new endeavour and who wanted to make use of their creativity and ingenuity. Their chosen work brought a level of excitement and adventure to their lives that was new to them. They now had paid employment and there was promise in the air for the future of their fledgling profession.

PART THREE

Building a Profession

Establishing Professional Organizations, Curative Workshops, and a Journal

POSTWAR GROWTH AND DEVELOPMENT

With our hands outstretched toward those who need us and a splendid army of
interested citizens back of us, there is no limit to what we may accomplish.

Edith A. Griffin, 1921[1]

In the years following the war, the future for ward aides, or occupational
therapists as many were starting to be called, was becoming uncertain.
Their work had been undertaken as a short-term solution to a wartime
problem. While it was clear that many veterans would require help for
years to come, with almost all of the injured soldiers having returned
home by the summer of 1919, even that work was sure to decrease. The
issue now was this: Is the work of the occupational therapist appropriate
for other populations and other settings? There is no evidence to suggest
that ward aides explicitly discussed among themselves whether or not to
continue; rather, they would have been concerned with how to go about
doing so. In order to move ahead in any fashion, an organization of some
sort was needed.

Never a very large cohort even when fully engaged, the ward aides
were dwindling in number significantly by 1920. Many who had become
ward aides because of the war returned to their previous lives, caring for
their homes and families and doing philanthropic work. As the military
hospitals and convalescent homes closed, some of the ward aides who
wanted to continue with the work took jobs in the United States, where
the profession was developing more quickly. In fact, the US surgeon general had explicitly invited occupational therapy aides who had been de-
mobilized from the Canadian services to come, saying they were urgently

needed. Many women acted on his invitation, thus decreasing the numbers of Canadian ward aides even further.[2]

The work of the reconstruction aides (as ward aides were called in the United States) was considered increasingly important, in part because of its expansion into orthopaedics. In this area, ward occupations were viewed as an essential adjunct to proper medical treatment in all military hospitals, and the work was now to continue with civilians.[3] Not surprisingly, the invitation from the United States prompted the sentiment at home that ward aides who had had their training at the expense of the Canadian government should stay and work in Canada.[4]

There was some growth in the work in Canada in terms of the settings in which it was carried out and the nature of the injuries seen. Specifically, work with people who had suffered industrial accidents was growing, along with work with special groups; for example, ward aides were beginning to work more with "crippled" children and people who were blind. In addition, "field service" (i.e., an early iteration of home care) was becoming popular for those not well enough to leave home for treatment, and curative workshops, staffed by occupational therapists, were being established for those who could work but not in a competitive environment. Tuberculosis continued to be a major health concern after the war, and occupational therapists were establishing their important role within treatment regimes for that population. Many of the aides had worked in mental institutions before and during the war, and that work would continue and possibly expand given the number of returned soldiers who suffered from war-related trauma.[5]

There was no organization to hold the ward aides together and no external supports to assist them in moving forward. It soon became clear that a formal association of some sort was needed. Perhaps the aides saw the National Society for the Promotion of Occupational Therapy (NSPOT, an American group) as a model and sought to emulate its success. Or perhaps Thomas Kidner, the Canadian who had overseen the ward aides' work while vocational secretary and had been one of NSPOT's founders, directly influenced the process in Canada. Now living and working in the United States and heavily involved with NSPOT, Kidner would have known many of the Canadian ward aides personally. In 1918, he was named chair of the International Committee of NSPOT and, in that capacity, likely invited other Canadians to join the American association.[6]

Within a few years of the establishment of NSPOT, two groups of Canadian occupational therapists emerged. They determined to keep the work going and see it established more permanently. One group was in Manitoba and the other in Ontario.

THE MANITOBA GROUP OF WARD AIDES

In June 1920, fifteen ward aides working in Manitoba formed the Canadian Society of Occupational Therapists of Manitoba (CSOTM).[7] Edith Griffin led the effort along with Jessie Stewart. In an undated letter to those trying to establish an Ontario society, Griffin responded to a request to describe how the Manitoba society had been organized. She described how all the ward aides in the province had met and decided to form a society. The society began with those aides and three or four other people who were in some way connected with the work. "After these preliminaries," she writes, "we were ready for other members and getting doctors, Superintendents of hospitals and some sustaining members who are people interested in any cause they feel worthwhile." At a later point in the letter, Griffin reflects on the postwar change away from working in the vocational branch: "We have been turned over to the Medical as I suppose you have. It makes some trouble in getting adjusted." With no further elaboration on this point, it is difficult to know whether she found the change welcome or not.[8]

In addition to organizing occupational therapists in Manitoba and establishing a curative workshop, the CSOTM sought to form a national association made up of the provincial societies. By 1922, the CSOTM had forty-four members.[9] Despite its small numbers, the Manitoba society was successful in raising funds for a curative workshop that was located in the Builders' Exchange Building in Winnipeg. While looking for an institutional structure to house the work, the society investigated the possibilities of working with the Social Service Commission of Winnipeg, a setting that must have felt welcoming to them.

The idea of occupational therapy aligning itself with the field of social work (as social services would soon be called) was appealing in many ways. Both social workers and occupational therapists worked with clients to decrease dependence. While each discipline used different means to achieve this goal, with the social worker focusing on society's resources and the occupational therapist focusing primarily on the individual's skills – giving agency to individuals was a key element in the work of both groups.

When social services made discharge plans for patients, they often found it useful to ask an occupational therapist to make home visits in order to improve the patients' level of productivity. Edith Griffin, who was leading Manitoba's efforts to organize the therapists, wrote about the economic contribution that occupational therapy could make to society and how that factor would, in turn, influence health. Although not using the same language as would be used today, Griffin – almost a century ago – was viewing employment as a "social determinant of health" and promoting occupational therapy's role in facilitating it. She was particularly interested in the ability of curative workshops to provide opportunities for those who could be productive but only if their work was protected – or "sheltered" – in some way.[10]

For reasons yet unknown, the Manitoba society was not able to continue in its efforts. Nonetheless, individual therapists remained active and continued to expand the work. In 1923, the *Winnipeg Evening Tribune* sang the praises of these therapists in an article entitled "Occupational Therapeutists: War Experiment Now Ranks as Profession."[11]

THE ONTARIO GROUP OF WARD AIDES

In Ontario, the ward aides were having better luck establishing a society. (Emily) Doris Stupart, who had graduated from the first ward aides course at the University of Toronto in 1918, helped to organize the Ontario Society for Occupational Therapy (OSOT). The name of the group (which was changed in 1968 to the Ontario Society *of* Occupational Therapists)[12] makes clear that its earliest goal was to promote the work rather than to serve the workers. This plan was understandable given the timing of the venture; without promoting the profession, there would be no work for the workers.

The Ontario society held its first meeting on 4 October 1920 at the University College Women's Union at the University of Toronto. Stupart was elected as the society's first president, and Mrs H.E.T. Haultain its first vice-president. Mrs Haultain was the wife of Professor Haultain, the vocational officer for Ontario who had organized the ward aides course at U of T. The secretary was Mrs Burrell, and the treasurer was Kathleen de Courcy O'Grady.[13] Meetings of local branches of the Ontario society were held in Ottawa, Kingston, and Hamilton, at around the same time as the provincial society held its first meeting.

The charter of incorporation was received from the Ontario government on 19 January 1921.[14] The signatories of the letters patent for the society were Doris Stupart, supervisor of ward aides, D Unit; Mabel Lyle Graham, supervisor of ward occupations at the Toronto General Hospital; Addie Gertrude Burrell, civil servant; Kathleen de Courcy O'Grady, ward aide, Christie Street Hospital; and Margaret Bickell, supervisor of ward occupations at Pearson Hall. Of interest, the letter from the Ontario government granting the charter was written not to Doris but to her father, Sir Frederick Stupart.

The three objectives that the society set forth in the charter were modest yet essential to any subsequent steps: (1) to study occupations suitable for the various forms of handicap and also to study their remedial effects; (2) to advance occupation as a therapeutic measure; and (3) to disseminate knowledge on the subject. No mention was made at this time of any notion to develop the work into a profession or to establish an educational program.

While seemingly off to a good start, within a few months the society decided that it could not achieve its goals without help. According to Stupart, the public had not thought about the "value of occupation of mind and hands as a means to health" outside of the context of war and would need to be educated.[15] The strategy that OSOT decided upon was to engage the help of those with influence in government circles and the medical establishment. Many of the ward aides had powerful connections; they knew people who were politically and socially prominent, and perhaps more importantly, they knew physicians who had come to value their work. It would help to have physicians as allies. Given their gatekeeper role, if they approved, occupational therapy would grow; if they disapproved, the growth of the work would be severely challenged.

OSOT invited a number of influential people to form an honorary advisory board. Once formed, the board was composed of twenty-one individuals, just three of whom were women – one was a ward aide (Miss Jean Gunn), while the other two were wives of prominent men of Toronto (Mrs James Ince and Mrs Arthur Vankoughnet). Of the remaining eighteen members, ten were physicians and eight were prominent men of varying backgrounds.[16] The lieutenant-governor of Ontario, Lionel J. Clarke, became OSOT's honorary president, Dr Goldwin Howland was the honorary secretary treasurer, and Sir Robert Falconer, president of the University of Toronto, was the honorary vice-president. Dr Alexander Primrose, the dean of the Faculty of Medicine at the University of Toronto, took on the important role of chairman of the board of management. How OSOT managed to enlist the help of such a stellar roster of individuals remains something of a mystery.

Before proceeding further with the organization, Dean Primrose, as chair of the board of management, decided to appoint a committee of physicians to gauge the medical profession's current support for occupational therapy. He asked the committee to "determine, from the Professional standpoint, the value of Occupational Therapy in the Wards of the civilian hospitals, in the Out-patient department and in connection with Public Health work, both City and Provincial."[17] The minutes of that meeting recorded the significance of the physicians' task. They were to decide "whether they should recommend the support and advancement of Occupational Therapy to the Medical Profession."[18] Had the decision been negative, OSOT would have been stopped, at least temporarily. Indeed, the society might have disappeared, or at the least, might have had to take a very different approach.

Primrose 's special committee of physicians and their role in determining the work of occupational therapists provides a good example of the power that physicians had over the nascent profession of occupational therapy from the outset. However, OSOT may not have been counting on giving over control of their destiny to physicians. It is not clear whether OSOT decided to involve physicians for tactical reasons, just to help the organization get started, or whether it consciously intended that the focus of the work be shifted toward a more medical approach. In some instances, physicians may have lent their support simply because of their own positive experiences with occupational therapy during the war. However, within a few short years, the engineers, teachers, architects, social workers, artists, and vocational educators who had been so involved with occupational therapy early on had withdrawn and prominent medical men had taken over.

A similar process occurred when physical therapy was being established, albeit with mostly different players, and at a slightly later time. These new players had a more direct link to medicine; their antecedents were found in the work of masseuses and of physicians who called themselves "electrotherapeutists." Physicians were (relatively) quick to see physical therapy as an adjunct to their own work, and they were anxious to keep physical therapists under their wing lest they become a threat to the physicians' own scope of practice.[19] Occupational therapy, on the other hand, had been grounded in social and vocational work, as well as in artistic ventures, and its link with medicine was much less obvious.

Once the decision was made to move forward, physicians took on the task of promoting occupational therapy within their own medical literature and in the popular press. For example, Dr Alexander Primrose frequently contributed articles about the profession to the *University of Toronto Monthly*. In 1923, he wrote about the potential growth of occupational therapy: "[T]he day is not far distant when every large general hospital will consider a department of this sort as one of the essential parts of its equipment."[20]

Occupational therapists in the 1920s seemed able to garner the attention of the popular press with ease. The open meeting of OSOT held at Government House on 1 May 1925 and hosted by the lieutenant-governor and Mrs Cockshutt was written up in the *Evening Telegram* the following day. Dr Primrose presided over the meeting, and more than 250 people attended. Distinguished speakers attested to the value of occupational therapy, especially in psychiatry, but also for those with tuberculosis and children with disabilities. Maurice Hutton, the principal of University College at the University of Toronto brought the meeting to a close by describing occupational therapy as the "gospel of Practical Christianity."[21] As Hutton himself was a deeply religious man, his statement is a reminder of the ongoing religious sentiment that pervaded what were perceived as "good works." Being an occupational therapist was now seen as one way to live a meaningful life.

Occupational therapy was slowly spreading across the country in civilian settings, yet it generally required additional financial support to do so. With no system of state-supported health care at the time, new work in hospitals often required financing through bursaries. Funds to support patient care and staff salaries were raised by philanthropic groups such as the Imperial Order of the Daughters of the Empire (IODE), Kiwanis, the Junior League, the Rotary Club, the Girl Guides, and Big Sisters. Some ward aides may have been members of these philanthropic groups (e.g., Cybel Lighthall was a prominent member of the Junior League), and other personal contacts with the members would have helped direct fundraising efforts to this purpose. The funds paid the salaries for occupational therapists who could then demonstrate the work in a new setting on a temporary basis; evidence of the work's success would be used in requests to permanently expand occupational therapy positions.[22]

Using a bursary system to fund new work was deemed more acceptable than offering services on a volunteer basis. The practice of having qualified therapists work without pay was called into question – in the United States as well as in Canada – as possibly harmful, for it appeared to demean the service and might inadvertently lead to lower pay for the work.[23] It is unlikely that the ward aides were concerned about protecting their "unique body of knowledge" from the hands of untrained volunteers, as they had not yet established their scope of practice, except in the broadest of terms. However, it was clear that they did not want to be thought of as volunteer do-gooders – despite any claims of "practical Christianity."

CURATIVE WORKSHOPS

A major undertaking of OSOT (as it was for the Manitoba group) was to establish a curative workshop where patients could perform work-like activities outside of the hospital and away from home. Initiated in vari-

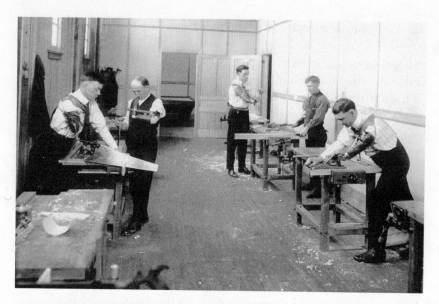

Soldiers with amputations making prosthetic limbs at a workshop in Camp Hill Military Hospital, Nova Scotia, 1920. CAMH Archives, Toronto.

ous forms in the United Kingdom in the 1800s and culminating in the establishment of the Lord Roberts Memorial Workshops in 1904, the workshops were brought to new prominence by the orthopedic surgeon Sir Robert Jones during World War I.[24] He supported both direct and indirect curative work: for example, a person could saw wood to exercise the shoulder or elbow directly, or he could saw wood and unconsciously use a stiff ankle joint as he became interested in the work his hands were doing. Jones pointed out that psychologically it is better to engage the man in productive occupational treatment than to give him a mere exercise with tools. "An ingenious tutor," he said, "can generally manage this."[25]

A major goal of curative work overseas during the war was to make men fit to return to the front as soon as possible. Soldiers treated in curative workshops often included those who suffered from mental trauma or "war neuroses" brought on by actual, as well as anticipated, war experiences. These soldiers were of particular interest to the military command; with their bodies intact, they were physically fit and thus had great value as soldiers – if only they could be helped emotionally to return to the front. The curative workshops at hospitals in England and France relieved soldiers of the stress of combat and, at the same time, provided them with the assurance that they would be able to cope upon returning to the front lines.[26]

In the postwar years, curative workshops helped physically disabled soldiers move from dependence – with its connotations of femininity – to employment and a much-desired return to masculinity. They marked a stage along the path that took the soldier forward from making objects in a hospital workshop to a paid position in a civilian workplace.[27] Established in many settings in North America, curative workshops were soon seen to be an early phase in return-to-work programs for civilians. They were intended to speed the transition from invalid status to economic independence while also saving money for insurance companies and industrial plants in the long run.[28]

In order to build its curative workshop program, OSOT needed financial support. The IODE was an ideal group to approach because it had branches across the country and, while OSOT was a provincial society, it was planning work that could become dominion-wide. In an appeal to the IODE in 1922, Stupart, on behalf of the executive of OSOT, wrote about various new services that occupational therapists could provide to men and women disabled in civilian life from tuberculosis, heart conditions, and all forms of mental and nervous disease. She noted that the work had a preventive aspect, as it would provide opportunities in art that could widen the interests of those "who might otherwise lead unhealthy and uninteresting lives." OSOT also envisioned travelling aides going to smaller towns and villages to give courses, thus "affecting the development of the artistic sense throughout the country."[29] Ruskin and Morris, as well as the members of the Canadian Handicrafts Guild, would have been pleased with this new plan indeed.

In stating her reasons for asking the IODE for support, Stupart described the proposed central workshop as follows: "1) it is a great and good movement, 2) it is peace work that is necessary, 3) IT WILL FORM A NEW AND PERMANENT OCCUPATION for women, and 4) it is a splendid means of developing Art in Canadian homes, particularly in improving the lives of those in the country and small communities" (Stupart's capitalization).[30]

Curative workshops became established in the early 1920s in Toronto, Vancouver, Winnipeg, and Montreal.[31] Occupational therapists and physicians urged the community to raise funds for the workshops. In a booklet entitled "Honour the Dead by Helping the Living, Ontario Society for Occupational Therapy Curative Workshop," Dean Primrose, in his capacity as chairman of the advisory board of OSOT, set out how these funds

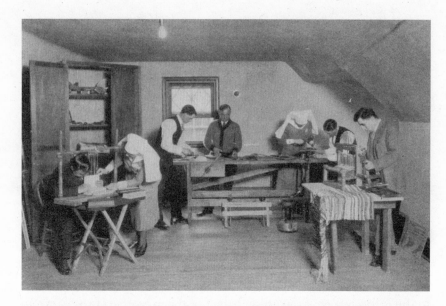

Curative Workshop in Toronto, c. 1929. This workshop provided fieldwork experiences for occupational therapy students and operated as the headquarters for the Ontario Society of Occupational Therapy in its early years. Courtesy CAOT Publications ACE.

would be used.[32] Funds were needed not only to operate the workshop, but also to transport patients from home to the workshop. In the event that transportation was not possible, the patient would be treated in the home as part of the field service program. Patients could be referred for home visits by doctors, clinics, the Department of Public Health, the Neighbourhood Workers Association, social services, and the Victorian Order of Nurses. Private patients would pay for their own treatments, while public cases would be paid for by a bursary program. A bursary of $100 provided treatment for one year for a patient able to attend the workshop, and a bursary of $150 provided treatment for a patient taught at home. A bequest of $2,000 provided a life bursary for hundreds of afflicted people. In this way, the booklet stated, one could "help some unfortunate to learn a useful occupation and so assist them to pass happy hours, forgetting their misery."[33]

Primrose extolled the virtues of occupational therapy for civilians and explained how occupations helped. The medical slant to the work was apparent in his description of how people could learn new skills and become productive while improving the function of their muscles and joints. He was careful to add that the work was "carried on under the direction and guidance of the doctors of the Advisory Board, and all patients attending the workshop must have a doctor's prescription."[34]

Primrose also stressed the psychological benefits of the work. Echoing the wartime rationale for occupations as a means of preventing the negative consequences of idleness, he noted how patients with nothing to do became lethargic and despondent, while those who were kept active recovered more quickly and went back to work.[35] True to the early work-oriented tenets of the profession, Primrose noted that articles produced in the curative workshop often had economic value and could start the patient on a road to productivity.

Some philanthropic groups raised funds to pay for a particular patient or the salary of a therapist. This approach generated good publicity for the profession, while the hospital benefiting from these funds came to the conclusion that it could not do without the therapists.[36] In a further iteration of this fundraising, crafts made in the Toronto Curative Workshop were used to support occupational therapy in the Hospital for Sick Children.[37]

"Street Fairs" run by the Bursary Committee of the Toronto Association of Occupational Therapy gave the profession a public face and much publicity. These weekend-long events were held in the 1930s on Devonshire Street – coincidentally to be the home of Physical and Occupational Therapy (P&OT) some thirty years later. A large number of sponsors supported the fairs, including the Toronto Daily Star, the Junior League, the IODE, and a number of hospitals, while individuals gave their time to act as judges, present prizes, or make announcements. The lieutenant-governor of the province opened the fair by cutting green and white satin ribbons. These events were described in broadsheets provided on the day and written up in the daily news.[38] The early occupational therapists certainly benefited from having partners to help them develop their work: private individuals provided the much-needed services, and philanthropic groups gave the financial support.[39]

Curative workshops adjusted to address the needs of people who sustained work-related injuries during the industrial boom of the 1920s, and they continued to offer services during the economic depression of the early 1930s. During and after World War II, treatment in curative workshops was directed, once again, toward helping injured soldiers return to work.

THE QUEBEC SOCIETY OF OCCUPATIONAL THERAPY

The Quebec Society of Occupational Therapy (QSOT) was founded in 1928, and the Montreal Branch held its inaugural meeting at the Mount Royal Hotel in Montreal on 8 February 1929. Over a hundred individuals "interested in the subject" attended. Mary Caton, a graduate of the School of the Museum of Fine Arts, Boston, and the Boston School of Occupational Therapy and a member of the American Occupational Therapy Association, was the secretary of QSOT, and Cybel Lighthall (see chapter 8) was on the advisory board. Here again, medical men took on a leading role with Dr John Meekins, professor of medicine at McGill University, being elected as president of the society. The founding event was reported in the American journal *Occupational Therapy and Rehabilitation* in 1929 in recognition of the close working relationships among the practitioners of the profession in the two countries. The report also noted that a training course was contemplated for McGill and that the École des beaux-arts would cooperate. However, such initiatives were dependent on funds, which, it turned out, would not be forthcoming until 1950.[40]

QSOT was clearly anglophone in its membership. While excellent work was being carried out in many francophone settings, including asylums, sanatoriums, and general hospitals, there is no record of a parallel society being formed in the province. Occupations were generally carried out by nurses, and in Quebec these nurses were often members of religious orders. For example, nurses who belonged to the Sisters of Providence were providing occupations, generally work-related, for patients in Montreal's Saint-Jean-de-Dieu Hospital by the end of the nineteenth century. Indeed, the term *ergothérapie* was used in an article published by Eva Reid in 1914 in the *Boston Medical and Surgical Journal*. Reid was an American physician who extolled the virtues of work as treatment for mental disorders.[41]

FOUNDING A NATIONAL ASSOCIATION

Founding a national association was a gradual process, with steps that took a number of years. The need for such a group had been apparent since 1920 when the ward aides in Manitoba had originally tried to organize themselves as part of a national group. Once the Ontario Society for Occupational Therapy was established, it took on the founding of a national organization as one of its early tasks, and therapists from across the country joined in the effort.

The Canadian Association of Occupational Therapists (CAOT) came into existence in 1926. The structure included a board of management and occupational therapists representing each province. There is no record of elections for the various executive positions, but it must have been agreed upon in some fashion that Dr Goldwin Howland would be the CAOT's first president. Dr Primrose took on the position of vice-president, Mr W.J. Dunlop that of secretary. Dunlop was at the time the director of the Department of Extension in the University of Toronto, and he would oversee the occupational therapy program established there that same year. Members of the board were Dr Gilbert, Dr Faulkner (the minister of health of Ontario), Dr Jabez Elliott, Dr R.E. Gaby, Dr Robert Armour, Dr T.G. Heaton, and Dr Ruth Franks. Dr Franks, a psychiatrist, was to be a strong supporter of occupational therapy for many years, particularly in regard to the profession's role in mental health.[42]

The minutes of a meeting of the CAOT held on 20 November 1930 show that committees were appointed to deal with four priorities: education, a registry, development of the organization, and a charter.[43] Within these priorities, there was also recognition of the need for a (paid) full-time executive consultant and a professional journal.

Her Excellency Viscountess Willingdon, the wife of the governor general of Canada, had agreed to act as patron of the CAOT. Having a royal patron as a champion of an organization was a common British practice at the time and would not have seemed unusual. The viscountess and her husband, the governor general, had an interest in the arts, and this might have been a factor in her willingness to serve the association in this capacity. In addition, their son had been killed in World War I, and the viscountess may have known about the wartime work of the occupational therapists. The custom of having patrons continued at the CAOT until 1984, with successive governors general or their wives holding that position.[44]

In the fall of 1931, at the invitation of the Canadian and American Hospital Associations and in conjunction with OSOT and the AOTA, the CAOT held its first convention. The venue was the Automotive Building at the Canadian National Exhibition grounds in Toronto. By holding its annual meeting in Toronto at the same time, the AOTA was endeavouring to "prove" its friendship to its Canadian cousins and show gratitude to Canada for developing the use of occupational therapy during the

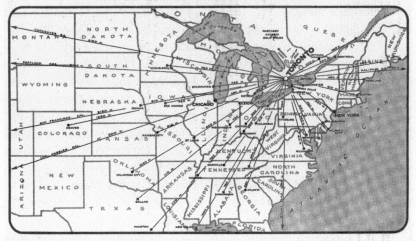

Map used to advertise the Fifteenth Annual Convention of the American
Occupational Therapy Association to be held in Toronto in September 1931.
Courtesy Archive of the American Occupational Therapy Association, Inc.

war. An editorial entitled "On to Toronto" in the journal *Occupational
Therapy and Rehabilitation* urged members to show their gratitude in particular to T.B. Kidner, the person who was so involved with the work in
Canada. It was noted how Kidner was "borrowed" by the United States
and had since become one of them, leading the advancement of the association in his adopted country.[45] Accounts of that first convention suggest that it was well attended and that the speakers and other events were
stimulating and provocative.[46]

In 1932, Mr Ross Gooderham (then vice-president and general counsel
for the Manulife Insurance Company of Canada)[47] was asked to apply
for a dominion charter for the CAOT. The charter was finally granted
in 1934, the charter members being Dr Howland, Mr Dunlop, Dr Gaby,
and two occupational therapists, Miss C. Helen Mowat, and Miss K. de
Courcy O'Grady. Affiliated members of the CAOT included members of
the Quebec Society of Occupational Therapy and all members of OSOT.
Each local association or society became a member, and all association
presidents became vice-presidents of the CAOT.[48]

The Depression of the 1930s limited any ideas of expansion for the profession. This was made evident in 1932 when, without any consultation with the medical officers, the federal government announced the closing of occupational therapy departments in veterans' hospitals. However, in an example of successful lobbying for the profession, the board of the CAOT met and passed a resolution that was sent to Prime Minister Bennett. A "letter-writing campaign" was launched and organizations such as the Canadian Red Cross and the Local Council of Women, which were also concerned about the welfare of the veterans, were invited to join the campaign.[49] A meeting then took place between physicians from Ottawa and representatives of the CAOT board. The result was that occupational therapists continued their work and the veterans' hospitals agreed to provide two internships for students, thus expanding the work even further.

The CAOT followed the practice initiated by OSOT and established an honorary advisory council. It was comprised of seven members from Ontario, five from Quebec, three from Alberta, three from British Columbia, two from New Brunswick, one from Manitoba, and one from Saskatchewan, as well as two members from New York City and one from Scotland. Of the twenty-five members, eighteen were physicians, including the soon-to-be famous neurologist Dr Wilder Penfield.[50] The composition of the honorary advisory council, like that of OSOT, was predominantly male and medical.

STARTING A JOURNAL

The CAOT had wanted to publish professional material for some time but had been undecided as to the format. In the United States, articles dealing with occupational therapy were published in different ways: first in a column (with varying titles) in the journal *Modern Hospital*, and then in the *Maryland Psychiatric Quarterly*. The AOTA established its own journal, *Archives of Occupational Therapy*, in 1922. The name of the journal was changed to *Occupational Therapy and Rehabilitation* in 1925, and in 1947, it became known as the *American Journal of Occupational Therapy*. It remains the most widely read occupational therapy journal in the world.

The CAOT appointed a committee in April 1933 to consider the idea of publishing its own journal. The committee, chaired by Dr T.G. Heaton, included Drs Hyland, Elliott, Franks, and Faulkner, and four occupational therapists, Misses Perigoe, de Courcy O'Grady, Wright, and Minty. They favoured a quarterly journal whose costs could be defrayed through paid advertising and recommended that the first issue of the new journal, to be called the *Canadian Journal of Occupational Therapy* (CJOT), be published in September 1933 with two thousand copies.[51] While this number far exceeded the number of practising occupational therapists, the intent was to use the journal to increase awareness of the profession. Copies were sent to superintendents of hospitals, sanatoriums, and institutions that had more than twenty-five beds, to all medical staff and boards of hospitals who had already adopted occupational therapy, and also to other entities where it was felt there was potential for developing the work. This first publication of the journal included a separate introductory letter from Howland.[52]

The membership of the original committee, tasked with determining the feasibility of a journal, became the editorial committee of CJOT, with Dr Heaton as the journal's first editor. Dr Howland wrote a three-part editorial for the first issue, beginning with a dramatic statement: "Occupational therapy, in the broad sense of the term, has become the most serious problem before the statesmen of every nation in the world at the present time."[53] It was 1933, and Howland was referring to the problem of unemployment with its economic, social, and emotional consequences. He drew a parallel for people who were sick, blind, paralyzed, or mentally infirm and whose lack of employment had negative consequences not only for themselves but for all of society. Occupational therapy, he argued, could keep the mind occupied and help restore "maimed limbs and minds to health."[54]

In the second section of his editorial, Howland discussed the need for advocacy by members of the occupational therapy community; they needed to explain the profession to physicians, to members of boards of hospitals, and to the public. To that end, he requested articles "from the pens of men and women through Canada who will tell of their experience with occupational therapy in the widest and most varied fields."[55]

Howland concluded his editorial with three news items. He described the work to be started at the Astley Ainslie Institution in Scotland by Amy DesBrisay, noted that every general hospital interested in providing occupational therapy must have a workshop, and advised that the CAOT required a field secretary if the work was to move forward.

Heaton stayed on as editor of the journal until 1936 and was followed by Dr Ruth Franks, who held the position for ten years. In an early editorial, Franks challenged occupational therapists to provide monetary support for the journal and for their work, pointing out that if women's philanthropic groups could raise funds for occupational therapy, then occupational therapists should be able to do so themselves.[56] Economic problems threatened the existence of CJOT in 1937, but the journal found a temporary solution in partnering with physical therapy for two of its four annual issues. In 1939, the journal published on its own again.

Up to this point, the professionalization of occupational therapy was following the path described by Freidson in his exploration of how professions come to be: the practice had preceded the profession – that is, the workers "did" occupational therapy and then decided to organize it and educate for it. The educational program was needed not only to produce future therapists, but also to allow its "graduates" to claim "a prolonged specialized training in a body of abstract knowledge," one of two components that constituted the classical definition of the "core characteristics" of a profession. Occupational therapy already possessed the second component, which was "a collectivity or service orientation."[57]

Prior to World War I, when nursing and medicine were the only health professions for which there was formal training, the steps taken toward the professionalization of occupational therapy were impressive indeed.

12

Establishing an Educational Program

Behind all other tools and media of treatment, is the basic tool, the occupational therapist.
Helen Primrose LeVesconte, 1948[1]

When Doris Stupart, the first president of the Ontario Society for Occupational Therapy (OSOT), reported on the work of the association in 1921, she noted that to be viable the profession would need to establish a permanent course of training, preferably within a university.[2] This need had also been identified by the Manitoba group and was likely recognized by occupational therapists practising across the country. If more therapists were not trained, the fledgling profession would disappear; if new therapists were not trained at a university level, standards would be difficult to uphold.

With the establishment of the occupational therapy course at the University of Toronto in 1926, the profession became viable in Canada. Although there were times when the program's future was uncertain and its structure was to take on different forms, it was this educational program that facilitated the growth and development of the profession.

A DIPLOMA COURSE IN OCCUPATIONAL THERAPY AT THE UNIVERSITY OF TORONTO

By the early 1920s, soldiers with chronic conditions were still in care and new areas of work were still opening up. Physicians across the country had become accustomed to having occupational therapists in their medical wards, their psychiatric hospitals, and their TB sanatoriums. The Workmen's Compensation Board had seen the value of referring its cases to curative workshops, as did various other social services. But with no new therapists being trained, many marrying and leaving the workforce, and others moving to the United States to work, the numbers of practising therapists were rapidly falling.

Although there is no documentation of OSOT's plan for garnering support to launch a permanent training course, several steps appear to have been taken. OSOT first prepared the way by building awareness of the work within the university and among the general public. Primrose wrote about OSOT's activities regularly in the *University of Toronto Monthly*. In 1922, OSOT arranged for the University of Toronto to host a series of ten open lectures on occupational therapy. The story in the *Varsity*, the U of T student newspaper, noted that although the lectures were "designed to appeal to one engaged in Occupational Therapy, they will be open to the public."[3]

There was also publicity for the profession in the popular press. *MacLean's*, for example, ran a story in 1922 entitled "God Bless the 'Girls in Green'! Story of a New Vocation for Women – Occupational Therapy – in Which Dominion of Canada Leads the World."[4] Activities organized to raise funds for patients in hospitals and curative workshops were also written up in the press and attracted the public's attention.

In 1924, OSOT brought forward its first proposal for an educational program.[5] However, there was presumably more work to be done, and in 1925, the society presented a revised proposal to W.J. Dunlop, the director of extension at the University of Toronto, for his consideration. The university had created the extension department in 1920 to provide lectures to the community in an effort to share knowledge outside the "ivory tower." The department also served as a temporary holding operation for courses – like occupational therapy – whose future was uncertain.[6] On 8 January 1926, the Committee of Extension, headed by Dunlop, submitted a report to the university senate stating that the Ontario Society for Occupational Therapy was requesting a permanent two-year course under the direction of the university. The committee noted that occupational therapy was considered a "necessity in Government institutions, asylums, Homes for Incurables and general hospitals." It further noted that "the Workmen's Compensation Board of Ontario has asked for the assistance of the Society in dealing with a stipulated number of patients every month. This is an indication of the need for training now asked for."[7] OSOT had clearly done its homework and had been ready with evidence of the need for the program.

Having the report from Dunlop accepted had been but a step in the process, and OSOT soon realized that gaining full approval for a new course for women at the University of Toronto would not be easy. At a time when female students were still few in number, when women had only just achieved the right to vote and were only tolerated in the work world, OSOT would require help to make their voices heard. The society turned to the group of prominent and influential men who were acting as its advisory council.[8] Dr Goldwin Howland, the honorary secretary treasurer of OSOT, asked Dr Primrose, then the dean of the Faculty of Medicine and also the chairman of OSOT's board of management, to present the proposal to the Senate and to Sir Robert Falconer, the president of the university. Falconer, it should be noted, was the honorary vice-president of OSOT. In this way, the matter was quickly and satisfactorily dealt with![9]

The program for the two-year diploma course was advertised in the University of Toronto commencement booklet for June 1926. The entrance requirement to the university was junior matriculation (normally achieved by age sixteen or seventeen), as it was for any Canadian university at the time. However, applicants to occupational therapy were to be at least eighteen years of age, which indicated that they should have some additional education or experience. The course was described as a "new course for young ladies who are anxious to be of service in the healing of the sick and maimed and convalescent."[10]

The first class opened with twenty-five students. The course was popular for many of the same reasons that had made it appealing to the ward aides: it drew on what were perceived as women's caring instincts as well as their ability to nurture and teach. It also tapped into their artistic abilities and creativity. The course still tended to attract women from upper middle-class families, often with previous post-secondary education – women who did not want to be nurses or teachers or social workers and were intrigued by this new profession.

The occupational therapy course was a new option for women who wanted a university education. While the attendance of women at university was no longer considered "unnecessary" as in earlier eras, many of the traditional notions about "a woman's place" were far from settled. There had been some thought that education might help women to be better mothers, but there was also an ongoing concern that a university education might hinder women from fulfilling that role, as it would drain them of needed energy.[11]

THE CURRICULUM

To prepare for the Canadian program, OSOT studied the best curricula in the United States and adapted them for Toronto. The courses offered in Year 1 were English, French, psychology, hygiene, physiology, anatomy, physical drill, sociology, art, and applied arts. There was also training in a number of crafts, including woodworking, weaving, basketry, needlework, and leatherwork. In Year 2, psychology, sociology, French, and English classes continued. New courses were kinesthetics and remedial exercises. The craft courses included art, metalwork, bookbinding, modelling, and cord work.

That first program was led in an unusual manner. Florence Wright, a graduate of the Ontario College of Art in 1906 and of the ward aides course in 1918, was considered the supervisor of the program, but she was also enrolled as a student in the program she was leading and in 1928 received her diploma along with the other students.[12]

The liberal arts courses included in the curriculum would have supported the overall purpose of the program, but some courses, like English and French, would have been added to provide an education comparable to other undergraduate programs at the university. Concerned about the need for liberal arts courses in professional curricula at the university, President Falconer noted that "even in the utilitarian environment of the professional schools this idealism was possible, for the student could both attain 'a wide and liberal knowledge of the subject' and acquire the sense of a 'vocation for service.'"[13] As the numbers in professional faculties were becoming equal to those in liberal arts, there was concern for keeping a focus on the humanities.[14]

In an effort to ward off potential criticism that the new program was marshalling more federal resources for Ontario, and for Toronto in particular, than appropriate, the first letter to the Senate requesting the program noted that the course was to be "the headquarters for the Dominion of Canada, so that pupils will not be of Provincial origin alone, but will come from all parts of the Dominion."[15] Indeed, this intention came to be realized out of necessity: as the only program in occupational therapy in Canada until 1950, the U of T program drew students from across the country. Nonetheless, the majority of students came from Ontario, where the financial expenses and emotional concerns about sending a daughter off to university could be more easily borne. The U of T program became instrumental in defining the profession in Canada as graduates returned to their home provinces, spreading the U of T vision of occupational therapy through their practice. In addition, when new educational programs developed, they drew on U of T graduates for faculty, who then influenced the direction of education in those settings. New programs opened across the country, beginning with McGill University in 1950 and following, in 1954, with the Université de Montréal, which offered the first French-speaking occupational therapy program in the world.[16]

Clinical work in hospitals and asylums took place periodically during the year and as block sessions during the two summer months. Students' clinical work required supervision by qualified occupational therapists, and as a result, most fieldwork placements were in provincial asylums, which were the main employer of occupational therapists at the time. The desirability of having occupational therapists in the asylums and the shortage of them was such that asylums appointed some occupational therapy students as "summer staff" to help meet the demand for service. Internships, as they were called, were also provided by the Canadian National Institute for the Blind, the School for Crippled Children, civilian hospitals, curative workshops, and TB sanatoriums.

Despite the fanfare that had accompanied the launching of the program and the many stories about it in both the popular press and the university press, there was an air of uncertainty about the continuation of the program from the start. At the first graduation in 1928, W.J. Dunlop, the director of extension and the person responsible for administering the program, sounded the first alarm: "[W]hether or not the demand for a course will continue, the authorities cannot tell at the present, so the classes are under the Extension Department until they can be thoroughly proved and incorporated in the university proper."[17]

Like the ward aides before them, graduates of this new program also worked for a few years, married, and then left the profession, rarely to return. In 1933, the lieutenant-governor of Ontario, H.A. Bruce (who was also a surgeon and a supporter of occupational therapy), reflected on the war years and the fate of the ward aides: "I found that one of the greatest difficulties was that matrimony thinned the ranks of the aides at an appalling rate – and still does!" Bruce went on to say, "Might I suggest to young ladies who seek an opportunity of practicing the home-making arts, that occupational therapy seems to offer a splendid opportunity to achieve this ambition."[18] Bruce's comment was no doubt met with laughter and also some discomfort.

The University of Toronto program developed and maintained a close connection with educational programs in the United States, and through the program, the university joined an elite North American group of schools in 1935. The American Medical Association (AMA), which was the accrediting body for occupational therapy programs at the time, recognized just five schools in all of North America: the schools were in Boston, St Louis, Philadelphia, Milwaukee, and Toronto.[19] In its review of the program at the University of Toronto, the AMA noted that it had the best of lecturers in anatomy, physiology, medicine, and surgery while also keeping its focus on "the arts and crafts required and the therapeutic side."[20] The AMA, somewhat erroneously, took this finding as evidence that the occupational therapy program was an integral part of the university.

Though the profession in Ontario did not set out to work within social services as did the group in Manitoba, meeting social needs was a key focus in the early curriculum and influenced recruitment strategies. In a paper written for the journal *Social Welfare* in 1928, Dunlop referred to the course as "a pleasant and a profitable phase of Social Service."[21] Indeed, courses in social services were included in the curriculum during the first few decades of the program. Occupational therapy students wrote exams in casework methods, social casework, social welfare, and social legislation.[22] It is not surprising that this emphasis on social services existed, given the university's concern for the social problems in its geographical area and its determination to actively support social reform. In fact, occupational therapy students were expected to do volunteer work, and many recorded in their yearbook entries that they had been volunteers at the University Settlement House.[23] The relationship between occupational therapy and social services programs at the University of Toronto was somewhat reciprocal; for example, a special mental hygiene program in social work included three hours per week in occupational therapy.[24] The focus on social welfare disappeared over the years with the growing dominance of the medical model and the perceived need for more medically oriented subjects.

In 1929, when the University of Toronto launched a course in physical therapy, the student newspaper commented: "Basket-making was instituted as a course a few years ago. This year sees the opening of a course to train expert masseurs. Whether or not a tonsorial course will be started next, we do not know." The story was picked up by the *Mail and Empire*, which asked if the university was becoming a trade school. They interviewed Dunlop, who pointed out that the physical therapy program was "in no sense ... a trade course" and that the logical conclusion to the criticism was "that the university should give nothing but arts courses." In the same article, the university president, Sir Robert Falconer, commented that physical therapy "was established at the instance of outstanding physicians and surgeons." Dean Primrose weighed in on the discussion and pointed out that "basket-making and the course in massage were a very minor part of the curriculum and both were practical." Florence Wright, the director of the occupational therapy program, was reported to have thought the criticism not worth noticing.[25]

The sense of impermanence around the program, sometimes unfounded and sometimes real, continued. This must have given an ongoing sense of not belonging to both students and faculty. In 1930, a story in the *Varsity* speculated that the course was to be abandoned, but when asked about it, Dunlop denied the rumour: "[T]his same rumour seems to be spread abroad every year. I am anxious to know where it originates."[26] Five months later, a story in the *Toronto Evening Telegram* reported that there had been discussions at an OSOT meeting about there being too many graduates for the vacancies in Toronto, while openings in Alberta could not be filled. In discussing solutions to the problem, Dunlop (adding grist to the rumour mill) said that if something were not done to develop the work, the course would have to be dropped. Primrose responded that Dunlop was too pessimistic, and another OSOT member suggested that it was up to the doctors to demand more aides in hospitals.[27] While differences in geographic demands were of concern, they were not as serious as problems brought by the Depression of the 1930s, which necessitated halting admissions to the program in 1932 and 1933 when jobs of all types disappeared.

In 1946, when the program in occupational therapy was lengthened to three years, concerns about it being a "technical course" reappeared on the campus. The *University of Toronto Monthly* noted that "while the curriculum provides specific training for a profession, it is of broad educational value to the student."[28] With the lengthening of the program came the return – in both the first and second year – of courses in English that had been included in the original diploma course and later discarded. The heaviness of the course load in occupational therapy had been apparent for many years. It was likely due to early concerns about meeting the needs of both a professional training program and what was then considered a *bona fide* university education.[29]

From its inception in 1926 until 1949, the program was overseen by Dunlop, a supportive but apparently paternalistic and somewhat possessive man who, according to those who worked with him, exercised considerable control.[30] With the place of female academics still questioned and the occupational therapy program considered less than permanent, the voices of the very small number of faculty members remained soft if not mute. It was as if they feared that saying the wrong thing might see them turned out altogether.

When plans were being made to combine occupational therapy and physical therapy in one course in 1949, it was understood that the planning committee's task was to work out the details of the new program rather than to consider its appropriateness.[31] There was little to no consultation prior to the decision by the Faculty of Medicine to combine the programs and take them in. Occupational therapy was not alone in finding itself not consulted before a major change; other helping professions with a preponderance of women – like nursing and social work – also lacked direct access to sources of power. Thus, there was an ongoing sense that participation by the members of these disciplines was not valued by the rest of the academic community.[32]

HELEN PRIMROSE LEVESCONTE

The most illustrious graduate of that first course at the University of Toronto was Helen Primrose LeVesconte.[33] Her legacy is seen across a wide spectrum of the discipline's core values and ideals, in clinical practice, and in education programs. LeVesconte promoted the profession enthusiastically and tirelessly, determined that there should be no limits to what could be achieved. LeVesconte was a fearless pioneer. Her career provides a glimpse of the work as it was evolving and yet another story of a woman who chose the profession – and helped shape it – when it was still in its infancy.

LeVesconte came from a privileged background. She attended two elite private girls' schools – Havergal College and the Margaret Eaton School of Expression. Her father was prominent in legal and military circles. Many in her mother's family had attended university, including her aunt, Charlotte Ross, who had been one of the first women to graduate from the University of Toronto. A cousin had founded *MacLean's Magazine*;

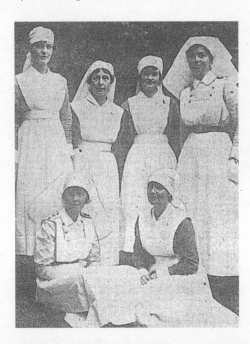

Amelia Earhart as a VAD at the Spadina Military Hospital in Toronto. Next to Earhart (*back left*) are fellow VADs Jenne Lewis and Helen LeVesconte, both of whom went on to graduate from the first diploma course at the University of Toronto in 1928. Photographer/GetStock.com.

Canon Cody, who was president of the university from 1932 to 1945, had confirmed her; she had sat beside the Hollywood actor Raymond Massey in grade school; and many of her male friends had become doctors.[34] Thus, her family and social circle included people of influence and strong role models.

Unlike many of her peer group who married and became involved in philanthropic work, LeVesconte decided to pursue a career. She followed her initial training with employment as a physical education teacher but soon became dissatisfied. She volunteered at the Spadina Military Hospital as a member of the Voluntary Aide Detachment (VAD) during World War I and was greatly impressed by the work of the ward aides.[35] One of her co-workers was Amelia Earhart, and LeVesconte kept up a friendship with her for some time.[36] By 1926, she had decided to enter the newly established course in occupational therapy. She enjoyed the program and years later marvelled at the calibre of teaching that had been provided, saying that she felt privileged to have been at the university.[37]

LeVesconte never married and was thus protected from the most common cause of attrition in the profession. After graduating in 1928 (at age thirty-two), she was appointed to a series of positions, seemingly without her involvement in the process. Her leadership skills soon became

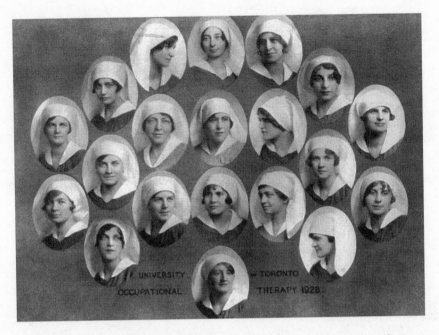

First graduates of the diploma program at the University of Toronto, 1928.
Helen LeVesconte is at bottom right. Courtesy Department of Occupational
Science and Occupational Therapy, University of Toronto.

evident, and by 1933, she was simultaneously holding the positions of
part-time director of the U of T program, consultant for the Ontario Department of Health, and director of occupational therapy at the Toronto
Psychiatric Hospital. In 1945, she became the full-time director of the
program at the University of Toronto, where she remained until her retirement in 1967.[38]

LeVesconte's clinical work was primarily in the area of psychiatry and
her interest in mental health was sustained over the length of her career.
She particularly enjoyed her work at the Toronto Psychiatric Hospital
and her relationship with Dr C.B. Farrar, who was already a strong supporter of occupational therapy when she first came to work for him. In
1925, Farrar addressed an open meeting of the Ontario Society for Occupational Therapy and was quoted in the *Evening Telegram*: "Next to
proper housing and proper feeding, occupational therapy is the most important factor in the cure of nervous patients. The rest cure, so long ordered for these patients, has been supplanted by work, and occupational
therapy provides this most necessary employment and effects the cure."[39]

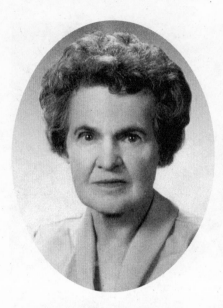

Helen LeVesconte, c. 1960.
LeVesconte directed the program
at the University of Toronto
from 1933 to 1967. Courtesy
Department of Occupational
Science and Occupational
Therapy, University of Toronto.

LeVesconte's philosophy of occupational therapy was developed through her clinical practice, her interactions with occupational therapists in other countries, and her work as an educator. It permeated the educational program that she ran and, through its graduates, the whole of the profession through the first half of the twentieth century. Her philosophy, which is clear from her writings, was particularly powerful in regard to the relationship between therapist and patient. LeVesconte was adamant that it was the therapist's job to see to it that the patient was engaged in the treatment process. For her, there would be no "unmotivated" patients, save when the occupational therapist failed to do her job. She saw the relationship as one in which the therapist initially held power and only gradually relinquished it. In her book *Guideposts of Occupational Therapy*, she writes, "So the wise therapist will first control and direct the patient. Then like the pilot and his trainee, both must share the controls. Only when the controls are taken over by the patient himself is he exerting his maximum capacities to achieve his maximum success."[40]

While she did not use the term "meaningful activities," LeVesconte noted that activities had to be related to the patient's sense of values if they were to spark interest and engage him or her over a sustained period.[41] All interventions were to be directed toward the triad of physical, psychological, and vocational function, with no arbitrary boundaries. She was "not in accord with those who believe that we can set boundaries to the field of occupational therapy, or who maintain that vocational training is not occupational therapy – for many it is the best therapy, because it means continued satisfactory adjustment to community life."[42]

Given her lack of formal research training, LeVesconte made an admirable effort to provide evidence for practice. She was involved in several studies, most notably one for which she was responsible for documenting treatment outcomes for epilepsy.[43] Writing in 1935 of the need to extend the length of the educational program to four years, she noted that additional time would allow for more emphasis on research methods.[44]

Mindful of the need to better portray the profession and help others understand its aims and methods, LeVesconte advocated for improved language skills in therapists' oral and written communications. She herself published a number of articles, which was unusual for occupational therapists at the time. She wrote well, demonstrating her own broad knowledge base as well as the research she had done prior to writing.[45] LeVesconte worked on a history of occupational therapy in Canada at a time when there was very little written history of the profession anywhere in the world.[46]

Over the course of LeVesconte's academic career, she taught some 1,850 students and inspired a number of them to follow her footsteps into academia. Among these graduates were two who went on to make significant contributions to the U of T program. Isobel Robinson graduated in 1939 and joined the faculty in 1943, taking over from LeVesconte as director in 1967. Thelma Cardwell graduated in 1942 and joined the faculty after serving overseas in World War II. LeVesconte, Robinson, and Cardwell all played major roles in the various professional associations – OSOT, CAOT, and the World Federation of Occupational Therapists.

LeVesconte's ideas continue to influence the occupational therapists of today, and she is fondly remembered by those who knew her. Being at the helm for so many of the early years of the profession, LeVesconte had an opportunity to make some of her own dreams come true, although not always at the time or in the manner she had planned.[47]

13

The Men in Front of the Women

We are too diffident a group, both individually and collectively. We are much
too timid in bringing our work to the attention of others. In short, we are ineffective
in selling our profession. It is time we learned to be vocal, to be enthusiastic,
to be competent, in representing the professional point of view of our discipline
and in interpreting our aims and functions.

Thelma Cardwell, 1966[1]

MALE LEADERSHIP AT THE START OF THE PROFESSION

Although occupational therapy has generally been considered a "female
profession," with less than 10 per cent of practitioners being male, men
were very influential in the founding of the profession and very involved
in its running for over forty years. On the one hand, there were men who
held positions that put the women in their employ. For example, Kidner,
as the vocational secretary of the Military Hospitals Commission (MHC)
was nominally in charge of the ward aides nationally; Haultain, as the
vocational officer of Ontario, oversaw the ward aides in his province, as
did the (male) vocational officers for all the other provinces; Burnette
was the head of the ward aides course at the University of Toronto for a
time; and when the diploma course was established there in 1926, W.J.
Dunlop, as the director of the Department of Extension, was in control.[2]
When it came time for the profession to form provincial societies and a
national association, to establish an educational program, and to publish
a scientific journal, the men took on the leadership tasks. The women
continued to do the behind-the-scenes organizing and, of course, the
front-line work.

These relationships were a function of the clear demarcation for
gender roles at the time. While stereotypical and not appropriate, they

are understandable. For the most part, the men in that era were highly educated and experienced, while the women were just becoming educated and employed. Fighting in the war was clearly seen as "men's work," and to the extent that women were involved, they were there to assist. Nurses and the women in the voluntary aide detachments (VADs) helped in hospitals at the front and at home, and women provided "soldier's comforts" in stations overseas. Providing occupations at the soldier's bedside or on the hospital wards in Canada was another way to assist. It was perceived of as caring and nurturing and, at the time, unquestionably a role for women, for whom these characteristics were thought innate. Women were thought capable of practising the art of caring (which came naturally) but not the science (which needed to be learned).

The men who oversaw occupational therapists in the work environment championed their cause, but they, along with other men, also became involved with occupational therapy in a completely voluntary capacity. These men held positions within occupational therapy organizations and lent their names and prestige to the work of occupational therapists, helping them in a variety of ways: bringing forward their requests to the appropriate authorities, writing about the work in academic and popular media, and advocating for their services in medical circles and other public and private forums.

Records show the continuing involvement of these men, who were mainly physicians, for some four decades from the start of the profession. These are the men of interest here. What motivated them to become so involved in this voluntary capacity? Why did the women keep the men, who were not occupational therapists, involved for so long? And what effect did this relationship have on the profession? Profiles of Dr Alexander Primrose, Sir Robert Falconer, Thomas Bessell Kidner, and Dr Goldwin Howland provide an opportunity to consider how the involvement of these men influenced the development of the profession.

DR ALEXANDER PRIMROSE (1861-1944)

Dr Alexander Primrose was particularly instrumental in helping to bring the profession forward at a crucial time. His work with the Ontario Society of Occupational Therapy (OSOT) over a ten-year period was of major importance.

Born in Pictou, Nova Scotia, Primrose received his medical training in Edinburgh before coming to the University of Toronto in 1888. Starting out as an assistant demonstrator in anatomy, he soon became known as an outstanding teacher. He made ambidextrous drawings on the black-board with coloured chalk, used diagrammatic sketches during surgery, and usually illustrated his case notes with careful drawings.[3]

Primrose had first-hand experience with the traumas of World War I. In 1915, then aged fifty-four, he joined the No. 4 (Canadian) General Hospital, moving with it to Salonika, Greece, where he lived in tents and operated under canvas in primitive conditions. While not injured him-self, he was witness to great suffering. Most significantly, he suffered the loss of his only son, Lieutenant Howard Primrose, to the war. At the age of twenty, Howard had gone overseas in June 1915 and served in England until, in May 1916, he joined the Fourth Battalion in France. He was sent to Ypres and within weeks was killed in action by enemy shellfire.[4]

After receiving the news of his son's death, Primrose took compas-sionate leave to be at home with his wife and three daughters. When he returned to the war in 1917, it was to serve as consulting surgeon to the Canadian Forces in England, advising on patient care in hospitals across England. It was during these experiences overseas that he came to see and appreciate the use of occupations with injured soldiers.[5] Primrose was called back home again in 1918 when his wife became ill. She had not stopped mourning for her son, and some relatives thought she was suffering from a broken heart. No doubt her weakened condition contrib-uted to her death in October of 1919, but, in fact, she died as a result of the Spanish flu.

In 1920, Primrose was appointed dean of the Faculty of Medicine at the University of Toronto. It was at that time that he was asked to join the advisory board of the Ontario Society for Occupational Therapy and assume the role of chairman of the board of management. There are no records to indicate why he was asked or, indeed, who actually invited him. However, Primrose had many personal connections with the male relatives of the women who had been ward aides. C. Helen Mowat, for example, a graduate of one of the 1918 ward aides courses, was the niece of Sir Oliver Mowat and his wife's second cousin. In his role as dean of medicine at the University of Toronto, Primrose would have known other academics involved with occupational therapy, such as Professor Hault-ain, whose wife had been a student in the ward aides course and who was involved with osot; and Sir Frederick Stupart, whose daughter Doris had been a founding member of osot. A fervent Presbyterian,[6] Primrose would have wanted to help the university to be of service to the broader community and must have seen osot's cause as worthwhile.

Dr Alexander Primrose, c. 1920,
dean of Faculty of Medicine
and chairman of the Board
of Management of OSOT.
University of Toronto Archives,
Department of Graduate Records,
A 1973-0026/368(86).

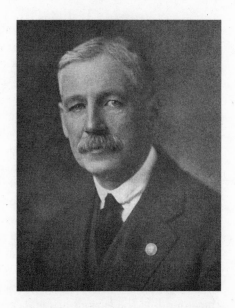

Having worked with many of his Toronto colleagues in the United
Kingdom and during the war in Salonika – for example, with Drs Gaby,
Elliott, Amour, Graham, and Wilson – Primrose was able to call on them
with ease to solicit their involvement.[7] He had the status that OSOT
needed at the time, being well connected medically in Toronto, within
the University of Toronto, and more widely in the United Kingdom and
the United States.[8] Primrose was also something of an entrepreneur and
not afraid of starting something new. In 1929, he joined a consortium of
doctors to finance the construction of the Medical Arts Building, which
provided the first purpose-built office space in Toronto for physicians and
surgeons.[9]

Primrose took on a very active role with OSOT, acting as its public voice
and advocating on its behalf. He drew the attention of the press when he
presided over an open meeting of OSOT at Government House. As written in the *Globe and Mail*, "Enthusiasm, optimism and a sincere faith in a
glorious future for the work marked this meeting – attended by over 250
people, presided over by Dean Primrose who pointed out the great role
occupational therapy played in the healing of both medical and surgical
cases and urging its claim to the attention of generous hearted Toronto."[10]

In addition to assuming a leadership role, Primrose took an interest in
the day-to-day activities of the profession. He was particularly involved

in establishing the curative workshop that served as a form of outpatient clinic as well as a place for sheltered employment, and he helped raise funds for that purpose. He also took an interest in the students and in 1927 wrote to the superintendent of the Christie Street Hospital asking that facility to employ two students over the summer to help them meet their financial obligations.[11]

It is difficult to know what would have motivated Primrose to be so involved with occupational therapy beyond the societal expectation that men of his standing should do their share in the work of social reform. His personality, along with his personal experiences in the war, likely contributed. In the obituary published in the *British Medical Journal*, he was described as "the sort of man to whom colleagues naturally turned for advice."[12] As for his particular interest in occupational therapy as a mechanism for helping, it is significant that Primrose had artistic leanings: he made drawings to illuminate his lectures, and his wartime diary included accomplished sketches and many detailed descriptions of the gardens on the grounds at the various hospitals he visited.

SIR ROBERT FALCONER (1867–1943)

Falconer was the fifth president of the University of Toronto, serving from 1907 to 1932. This was a period of increasing awareness of the need for social reform and of the duty of the educated population to do their part. In his inaugural address, Falconer emphasized the importance of civic service, stating that "the nation should look to the universities for distinct help in the present social conditions," and suggesting that the public must be concerned over the seeming "indifference on the part of the well-to-do to take up the burdens of civic and political life."[13] In keeping with his espoused ideology, Falconer became a founder of the University Settlement House in 1910, showing early in his tenure his sympathy for the plight of poor and immigrant families.

While there is some ambiguity about what he thought of the social gospel movement and its attempts to achieve "the Kingdom of God on Earth," Falconer did speak to the idea that "the Kingdom of God ... is to be realized by the redemption of men as a society of the sons of God."[14] Originally trained as a Presbyterian minister and having taught theology prior to becoming president, he believed in what was then termed "essential Christianity," which meant that he would support efforts to improve, directly, the lives of others.[15] It was, therefore, not surprising that he would have been a staunch supporter of efforts to help injured soldiers return to some form of work during and after World War I. In taking on tasks for the war effort, men like Professor Haultain and others in the University of Toronto community were responding to the challenge put forth by Falconer. Haultain's activities as vocational officer for Ontario and the efforts of the Faculty of Applied Science and Engineering to organize, house, and implement the new ward aides course in 1918 would have been openly supported by Falconer, albeit as only small parts of the myriad other activities the university undertook to aid the war effort.

By 1920, when the Ontario Society for Occupational Therapy was looking for people to support its cause, Falconer would have seemed an obvious, if not perhaps too lofty, choice. Who approached Falconer is not known, but by 1921, he had agreed to serve as the honorary vice-president of OSOT's advisory council. OSOT had recognized the need to establish a permanent course in occupational therapy at the University of Toronto and faced barriers in promoting its cause.[16] What better ally could OSOT hope for than the president of the University of Toronto? Falconer had approved the earlier ward aides course and could be expected to support plans for the new diploma course in 1926. That Falconer could see the value of occupational therapy beyond its wartime use attests not only to his broad interests in helping humanity but also to his philosophy on the nature of a university education. At a time when the place of professional schools in universities was under discussion, Falconer held strong views on how universities should serve society.

Falconer likely saw the new course as one that took a middle path, combining scholarship with practicality and introducing more vocational subjects.[17] A program in occupational therapy would have been appealing because it had the practical outcome of ensuring jobs for its graduates. In turn, the work of graduate occupational therapists had a practical outcome for its recipients – those who had been ill or injured – helping them return to the activities of daily life, including employment. Thus, the program could be said to support what Falconer saw as an ideal combination of "the spiritual and the practical, uniting the moral values of service to the community with the highest technical efficiency."[18] Knowledge *and* a vocation for service were needed from a professional school, and occupational therapy met those criteria.

Support for so-called women's professions had begun with the establishment of the Department of Social Service (i.e., social work) at the University of Toronto in 1914. This was followed by a course in public health nursing in 1920, in occupational therapy in 1926, in library science in 1928, and in physical therapy in 1929. However, these programs

all led to a diploma or, in the case of public health nursing, a certificate. The only women's profession that apparently warranted a degree
was domestic science. Established in 1907, domestic science was perhaps
considered of greater importance because its original goal was to prepare
women for their future roles as wives and mothers and was not seen as
threatening to the status quo.[19]

THOMAS BESSELL KIDNER (1866–1932)

Kidner's involvement in occupational therapy was somewhat unique, as it
encompassed both a paid position (overseeing the work of occupational
therapists) and, at a later time, a voluntary position with the American
Occupational Therapy Association (AOTA).

Kidner was brought to Canada in 1900 to organize and teach manual
training (see chapter 5). He maintained his involvement in this work
with successive moves from Nova Scotia to New Brunswick to Alberta.
He was recognized as an expert in the field when, at the end of 1915, he
was appointed vocational secretary of the Military Hospitals Commission
of Canada.[20] Kidner was responsible for the whole continuum of activities
that aided the injured soldier's return to work, and these included what
was now being called "occupational therapy." With the first hurdle in
recovery being to "restore the spirit,"[21] Kidner had embraced the idea of
bedside and ward occupations. Because of that stance, he was invited
to be a founding member of the (American) National Society for the
Promotion of Occupational Therapy (NSPOT) in 1917. When the initial
meeting was being planned, correspondence between its organizers, William Dunton and George Barton, indicates that Kidner was highly regarded and that having him involved was thought to be "a feather in our
[the organizers'] cap."[22] Barton asked Kidner to chair a subcommittee on
international relations, which made him the connecting link between
the United States, Canada, and Europe.[23] Becoming a founding member
of NSPOT – soon to be known as the American Occupational Therapy
Association – marked Kidner's transition from an employer of occupational therapists (i.e., ward aides) to a volunteer worker who would give
fifteen years of service to the profession.[24]

By 1919, Kidner had emigrated from Canada to live permanently in
the United States. Although the work of re-establishing injured soldiers
was far from finished in Canada, Kidner was ready for a change, and he
had found work in the area of his initial training for architecture with the
National Tuberculosis Association in New York City.[25] Tuberculosis was

a major health concern during the war, and Kidner had already given the area careful thought. He was interested in the use of graded occupations in the recovery of these patients and in architecturally appropriate housing for them that would include workshop space.[26]

Meanwhile, Kidner was becoming more involved with the AOTA. Despite his protestations that the AOTA should have a "medical man" as its president, Kidner served in that capacity for six one-year terms (from 1922 through 1928) plus an additional term as acting president in 1930.[27] While he was not a physician himself, his reverence for medical doctors and medicine in general appears to have influenced him to push the profession in that direction during his tenure in office. He may also have been influenced by the growing power of the medical model and the need to align the profession in order for it to survive.[28]

During the eighteen or so years he spent in Canada, Kidner had changed jobs four times. Each change meant a move to a new province and a new set of people with whom to interact. With his move to New York and his involvement with the AOTA, which had its headquarters there, Kidner seemed to find a permanent home – and something of an extended family. In fact, his own family had begun to disintegrate by this time. Although the move to New York had appeared to give him the opportunity to bring his family together after having been separated from them while he was in Ottawa, it had the opposite effect. In 1927, Mrs Kidner, who had been deeply unhappy in New York, returned to her home in England, taking their daughter and three granddaughters with her.[29] In 1929, Slagle told Dunton of her concern for Kidner's health, writing, "he seemed nervous and over-wrought and it is not to be wondered at with all the stress of mind and heart through which he seems to be passing all the time."[30]

By the time he took office as president in 1922, Kidner had worked with the first four presidents of NSPOT/AOTA (Barton, Dunton, Slagle, and Hall).[31] His relationship with Slagle and Dunton had become close, with the three writing to one another regularly and visiting one another frequently. Slagle was the secretary of the AOTA for all the years that Kidner was president, and the two worked closely together, putting in long hours. They appeared to enjoy one another's company and to have developed a level of trust such that Slagle was named as the executor of Kidner's will.

Kidner was considered friendly and outgoing and often the one to enliven a party with his songs and tales.[32] In 1921, Dr Herbert Hall (who was president of the AOTA from 1920 to 1921) wrote Dunton describing a visit

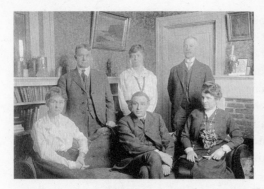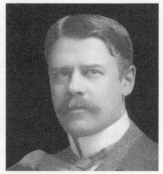

LEFT Founders of the National Society for the Promotion of Occupational Therapy, 1917. Seated (*left to right*): Susan Cox Johnson, George Edward Barton, and Eleanor Clarke Slagle; and standing (*left to right*): William Rush Dunton, Isabel Newton, and Thomas B. Kidner. Courtesy Archive of the American Occupational Therapy Association, Inc.; RIGHT Dr Goldwin Howland, c. 1920. Honorary secretary-treasurer of OSOT, chairman of OSOT's Educational Committee, and president of the Canadian Association of Occupational Therapists from its inception in 1926 until 1948. University of Toronto Archives, Office of the Registrar, A 1965-002/047P(23).

by Kidner and Slagle to his sanatorium, Devereux Mansion: "Mr Kidner, as usual, showing his excellent taste in the picking out of good looking girls [at the sanatorium] for protracted conversation."[33]

During his presidency, Kidner's main concern was to build a strong and accountable profession. He saw the development of standards of training and a registry for therapists as the means of reaching this goal. Once training standards were set, only those with appropriate education and experience would be entered into the registry, thus protecting the public and the profession.[34] Kidner was a strong promoter of the profession, speaking widely on the topic in various venues, including the radio.[35] He was highly respected as president and was described as an excellent presiding officer and parliamentarian.[36]

Kidner's voluntary contributions to occupational therapy stemmed from his role in formulating and overseeing the work during the war. For Kidner, there was a clear link between manual training (in the form of handicrafts) for educating children and manual activities (generally handicrafts) for treating injured soldiers at the bedside: just as manual occupations helped children learn and develop skills, so were they a good starting point in preparing injured soldiers for new jobs.[37] When he advocated for the profession, it was from the deep well of his own beliefs and experience.

In his official role with the AOTA, Kidner could rely on a number of people whose company he enjoyed and who cared about him at a time when his private life was in disarray. His death at age sixty-six brought forth an outpouring of feeling from members of the AOTA.[38] At the organization's annual meeting in Detroit in 1932, the evening session was given over to tributes to Kidner. Notices of his death appeared in various journals and newspapers, including the *New York Times*.[39]

DR GOLDWIN HOWLAND (1875-1950)

How Goldwin Howland first became involved with occupational therapy is not known, but that he was a major force for some thirty years is not questioned. His enthusiasm for the profession could be seen in his description of it "as one of the greatest agents in restoring normal health to countless numbers and making life acceptable to many of those without hope of total recovery."[40] The profession's affection, respect, and gratitude were evident from the obituary notice written by Helen LeVesconte that was published in the *Canadian Journal of Occupational Therapy*. There she commented on his forward thinking, stating, "His footsteps are still ahead of us in the trail he blazed." She went on to describe Howland as "a dynamic personality [who] radiated a drive for action, and an anticipation for the future which will continue to live in the heart and spirit of occupational therapy."[41] If there was a "father of occupational therapy" in Canada, that honour has most often been ascribed to Goldwin Howland. (There is no reference in the literature to a "mother of occupational therapy.")

One of six children, Howland was born in 1875 into a socially and politically prominent Toronto family. His grandfather was a father of Confederation, a successful businessman, and the second lieutenant-governor of Ontario. His father, William Holmes Howland, had also been successful in business and politics but left those fields behind to become an evangelical Anglican and a fervent social reformer. As the mayor of Toronto in 1886–87, he was largely responsible for establishing the reputation of the city as "Toronto the Good." When he died at age forty-nine, there were likely expectations that his son Goldwin, then seventeen and the new head of the household, would continue his father's good works.[42]

Howland graduated from the University of Toronto with a bachelor of medicine in 1900. An entry in the yearbook, *Torontonensis*, noted that "Goldie" was known for his "all round ability and for jovial good-fellowship."[43] He did postgraduate work in neurology in London and Berlin and had a special interest in what was then known as neuropsychiatry. From 1905 until 1948, he was the head of neurology at the Toronto General Hospital, and he was the first consulting neurologist to have that title in Canada.[44]

There is little evidence to suggest that Goldwin Howland's work with the profession was motivated by religious beliefs. His wife, Margaret Carrington, whom he met while studying in England, attended church regularly and volunteered with several charitable organizations; Howland, on the other hand "would appear at Christmas and Easter for church" but otherwise did not seem to be religious.[45] They had three children, but their daughter Doris died at age five in the influenza epidemic. Sometime after her death, they took in a little girl from a poor family living in Basingstoke, England. The child, though never formally adopted, was considered very much a part of the family; she went to private school along with the other Howland children and then became a nurse.[46] Howland's son William was to become the chief justice of Ontario.

Howland's interest in occupational therapy was likely sparked during his medical service in World War I. As a major in the Canadian Army Medical Corps stationed at Base Hospital, Medical District 2 (Toronto), he worked primarily as a neurologist. At the "Out-Door Department" of the Toronto General Hospital, he saw a great many "nervous cases" – that is, ailments with functional, as opposed to organic, causes. He appreciated the need for the occupational work carried out at the bedside by women, who were either trained nurses or with the VAD. In a description of the re-educational work for soldiers being undertaken by the University of Toronto, Howland is mentioned as a driving force as early as 1917.[47]

The first occupational therapy department in a civilian (general) hospital in Canada was established at Howland's hospital – the Toronto General Hospital – in 1919, no doubt at his urging.[48] The occupational therapy department appears to have been the outcome of Howland's work with Amy DesBrisay, a graduate of the 1918 ward aides course at the University of Toronto. It was perhaps through his connection with DesBrisay that he was asked to support the newly formed Ontario Society for Occupational Therapy and serve on its honorary advisory board.

As chairman of OSOT's Educational Committee, Howland worked to establish a two-year diploma course to be housed permanently at U of T. He was also instrumental in the creation of the Dominion [Canadian]

Association of Occupational Therapy (CAOT) in 1926. He became its first and longest-serving president, stepping down only in 1948.

Howland was a great advocate for occupational therapy, extolling its virtues in lectures and in print to the general public and to others in the health professions. He was described as "the most keen and enthusiastic fighter of all those who have worked so hard to bring this splendid curative work [occupational therapy] to its present position in hospitals, institutions and private homes in Canada."[49] Recognizing the need for occupational therapists to work alongside nurses, he promoted the work within the nursing profession. However, he knew that the real gatekeepers for the growth of occupational therapy lay in the medical profession itself. Toward that end, he wrote articles and letters and gave speeches to his medical colleagues on the profession's behalf. When the first volume of the *Canadian Journal of Occupational Therapy* was published in 1933, Howland saw to it that physicians across the country received a copy as well as a letter introducing the work.[50]

Concerned about equal access to health care, Howland thought occupational therapy should be available to everyone, regardless of means. He worked with practising therapists and philanthropic groups (and with Dr Primrose) to develop a bursary system for people who needed therapy but could not afford the service. Indeed, he saw occupational therapy as "a marvelous field for helping those less fortunate citizens who have fallen aside in life's current."[51]

Looking back, it is easy to see Howland's role in the development of occupational therapy as patriarchal. While he would have been working with an executive committee, there is little indication of collaborative planning and he seems to have taken it on himself to stake out the parameters of the profession. He may have done so out of concern for the brevity of service of most women in the profession, with so many leaving after a short time. In an address given during or just after World War II, he commented (as had Dr Bruce two decades earlier) on the success of occupational therapists in a way that would have brought a mixed reaction even then. He noted the excellent work of forty-one occupational therapists in uniform, stating, "So far, our girls have been very successful – nine of them are married already!"[52]

Like other supporters of occupational therapy, Howland appears to have enjoyed using his hands and had a number of hobbies. He was an avid gardener, loved the outdoors, and enjoyed spending time fishing in Algonquin Park.[53]

Howland grew up with an expectation that he, like his father, would devote his life to caring for others. He met this expectation in his work as a neurologist and through his role in occupational therapy. That it was also pleasant to lead a group of intelligent, creative, and committed women over a period of some twenty-eight years may have been a factor as well.

Primrose, Falconer, Kidner, and Howland were four men who helped the profession – in a voluntary capacity – to become established and move forward. Each man provided support in a different way and was likely motivated to be involved for different reasons. Many other men, primarily physicians, also became involved in a voluntary capacity but seemingly to a lesser extent. Drs C.K. Clarke, Edward Ryan, Herbert Bruce, Jabez Elliott, R.E. Gaby, Robert Armour, and C.B. Farrar were all strong supporters of the profession. The names of other prominent physicians, such as Wilder Penfield and Clarence Hincks, were found on the mastheads of the journal for some time. Much more is to be learned of the nature of the relationship between these men and the occupational therapists. Did the men, for example, actually lead the women, or did the women knowingly "use" the men to make their voices heard.

It is tempting to suggest that apart from supporting the profession for altruistic and religious motives, many of the men were drawn to it because they appreciated, at some level, the idea of engaging in work with their hands. Primrose liked to draw (and was a surgeon); Howland liked to garden; Kidner was a skilled craftsman; and Haultain, the engineer, liked to build wooden models. Dr C.K. Clarke, another strong friend and supporter of occupational therapy, also enjoyed making things with his hands. When Dr C.B. Farrar visited Clarke just before his death, he found him sitting up in bed, making a hammock. "He was one," Farrar said, "who did things with his hands as well as his head."[54] In the United States, two very strong supporters of occupational therapy, Dr William Dunton and Dr Herbert Hall, also liked to do things with their hands. Dunton was well known as an expert quilter,[55] while Hall enjoyed a myriad of crafts, including pottery and toy making. In a letter to Dunton in 1922, Hall rather humorously writes, "[M]y recreation at present consists in painting toys ... just completed a fleet of tugs, and steam colliers in unnaturally brilliant colors. I can paint a steam collier in fifteen minutes. This craft is about nine inches long and is intended for bath tub navigation."[56]

USING THE MEN

Writing in 1869, the philosopher John Stuart Mill said that "all women are brought up from the very earliest years in the belief that their ideal of character is the very opposite to that of men; not self-will, and government by self-control, but submission, and yielding to the control of others."[57] This mindset remained apparent decades later when the profession was becoming established. Gender inequality looked, in Jean Baker Miller's terms, "permanent" (i.e., rooted in fundamental immutable differences).[58] In the event, it turned out to be a "temporary inequality," more like the relationship between parent and child, where there is an assumption that the so-called lesser partner will be taught and will, over time, become equal.

The sociologists Maxwell and Maxwell have studied the professionalization of occupational therapy and the role played by what they term its "sponsors" – that is, the men of the social, economic, and medical elite who helped to move the profession forward.[59] While they attribute the rapid establishment of the training school to this sponsorship, they do not delve into the negative implications of the relationship beyond noting that when the sponsorship ended in the 1960s, the profession was forced to attend more closely to its public image and identity. In the introduction to their work, they stress the difficulties with identity experienced by occupational therapists without explicitly linking the two issues.

It is doubtful that the doctors on OSOT's advisory board thought that their patriarchal relationship with the profession was temporary, and it is not surprising that therapists had difficulty deciding whether, as the so-called lesser party in the relationship, they had as much intrinsic worth as the one deemed superior. Furthermore, if the women had been, in the words of the renowned Professor Higgins, "more like a man," the men may not have tolerated it, since this would have eroded what they saw as their role: to enact their moral duty and their belief in their own ability to effect change over a wide domain.[60]

The early relationship between occupational therapists and the men who volunteered their help appears, at first glance, to have been somewhat benign and clearly helpful. However, as time went on and the medical model became more prominent within occupational therapy, the relationship appears to have grown even more paternalistic. Over time, the actions of these men, though helpful, appear to have contributed to the women's diffidence and, with women being the overwhelmingly represented gender in the profession, to the diffidence of the profession. Despite the value of the help they gave, the men perhaps unwittingly entrenched the profession in the position of helpmate, of auxiliary personnel, of adjunct. In 1966, in her inaugural and oft-quoted address as the first occupational therapist and female president of CAOT, Thelma Cardwell gave voice to this concern: "We are too diffident a group, both individually and collectively. We are much too timid in bringing our work to the attention of others. In short, we are ineffective in selling our profession. It is time we learned to be vocal, to be enthusiastic, to be competent, in representing the professional point of view of our discipline and in interpreting our aims and functions."[61]

Cardwell knew, of course, whereof she spoke: she had been the vice-president of CAOT during Dr Norrie Swanson's tenure as president from 1960 to 1966. Swanson had been the third male physician to have taken the role, succeeding Dr Hoyle Campbell, who had served from 1948 to 1960 after Howland's twenty-two-year term. Swanson had apparently urged Cardwell many times to stand for president but she had refused. Eventually, it is said, he resigned in a conscious effort to force her, as his vice-president, to take over.[62]

Given the times, it is likely that the male (and medical) backing of the profession led to a more rapid development than would have occurred if occupational therapy had been led solely by women. The doctors may have been paternalistic, but they worked hard to showcase occupational therapy skills, spoke out in public circles, stayed loyal, and attended meetings regularly. In addition, the doctors were said to have been "nice guys," and the occupational therapists were happy to have them around.

The occupational therapists' reaction to the pervasive influence of men and, in particular, male physicians was, eventually, to resist. Gradually, male – and physician – influence decreased. As "second wave" feminists, occupational therapists in later generations (from 1960 onward) decided that they should go it alone. Physicians were not needed for the curriculum, nor did they need to be asked for support. Occupational therapy seemed determined to steer its own course without any help from friends in high places.

14

Conceptual Conflicts

I have an uncomfortable feeling that we have run away from the hard work in the field of mental diseases to holiday in the by-paths of orthopedics and social service. These things are undoubtedly laudable but I have a suspicion that they are also easy.

Norman Burnette[1]

Between 1890 and 1930, many changes had occurred in Canada in terms of its size, population, and economy. While the country had suffered major losses in the Great War, some would say it had also gained an identity. Having entered the war as a colony of Great Britain, Canada emerged with great pride in its soldiers and a new sense of independence.

By 1930, Canada included nine provinces and two territories, stretching from sea to sea to sea. The population of just over ten million had been growing rapidly in most parts of the country but showed some decline in Prince Edward Island and Nova Scotia. Fifty-four percent of Canada's inhabitants were now living in urban areas, marking a major shift from the primarily agrarian society found at the beginning of the century. The majority of the population was still British (52 per cent), followed by French (28 per cent). Other European immigrants were gradually growing in number, while what was considered the Native and Inuit population comprised 1 per cent.[2]

Religious groups, led by Roman Catholics (who comprised 40 per cent of the population), as well as the many philanthropic organizations (such as the "Y," the Imperial Order of the Daughters of the Empire [IODE], the Red Cross, and the various settlement houses) continued to play the primary role in meeting the needs of poor and immigrant populations and caring for those who were ill or disabled. Recognizing the socialist strand in Canadian politics, a number of left-leaning individuals founded the Co-operative Commonwealth Federation (CCF) Party in 1932. Built on the foundations of the social gospel and led by J.S. Woodsworth, formerly a Methodist minister, the CCF promoted the idea that government should play a major role in providing for those in need. However, social welfare schemes would not be in place for many years to come.

While social and political changes in Canada affected the context in which the profession of occupational therapy grew, the most profound change would come from within the ranks of the women themselves. First-wave feminism, roughly defined as the period from the mid-nineteenth century through to the early twentieth century, saw women emerge from their sheltered, somewhat narrow, and predetermined lives into a world of far greater opportunity. Their own struggles as women had been bound up with their pursuit of social reform – for the right to vote, for better labour laws, for the protection of women and children, for temperance, for public health measures, and for greater educational opportunities. Fortified with their newly developed leadership skills and highly commended for their work during the war, women were developing a new identity. Although there were many battles yet to come, women had reached a new place by 1930.

Occupational therapy offered women a new profession in which to move forward; however, the direction in which the profession was to move was by no means clear. While the philosophical foundations of occupational therapy in Canada were apparent by the beginning of the twentieth century, they had not been transformed into a cohesive base. The movements that contributed to the foundations of the profession each strove to help society in a different way: the mental hygiene movement to help patients through their mental illness and make their lives – and the lives of those who cared for them – more tolerable; the settlement house movement to build healthy communities and to help immigrants and the poor gain jobs and skills; the arts and crafts movement to restore the soul after its battering by the Industrial Revolution and the new fast pace of life; and educational reform to show a better way of learning through manual arts. Each movement lent purpose and methods to the developing discipline, but as work in these areas unfolded, their seemingly disparate approaches meant that occupational therapy might take any one of several directions as it moved to create a place for itself.

With limited opportunities for communication before 1930 beyond letters, telegrams, or visits that involved lengthy travel, and with the organizational structures for the profession barely in place, there had been little hope of opening a dialogue among members and building a unifying approach. Indeed, the Canadian Association of Occupational Therapy (CAOT), having formed just four years earlier, was about to hold its first annual conference in 1930, and the first issue of the *Canadian Journal of Occupational Therapy* was yet to be published.

From a practical perspective it was unclear whether the profession should work from within other disciplines as a subspecialty or continue to create an entity of its own. There were strong reasons to align occupational therapy with nursing or public health or with social work. Similarly, the teaching skills that marked the methods of early craft and settlement house workers suggested an alignment with teaching and education, and the creative aspects of the work provided an option for involvement with the world of art. In the aftermath of World War I, there were compelling reasons to align occupational therapy with vocational training, and by the 1930s, occupational therapists working with civilians with physical illness and disability could see an affinity with physical therapy and rehabilitation.

TEACHING AND THE ARTS

Both teaching and the arts were compatible with occupational therapy. In the early years of the profession, most occupational therapists saw themselves as teachers. Indeed, many had gained formal teacher qualifications prior to becoming occupational therapists. Their knowledge of educational philosophies and methods made them expert teachers of handicrafts, particularly when they also had experience in the techniques of manual training. Their role was to instruct – albeit with knowledge of the patient and his or her capabilities in mind – and to stimulate interest. Hilda Goodman and Cybel Lighthall (see chapter 8) were among those who entered the profession with prior qualifications as teachers. Susan Johnson, one of the founders of the National Society for the Promotion of Occupational Therapy (NSPOT) in the United States, made a strong plea for taking the profession forward within the discipline of education.[3] The links with education can be seen today, where instruction in the activities of daily living for people with disabilities is a major area of practice. Work with special-needs children occurs within the school setting and is aimed at enhancing the ability to learn, and assessment and ongoing evaluation are major components of all interventions. Because of these links, many occupational therapists do their graduate work in the field of special education.

Artistic ability characterized many early occupational therapists. Many had been trained at well-known art schools such as the one at Mount Allison University or the Ontario College of Art and Design, as well as the Pratt Institute in the United States. In addition to their art school training, some had specialized in craftwork (e.g., Jessie Luther, Alice Peck, and "Miss Scott"; see chapter 6). These women were interested in using activities that would stimulate creativity and potentially lead to a form of work. Exhibitions that showed the artistic merit of work produced by patients helped bring attention to the profession, but the profession's link with the art world remained tenuous as the years went by. Had it been maintained, occupational therapists would not have given up their potential role in art therapy, and they might have been more comfortable using other creative arts in treatment, such as music therapy and psychodrama.

NURSING

The early work of occupational therapists in asylums was clearly aligned with nursing. The purpose of occupational therapy was, primarily, to help institutions manage patients' behaviour and, secondarily, to provide a means of relieving the tedium of lengthy stays. Some institutions employed craftworkers as instructors, but in many instances the work was carried out by nursing staff and attendants. Susan Tracy, an American nurse, is often credited with having started occupational therapy in 1906 when she gave a course at the Adams Nervine Hospital near Boston. Her book, *Invalid Occupations*, published in 1910, was meant to be a resource for nurses and attendants, providing instructions and the rationale for various activities. A course on occupations for asylum attendants was offered by the Chicago School of Civics and Philanthropy in 1908, and the book *Occupation Therapy: A Manual for Nurses*, by the psychiatrist W.R. Dunton, was another indication that nurses were expected to use occupations with their patients.

In Canada, almost two decades later, the work of the occupational therapist and the nurse remained intertwined. In an address to the class taking the graduate nurse extension course at the University of Toronto in 1926, Howland, who was by then the president of the newly formed Canadian Association of Occupational Therapy, referred to occupational therapy as one of three branches of nursing, the other two being public health nursing and social service nursing. He felt strongly that nurses should be the ones to "re-awaken interest in patients" and that training for all nurses should include classes in occupational therapy. He may have exasperated his audience, however, when he went on to say that he considered such classes to be of more value to nurses than a lot of "the highly scientific subjects."[4]

In explaining why he thought nursing was the best preparation for occupational therapy, Howland described the problems with the other options, saying that an art school graduate would be too concerned with art and a university graduate would not be not practical enough. The best aides, he observed, were those "who do not know too much to start with along any line, but together with the artistic sense, have the altruistic desire, to help others, which you will claim is a compendium of the basis of a nurse and the basis of an artist combined."[5]

While there was a strong working relationship between nursing and occupational therapy, it may not have been very congenial. Cybel Lighthall's lectures to students in the ward aides course at McGill University in Montreal in 1919, for example, placed nurses at the top of the administrative hierarchy within hospitals and warned students to ignore nursing procedures at their peril.[6] This idea that nursing skills were paramount was evident in psychiatric institutions in 1930, when the director-general of mental hospitals in the Ontario Department of Health insisted that trained occupational therapists could only be employed as paid workers after they had completed at least six months of work in the nursing division.[7] With such an arrangement, physician control over nurses would certainly extend to occupational therapists.[8]

SOCIAL SERVICES

While the relationship between occupational therapy and nursing developed primarily as a procedural matter, the relationship with social work was one born of complementarity. Both professions had strong links with the settlement house movement (see chapter 4) and were interested in building healthy communities. The links between social work and occupational therapy had been apparent from the time of Octavia Hill's work in the mid-1800s through to the settlement house movement at the turn of the twentieth century. The idea of helping poor and immigrant populations manage their daily activities and become productive citizens had informed the developing philosophies of both social work and occupational therapy. In the early 1900s, the Canadian Handicrafts Guild set out to help Native and immigrant groups become self-sustaining through sales of their handiwork, and Jessie Luther brought her settlement house experience to her community development work at the Grenfell Mission in St Anthony, Newfoundland (see chapter 6).

With the two professions sharing the goal of decreasing dependence, the goals for patients receiving services from either program included learning to manage their homes and their various activities of daily living and becoming employed or productive in some manner. Social workers and occupational therapists needed each other – particularly in home-based care, or field service, as it was then known. Both professions understood that many medical problems had wide-ranging individual and family ramifications and could not be considered solved just because the physician had discharged the patient from hospital. LeVesconte noted this broader context of care: "[A] medical problem is equally a social and community problem and it is the point of contact at which the physician, the social worker and the occupational therapist should join forces in constructive and co-operative planning."[9]

Burnette, who had led the ward aides course at the University of Toronto and served as acting vocational officer for Ontario at one point, was keenly aware of these wider ramifications of disability. Looking back at the lessons learned during the war, he commented that there was a new awareness "on the part of society that disability is no longer to be regarded merely as a personal misfortune, but also as an interference with the capacity for useful production, and therefore, as a social loss."[10] In order to increase productivity among those with disability, Burnette suggested that occupational therapists be added to the social service staff of hospitals so that they could not only provide bedside and ward work, but also carry the work into the home through the social service's after care branch.[11] This organizational structure was evident in some quarters in the 1920s; for example, occupational therapy at the Toronto General Hospital was set up within the existing Department of Social Services. On a larger scale, the Social Service Commission of Winnipeg was initially considered as the home of choice for occupational therapy within the province of Manitoba.

Students in occupational therapy often came to the profession from a background in social services, whether in a paid or voluntary capacity. The attraction was such that W.J. Dunlop, the director of the Department of Extension, which housed the occupational therapy program at U of T, chose to recruit applicants from among those interested in social services. Writing in the *Journal of Social Welfare* in 1928, he observed that occupational therapy was "a pleasant and a profitable phase of Social Service" and that it would appeal to women who wished to "render an important public service."[12]

VOCATIONAL REHABILITATION

Occupational therapy before, during, and just after World War I had a strong focus on work. The role Kidner played as vocational secretary of the Military Hospitals Commission and his continuing involvement with occupational therapists exemplified that connection. In the aftermath of the war, work could have become the one outcome around which occupational therapy might have developed as a cohesive entity. Burnette underscored the relationship between vocational rehabilitation and occupational therapy when he commented "that providing occupation to meet the needs of invalids was an offshoot, not of the practice of medicine, but of the vocational training scheme."[13]

The very name of the ward aides' main employer during the war, the Department of Soldiers' Civil Re-establishment, signified an alliance with work, as did the term "occupational therapy" itself. In English, the name makes the profession's connection with work explicit (much to the chagrin of those practitioners who try to explain why occupational therapy is not about work). The French name for the profession, *ergothérapie*; the German name, *Beschäftigungstherapie*; and the Swedish term, *Leg.Arbetsterapeut* (where *Arbet* means work or vocation) are all clear examples of the connection of the discipline to the idea of work.

It was recognized early on that care for the individual patient should include economic well-being and that the occupational therapist's work was not done until the patient was reintegrated into the community and had become productive in some capacity. Whether work came in the form of paid employment, in curative or sheltered workshops, home (or cottage) industries, or a hobby, it was recognized as a desired goal. However, there were still some who could not see the relationship between employment and health and did not see employment as a significant outcome of therapy.[14] For Kidner, the connection was straightforward. Speaking as the president of the American Occupational Therapy Association (AOTA), he said that all medical, nursing, and auxiliary treatments had "but one aim in view; that is, to enable the sick person to go to work again. That is the objective of occupational therapy and that should be its motivation throughout."[15] The war, with its large number of disabled soldiers, brought home the fact that the health of society was also at risk when people did not work.

There were conflicting views on how to incorporate work as treatment. While work in asylums provided an economic advantage to the institution when patients tended the fields, cleaned hallways, or mended clothing, it was incompatible with altruistic ideas about work as treatment. When the usual items produced in occupational therapy workshops happened to be sold, the proceeds would go to the institution ostensibly to cover costs of materials, but when patients became particularly skilled and produced saleable items, the goal of increasing patients' economic independence took over and they were generally allowed to keep any profits that were realized.

The return to work was a multi-stage process. It was accepted that occupational therapists would prepare patients at the early stage; they were clearly needed to build the patients' morale and self-confidence and to help them build or rebuild skills. But it was unclear where the role of the specialist in vocational training began and that of the occupational therapist ended. Occupational therapy appeared to be more concerned with the preparation for work, and vocational rehabilitation with the job itself.

Any potential for occupational therapy aligning with vocational rehabilitation was averted not only by those who were concerned with the profession's seemingly limitless boundaries but also by those concerned with the standing of vocational training in the public eye. Vocational rehabilitation was perceived as separate from health care and lower in status. Despite the fact that occupational therapy might never have advanced had it not been seen as the precursor of vocational rehabilitation during the war, occupational therapists soon turned away from vocational training, favouring instead the medical model.[16]

The professions of teaching, art, nursing, social work, and vocational rehabilitation all provided compelling reasons for occupational therapy to become aligned with them. However, none of the relationships with these disciplines were strong enough to counter the attraction of medicine, a field in which occupational therapy had had no prior involvement in terms of the types of interventions it provided.

PHYSICAL THERAPY AND REHABILITATION

It is curious to consider how occupational therapy came to be aligned with medicine when its beginnings – in the arts and crafts movement, the settlement house movement, and educational reform – made no claims to such a liaison. Even in the role played by occupational therapy in mental health – the place where it had been established over the longest period – the relationship was not within medicine. Not only was psychiatry itself seen as somewhat separate from the rest of medicine at the time, but occupational therapy provided in those settings was never aimed at addressing pathology – notwithstanding the existence of theories suggesting that engagement in specific occupations might indirectly affect pathology. The psychobiological model proposed by Meyer and others early in the twentieth century saw occupational therapy as a means of establishing balance and rhythm in daily life.[17]

Despite the fact that there was nothing medical about the work of early occupational therapists, by the 1930s the profession was becoming ensconced within the medical model. Although occupational therapists benefited from having increased medical knowledge, their greater familiarity with medicine was intended to help them understand their patients and their capabilities, not to enable them to treat their impairments. Like the great Canadian physician and teacher Sir William Osler, they thought it more important to know what sort of patient had a disease than to know what sort of disease a patient had. Thus began what Hooper and Wood have referred to as the "long conversation," where pragmatism (representing the restoration of people to satisfying lives) began to give over to structuralism (with its knowledge of how to fix body parts).[18]

An insidious change in the profession came with the notion that occupations should be *prescribed* by physicians. It is difficult to trace the rationale for this idea back to anything other than the new profession's need for a medical stamp of approval, the corollary being the physicians' desire to have control over the new profession. Physicians who supported occupational therapy saw themselves as arbiters of its use and were adamant that occupational therapy only be given with a doctor's approval. As Kidner, the non-physician, became increasingly involved with occupational therapy in the United States, he too supported this view of the physicians' role in the profession. As if to compensate for his own non-medical background, he seemed even more intent on promoting the relationship. However, he may simply have seen a greater opportunity for the fledgling profession's survival if it allowed itself to come under the wing of the physician. Canadian occupational therapists, like those in the United States, were quick to align themselves with medicine, effectively joining physicians as auxiliary helpers.[19] Even occupational therapists like LeVesconte, with her otherwise strong and independent views on the profession, joined in the chorus. Having revered those in the medical profession since her student days, she supported a subservient role for occupational therapy, stating that it must be "medically prescribed, medically supervised, and medically controlled."[20]

The growing influence of medicine on the profession could be seen in the proceedings of the 1932 annual meeting of the AOTA: "The large number of medical men present indicated the increasing interest in the scope of occupational therapy, its relation to educational training or to job objectives, and to its increasing use in mental and orthopedic hospitals."[21] With orthopaedic surgeons' growing interest in adapted and remedial activities to strengthen muscles and increase joint range, occupational therapists began to change their interventions so that they could more directly address pathology. They showed "a willingness to fit in."[22]

It has been suggested by historian Julien Prud'Homme that occupational therapists, like social workers, had to change their ways in order to become recognized as "health professionals" working within the ever-expanding hospital system. Both disciplines had to work hard to make their skill sets relevant to populations now labelled as having health – rather than social or psychological – problems.[23] For occupational therapists, it was a radical change to move from restoring people to productivity to fixing their broken parts. With the possession of a distinct body of knowledge being a prerequisite of professionalism, the reductionist ideas of the medical model were particularly attractive and soon overlaid the original foundations of the profession. Before long the change in orientation had an effect on the curriculum, with increased content for the sciences and decreased content for the arts and humanities.

Accompanying the new emphasis in occupational therapy for physical dysfunction was a perceived overlap with physical therapy. Because of that overlap, both Howland (in 1929) and LeVesconte (in 1935) suggested that the two educational programs be combined into one. The two were eventually combined in 1950 (an arrangement that was abandoned in 1971).[24] This particular alignment of disciplines remained of interest in the United Kingdom as late as the 1980s, with a report commissioned by the College of Occupational Therapists suggesting that combined training would be useful, as there was so much overlap in education and in practice.[25]

Two factors in particular had influenced the growing perception of similarity in the disciplines. The first was the introduction of activities in the treatment of people with tuberculosis. By the early 1930s, rest, fresh air, and good food had been augmented first by activities designed to provide psychological benefits during convalescence and then by graded activities. Elaborate schemes for improving physical tolerance through graded activities were developed according to the disposition of the patients, who were classified as bed, porch, exercise, or workshop cases.[26] Graded activities were originally concerned with how much hill climbing a patient could do, the distance being gradually increased. With the use of graded activities to increase strength and activity tolerance, occupational therapy took a large step toward the medical model of addressing pathology.[27]

The second factor was the treatment provided to injured soldiers at Hart House, at the University of Toronto, early on in the war (see chapter 9). There, the psychologist Dr E.A. Bott introduced what he termed "mechanotherapy."[28] Whereas adaptations had been made previously to accommodate physical dysfunction and facilitate engagement in occupations (e.g., the small looms used by Peck to enable patients to weave while confined to bed), Bott used adaptations to facilitate exercise. He used adapted games (e.g., bowling for amputees to encourage weight bearing on the prosthesis) and mechanical devices (such as pulleys and weights) to help soldiers move injured limbs in an activity. Bott had observed that when patients became interested in the work, they would forget their condition and work longer than they would at straight exercise. Mechanotherapy was seen by many as occupational therapy.[29]

This approach to treatment – considered as "remedial work" – appealed to occupational therapists. As an example, the activity of moving the beater on a loom to increase elbow flexion could take the place of physical exercises for the same joint. The process of designing the activity and gradually adding resistance was fairly straightforward. In the 1930s, Jean Hampson, an occupational therapist with previous training as a teacher, described her work at the Wellesley School for Crippled Children: "I fear my work is such a mixture of occupational therapy and physiotherapy that to overcome any difficulties which may arise, I always speak of it as remedial work."[30] Several decades later, however, even this semblance of engagement in occupations was lost and the era of "moving cones" came into play; in this treatment, the patient could achieve shoulder movements (e.g., abduction and adduction, flexion and extension) by moving plastic cones and there was no relationship at all to meaningful occupation. As occupational therapists performed more of these tasks, their work in some settings came to resemble that of physical therapists and efforts to distinguish the two became ever more difficult.[31]

Burnette voiced his concern about the profession's change in direction, stating somewhat prophetically, "I have an uncomfortable feeling that we have run away from the hard work in the field of mental diseases to holiday in the by-paths of orthopedics and social service. These things are undoubtedly laudable but I have a suspicion that they are also easy."[32]

When the Faculty of Medicine decided to combine the programs in occupational therapy and physical therapy at the University of Toronto, the dean of Medicine, Dr MacFarlane, defended the decision in an article published in 1950 in the *Canadian Journal of Occupational Therapy*. He noted the overlap in these services after World War II and explained that, within the newly created hospital departments of physical medicine, the plan would save the cost of establishing two therapies where one would do. The educational program would now provide a general course that would set out basic principles, the idea being that graduates could go on to specialize in a particular area, such as psychiatric work. MacFarlane concluded by stating that "the course as planned will give her [the graduate] the necessary training and background and will enable her to take her place with confidence in this increasingly important – but ancillary – service of medicine."[33] If there had ever been any doubt as to where occupational therapy stood, MacFarlane's description of it as an "ancillary service of medicine" soon put the profession in its place.

The move to a combined course in physical and occupational therapy was preceded by battles for control over the rehabilitation of the new population of injured soldiers after World War II. In major centres throughout North America, orthopaedic surgeons and the new specialty of physiatry (i.e., doctors of physical medicine) vied for the territory. In the end, the physiatrists took over the supervision of rehabilitation workers and set up departments of physical medicine and rehabilitation.[34] Many universities in North America followed suit and established the same organizational structure – a department of physical medicine and rehabilitation with occupational therapists, physical therapists, speech therapists, and physiatrists. However, very few educational programs actually combined physical therapy and occupational therapy into one program, as had been done at the University of Toronto.[35]

While it was agreed that the merging of occupational therapy and physical therapy brought economic benefits, these benefits were outweighed by the fact that different types of people were attracted to the distinctive demands of each profession and that a special viewpoint for each discipline needed to be developed from the beginning. Philosophically – and historically – there was little commonality between the two disciplines. That the combined programs were successful, even for a limited time, was symptomatic of the distance occupational therapy had travelled from its foundations. Fitting occupational therapy into a narrow rehabilitation model, where it overlapped so greatly with physical therapy, meant that its scope had also narrowed. The concept of the centrality of occupations in life was soon lost. Not enough attention was paid to employment and issues of productivity, to family and community integration, to psychosocial issues, or to mental health itself. The more medicalized occupational therapy became, the more constrained it was from doing what it had originally set out to do.[36]

Ultimately, the ever-expanding knowledge base in each discipline would make the so-called common denominators less stable. Nonetheless, the diploma in physical and occupational therapy at the University of Toronto continued until 1971 when the two programs separated and each became a four-year degree program (with a first year in arts and science). In 1974, the BSCOT degree, first discussed in 1935, was finally conferred.[37]

ON THEIR OWN

Over the years, occupational therapy has professed to take a holistic approach in its work. To the extent that it does so, it is a result of the foundations upon which it was built. That an alliance with any other profession would not be compatible with the goals of occupational therapy is not surprising. That the profession succumbed to the lure of the medical model is also not surprising, but that this alliance changed the profession's broader focus as a result is unfortunate.

There was (and is) an opportunity for occupational therapy to influence the medical model and help it see the patient in a broader context where change in one area (e.g., productivity) can affect changes in other areas (physical well-being and health).[38] Indeed, the very presence of occupational therapists on health care teams challenges physicians to extend their concerns beyond the medical treatment of the disease to the patient's psychological and social adjustment, economic well-being, and community integration.[39]

Issues of belonging have continued to trouble the profession.[40] Now there are questions about what the right home is for an academic program in occupational therapy: should it be in a faculty of medicine, a faculty of education, a faculty of health sciences, or within a free-standing school of rehabilitation? With different models now established across the country, the question remains. While there can be many viable options, if the best and most nurturing fit is to be found, the philosophical underpinnings of the discipline must be acknowledged.

15

Enduring Values, Ongoing Challenges, and Opportunities

Only that shall happen / Which has happened,
Only that occur / Which has occurred;
There is nothing new / Beneath the sun.

Ecclesiastes 1:9

The profession of occupational therapy has expanded and evolved since its beginnings in the early twentieth century. Many of the values embraced by therapists at that time remain in place today despite new discoveries in health care and the shifting conditions of practice. That many values have remained is likely a testament to how robust they were at the outset. These values bear restating because they are powerful reminders of the essence of the profession. Other values, ones that have wavered over the years, also bear revisiting.

HELPING AND COMPASSION ARE OKAY

The primary motivation for occupational therapists remains their desire to help those in need. There is an assumption that occupational therapists feel compassion for people who struggle to overcome adversity. American anthropologist Gelya Frank has described the founding of occupational therapy as "a historic achievement of women who entered the workforce to do good works."[1] As the field developed and doing good works took on a more professional guise, the value placed on helping, though threatened, remained. Occupational therapists should feel deeply proud of the humanitarian aspect of their work. The term "enabling," now used to describe the work of occupational therapists, may suggest a less direct form of helping, but it too is directed at improving the lot of others, at both the individual and the societal level.[2]

SOCIAL AND OCCUPATIONAL JUSTICE

The idea that everyone – the mentally ill person, the injured soldier, the new immigrant, the child with a disability, the homeless person, the convicted criminal – should have the same access to resources and opportunities is another basic belief that has persisted.[3] In the past, attempts to provide opportunities to vulnerable populations meant not only advocating on their behalf but in many instances actually raising funds to pay for services that would otherwise not be available. Services for low-income patients had to be independently funded given the lack of any state-supported health care. Therapists envisioned new areas of practice on the basis of their assessment of what was needed to improve the daily lives of those in need. They connected with one another, with community agencies, with philanthropic groups, and with people in high places to achieve their goals.[4] Today's occupational therapists are encouraged to make alienation, deprivation, inequity, imbalance, exclusion, oppression, and marginalization in everyday life more explicit concerns in their practice and to take steps to engage in social change.[5] In recognition of our past roles in this regard, it has been suggested that we use our history to "empower new generations of occupational therapists to see the profession as a pivot for activism."[6]

HOLISTIC APPROACH

At an early stage in the development of the profession, occupational therapists were aware of the many spheres of life that needed to be considered in helping an individual or a community. The consideration of the spiritual side of the person, though often thought of as a modern addition to occupational therapy, was present early on. It was of major concern during World War I, when ward aides attended first to the broken spirit of the injured soldier, knowing that this step would dictate all future options. The triangular form of the badge worn by the ward aides during the war depicted the triumvirate of mind, body, and spirit, making the spiritual dimension an equal component of the whole person. Ward aides spoke of the spirit in relation to the internal strength needed to fight against the adversity of illness and disability. "Spiritual rehabilitation" was seen as an underlying goal, as a way to maintain self-respect and develop ambition and initiative.[7] The spirit continues to be thought of as associated with energy, will, and resilience.[8]

The inclusion of spirituality as one of the four components of the "occupational performance model," first described in the Canadian document *Guidelines for Client-Centred Practice* in 1983, formally recognized the importance of connecting with this essential aspect of human beings.[9] It also meant that therapists needed to find ways to work with the spiritual side of their clients. Approaches entailing the use of narrative have been proposed,[10] and mechanisms for relating to another's spirit, including the therapeutic use of self, have been examined.[11]

Some occupations are thought of as particularly helpful in healing the soul and supporting spirituality. From the time of the arts and crafts movement, there has been an effort to equate engagement in art with health. The "art spirit" was considered inherent in all people. It could make daily life more meaningful and also provide refuge for a troubled soul.[12] The stresses of life have not abated, and people still seek refuge in occupations that allow for creativity.[13]

Artistic media have been used in occupational therapy for assessment purposes and as a means of enabling self-expression, particularly in psychiatric settings. Art classes and art studios are still found in outpatient units and community centres,[14] especially for people with chronic mental illness, the elderly, and those with dementia.[15] A keen interest in how art and creativity can be used to promote health is evident in many other arenas – for example, in public health research[16] as well as in business, where corporate workshops are designed to assist individuals and groups to activate their creativity and problem-solving abilities.[17]

The notion of a holistic approach has always been seen as more rhetorical than literal. Any one therapist would not have been able to help in all areas in the past and could not do so now; however, as a profession, occupational therapists are able to see the people and the populations with whom they work from this perspective.[18] Therapists today remain aware of the need to see their clients from all sides, in their various roles, and within their particular socio-cultural environments. Indeed, the role of the occupational therapist on inter-professional teams is often to bring this perspective to the attention of other team members, who might otherwise view the patient in a more restricted fashion.[19]

THE CENTRALITY OF OCCUPATION AND THE FORMS IT TAKES

The hallmark of occupational therapy remains a belief in the importance of engagement in occupations. Being engaged in occupations and
deriving the concomitant sense of agency are core values of the profession. At the end of the nineteenth century, educational reform provided
the profession with methods and a rationale for teaching a host of crafts.
While there was often debate about the end products of craftwork and
the possibilities for sale, it was the *process* of being engaged in occupations that was of greatest importance.[20] But for those who viewed work
as a major route to health, occupations that did not lead to real work
were criticized: for example, occupational therapy in the cement shop
at the sanatorium at Marblehead, Massachusetts (where the Canadian
Edith Griffin worked for a time), was criticized because "for several years
its only results were therapeutic." When the work became self-supporting
it finally earned praise.[21]

While occupations no longer include the widespread use of crafts,
the dilemma over whether occupations are used as a means or an end
is still apparent. There are currently rationales for using occupations as
both means *and* ends – that is, for developing the performance components and sub-skills needed for engagement in an occupation and also for
performing relevant occupations within relevant living environments.[22]
When occupational therapists work at the performance component level,
"turf" issues with other professions are more prevalent. For example,
using activities to build muscle strength or extend joint range will ultimately enhance performance but overlaps with the work of the physical
therapist, who uses exercise for the same reasons. However, many occupational therapists have difficulty working at the more abstract and broad-
based level of occupational performance (also known as occupational
engagement) and prefer more concrete and easily measurable interventions that address performance components. Thus, the dilemma remains.

There is a healthy and ongoing debate about the parameters of occupational engagement.[23] Moreover, interest in the field of occupational
science – and thus in the centrality of occupation itself – is deepening.
Within the Canadian context of occupational therapy, the focus on occupation is highlighted in publications written by leaders in the field
and supported by the Canadian Association of Occupational Therapists
(CAOT). Most recently, *Enabling Occupation II* has placed occupation
front and centre within the triad of the person, the environment, and

the occupation, and has established parameters whereby the profession's interest in the occupational person and the occupational influences of the environment is delineated.[24]

RELATIONSHIPS WITH PATIENTS/CLIENTS

Early occupational therapists clearly understood their responsibility to engage the patient in occupation. In Helen LeVesconte's view, the role of the therapist (see chapter 12) was to take a directive approach at the outset, then share the planning and decision making, and only gradually withdraw, leaving the patient in control.[25] The therapist assumed the overriding responsibility to engage the patient by conveying empathy and establishing a relationship.

Our contemporary view of client-centred practice recognizes the importance of the client's autonomy. Setting goals with clients means that they are invested in the treatment process. This works particularly well for clients who are motivated and able to get on with their lives following illness or injury. They are the ones who are referred to as "resilient" – the ones who, even in the most extreme conditions, cope and rise above adversity.[26] The spectrum of enablement skills that occupational therapists can use in working with these clients, as set out in the Canadian Model of Occupational Performance-Enablement (CMOP-E), is adequate. These skills include the actions of adapting, advocating, coaching, collaborating, consulting, coordinating, designing/building, educating, engaging, and specializing.[27] However, a more empathetic and directive approach is often needed with so-called unmotivated clients or those who are depressed and have lost hope. These clients require more time and a stronger therapeutic relationship, one that includes the skills of encouraging, stimulating, motivating, teaching, and supporting. These skills, which were expected in the past, are needed today in order to attain what is now considered "effective enablement."[28]

While the client-therapist relationship is considered a significant factor in the success of occupational therapy,[29] in this day of short-term involvements, where assessment is often the primary role for therapists,[30] there is little opportunity for expressing empathy and establishing rapport. Yet the motivating effect of the therapist's empathy – described in recent literature as "the enactment of the conviction that, empowered by someone's willingness to understand, the patient will gather the requisite measure of courage"[31] – remains powerful.

With the client's self-esteem often challenged, never in evidence, or severely damaged, interventions in the past were designed to re-establish in the patient the sense of possibility, the sense that he or she could do things, could undertake a task and see it through. The therapist's role continues to be seen in this way; that is, it is to help clients make an emotional investment in the therapeutic situation – to see it as important to their welfare.[32] Ideally, the therapist and client forge a therapeutic or working alliance.[33] The term "alliance" denotes the intent to move forward with an active, almost combative stance. It is more than a partnership or collaboration. It is a commitment on the part of therapist and client to stand together in the face of adversity and overcome it.

Motivational interviewing is one contemporary approach to treatment that focuses on helping individuals develop an internal drive to change.[34] This approach recognizes that motivation and resourcefulness lie within each individual and must be invoked rather than imposed; however, it also recognizes that people need help in getting "unstuck." Just as in the past, one way to help people get unstuck is to have them engage in occupations where they can see the possibilities for change.[35]

The starting place for a therapeutic relationship calls for an expression of empathy.[36] The relationship needs to be brought into play before the principles of client-centred practice can begin to be applied. For many clients, it is the therapeutic relationship they form with the therapist that provides the key to enabling their occupations.[37]

OCCUPATIONAL THERAPY IN THE COMMUNITY

The need for occupational therapists in the community was recognized in the very early days of the profession through the home visits provided by field service. However, the rapid increase in the number of hospitals paralleled society's growing belief that scientific medicine could produce health,[38] and the appeal of the hospital setting, like the medical model itself, was difficult to ignore. Work in the community was neglected until the 1970s, which saw the development of provincial home care programs and recognition of the important role that occupational therapy could play. For a time, there was a sense that the community setting might become the most appropriate place for the work of occupational therapists – that it was here that their role would be most valued.[39] Although hope for occupational therapy in the community flourished in the 1980s and 1990s, ongoing fiscal restraints and concomitant changes in the administration of community services have translated into a curtailment, not of the practice itself, but of the possibilities for the role.

Work in the community today tends to be limited in scope. Therapists have little time for the in-depth, holistic involvement that was once envisioned. When occupational therapists work in the community, they need to be able to do much more than replicate the work that used to be done in rehabilitation units of hospitals when patients had longer hospital stays. They must seize the opportunity to do the important work of addressing the demands of real life, helping clients find satisfying occupations and reintegrate into their homes and communities. Mental health treatment models, such as those found in assertive community treatment (ACT) teams, have acknowledged the need for broader and longer-term involvements for occupational therapists and exemplify the value that is gained by a more in-depth role for community practice.

The significance of the environment as a contributor to health and well-being is now well recognized. Today's occupational therapists can influence the initial design of communities and public spaces not only to improve physical safety and accessibility, but also to facilitate engagement and improve social interaction. This interconnectedness within communities is now widely accepted as important to health.[40] However, it was known to settlement house workers at the turn of the last century, and Jessie Luther strove to develop that interconnectedness in her community development work at the Grenfell Mission in 1906 (see chapters 4 and 6). Outside of the settlement house ideology, the benefits of interdependence and of connecting with and supporting others were not fully realized, neither within the profession nor in society more generally. The goal for most people, but especially the elderly and those with chronic illnesses and disability, is to maintain their autonomy and have some form of satisfying social and occupational engagement.[41]

PREVENTION AND HEALTH PROMOTION

Occupational therapists, like most health care practitioners, have difficulty acting in a preventive fashion, promoting health rather than providing health care. Not only is this a different way of working, but within the confines of current fiscal restraint and issues of third-party payers, it is difficult to achieve. However, occupational therapists have been familiar with the idea for some time. One example of prevention comes from the curative workshops that the Ontario Society for Occupational Therapy (OSOT) promoted in the 1920s. In a *Toronto Star Weekly* article describing the work, the society made the distinction between treatment and pre-vention, seeing the latter as directed at "that class of the population that was deteriorating mentally on account of monotony – the housewife, who has known nothing but the daily routine, the boarding-house class, the business girl or man who realizes their efficiency in the office, yet is con-scious that one side of their nature is starving." Hoping to engage the sup-port of the Imperial Order of the Daughters of the Empire (IODE), OSOT described the extent of its workshop program: "Occupational therapy offers the true element of pleasure – the development of the individual or whole from within – that makes for happiness and prevents disease, and so there will be classes for the sick, for prevention and cure."[42] This whole area remains undeveloped in occupational therapy as it is in health care generally.

Canada recognizes the need to implement preventive measures in part as a response to concerns over the sustainability of its publicly funded health system. Primary health care reform will go a long way to realiz-ing the goal of prevention by focusing on comprehensive and integrated services that go beyond diagnosis and treatment and extend to the de-terminants of health. Family Health Teams (FHTs) are another aspect of health care reform that can address prevention. In both cases, there are major roles for occupational therapy. Advocacy and good public relations are what make the potential contributions of occupational therapists known.[43]

EXPANDING THE MEDICAL MODEL

It has always been recognized that the occupational therapist must under-stand medical thinking; indeed, an understanding of the workings of the human body and mind has been essential to practice. Having the op-portunity to learn about the human body is also a major attraction of the field. However, occupational therapy was shoehorned into the medical model after World War I at a time when medicine saw health only as the absence of disease and its purpose only to eradicate disease. To ensure its viability, occupational therapy reorganized its use of occupations to ad-dress pathology more directly.[44] Occupations designed to reduce impair-ment replaced occupations intended to raise morale, build self-esteem, and develop skills. Differentiating the work of occupational therapists from other health care professionals in hospital settings became and re-mained problematic. At times, in order to be team members, the profes-sion compromised its traditional perspective of viewing the whole patient and its focus on helping people establish satisfying and productive lives. Few therapists were able – or chose – to raise their voices to challenge the reductionist approach.

The possibility – and importance – of being occupationally functional in the face of disability has been well articulated in the occupational therapy literature over the years.[45] Quality of life, balance, and recent discussions of occupational integrity have all become important distinctions within concepts of health.[46] Edith Griffin, an early occupational therapist who worked in Winnipeg, said as much in 1922 when she wrote, "[O]ften where the work of the surgeon, the trained nurse, the physiotherapists ends, our hardest work begins – the man is yet fitted into a useful place in the community ... we can see patients leave the hospitals equipped to earn a living, even better than before sickness ... we might call them cured, even if one leg is wood or the left hand has to do all the work."[47]

The idea that "health" can be defined in terms other than the absence of disease has now been promoted by many in medicine as well as in occupational therapy. Many physicians have recognized the narrowness of their approach and have tried to expand it.[48] More attention is being paid to the need to broaden the medical model so that it deals with the whole patient, over the whole continuum of care, and in the broader context within which health is determined as proposed some twenty years ago in Engel's paper "The Need for a New Medical Model."[49] As the scope of health and health care broadens, there is an important place for occupational therapy with its unique perspective on how to advance the health and well-being of those with illness and injury or social and economic needs.[50]

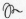

Much work remains to be done in promoting the vision of occupational therapy for the benefit of the profession, the recipients of the service, and the health and well-being of Canadians. In the words of Thomas Kidner, the profession must continue to "Organize, Agitate, and Educate."[51] There are great opportunities in occupational therapy today, even as there were in the beginning when observers of the nascent profession sang its praises so loudly.

ABBREVIATIONS

AMA	American Medical Association
AOTA	American Occupational Therapy Association
CAMH	Centre for Addiction and Mental Health
CAOT	Canadian Association of Occupational Therapists
CCF	Co-operative Commonwealth Federation
CEF	Canadian Expeditionary Force
CHG	Canadian Handicrafts Guild
CSOTM	Canadian Society of Occupational Therapists of Manitoba
DSCR	Department of Soldiers' Civil Re-establishment
DVA	Department of Veterans' Affairs
IODE	Imperial Order of the Daughters of the Empire
ISC	Invalided Soldiers' Commission
MDC	Milwaukee-Downer College
MHC	Military Hospitals Commission
NCMH	National Committee for Mental Hygiene
NCWC	National Council of Women of Canada
NSARM	Nova Scotia Archives and Records Management
NSPOT	National Society for the Promotion of Occupational Therapy
NTBA	National Tuberculosis Association
OSOT	Ontario Society for Occupational Therapy
QSOT	Quebec Society of Occupational Therapy
TB	tuberculosis
U of T	University of Toronto
UIC	University of Illinois at Chicago
UTARMS	University of Toronto Archives and Records Management Services
VAD	Voluntary Aid Detachment
WAAC	Women's Art Association of Canada
YWCA	Young Women's Christian Association

PREFACE

1 Townsend and Polatajko, *Enabling Occupation II*, 2.
2 In my program we learned to weave, make pottery, do metal work and leatherwork, sew, and do carpentry. In addition to learning how to do the crafts, we were taught about the motions required in anatomical terms and often about the craft's presumed affective characteristics.
3 From 1960 through 1963, I worked first in Fulbourn Hospital, a large state hospital in Cambridge, England, and then at the Toronto Psychiatric Hospital, the first university teaching hospital, established in 1925. I was blessed with directors who were wonderful role models in each situation: Rosemary Huggins at Fulbourn and Sheila Irvine at Toronto Psych.
4 See Brintnell et al., "The Fifties and Sixties," 27–8; Driver, "A Philosophic View of the History of Occupational Therapy in Canada," 53–60; and Robinson, "The Mists of Time," 145–51.
5 Bain, *What the Best College Teachers Do*, 25. Ken Bain is vice provost for instruction, professor of history, and director of the Research Academy for University Learning at Montclair State University in New Jersey.
6 Engel, "The Need for a New Medical Model," 37–53.
7 Levine, "The Influence of the Arts-and-Crafts Movement," 248–54.
8 The Muriel Driver Lectureship Award honours a member of the Canadian Association of Occupational Therapists who has made an outstanding contribution to the profession.
9 LeVesconte examined the origins of the profession from Greek and Roman times through to the 1980s and looked at the development of the profession in Canada, the United States, and the United Kingdom. Whether the sources of information for the manuscript were lost over time or simply never included, this situation made Isobel Robinson's further work very difficult. Nonetheless, the manuscript is a valuable resource. It now resides in the Canadian Association of Occupational Therapists collection at Library and Archives Canada.
10 Friedland, *The University of Toronto*.

INTRODUCTION

1 Wilcock, *Occupation for Health*.

2 Metaxis Quiroga, *Occupational Therapy: The First 30 Years, 1900–1930*. Of note also is a special issue of the *American Journal of Occupational Therapy* published in 1992, which was devoted to history.

3 For articles in the *Canadian Journal of Occupational Therapy* (CJOT), see Brintnell et al., "The Fifties and Sixties," 27–8; Driver, "A Philosophic View of the History of Occupational Therapy in Canada," 53–60; Friedland, "Knowing from Whence We Came," 266–71; Friedland, "Why Crafts," 204–13; Friedland and Rais, "Helen Primrose LeVesconte," 131–41; Friedland and Davids-Brumer, "From Education to Occupation," 37–47; Robinson, "The Mists of Time," 145–51; and Sedgwick, Cockburn, and Trentham, "Exploring the Mental Health Roots of Occupational Therapy in Canada," 407–17.

4 For historical vignettes celebrating the association's seventy-fifth anniversary, see sequential issues of *Occupational Therapy Now* for 2001. The early period is described by Friedland, Robinson, and Cardwell, "In the Beginning." Vignettes in the "OT Then" columns of this journal in 2006 include Head and Friedland, "Jessie Luther"; McQuay, "Dr. Goldwin Howland"; Trentham, "Occupational Therapy Street Fair"; McDonald, "Curative Workshops"; and Brackley, "Mary E. Black." An "OT Then" column for 2007 included Friedland, "Hilda Goodman."

5 In the *American Journal of Occupational Therapy*, Friedland and Silva, "Evolving Identities," 349–60; Friedland, "Diversional Activity," 603–8; and Friedland, "Occupational Therapy and Rehabilitation," 373–80. In the *British Journal of Occupational Therapy*, Friedland, "Thomas Bessell Kidner," 292–300. See also Friedland, "The Department of Occupational Therapy," 259–70, for reflections on the work in Toronto's first psychiatric teaching hospital.

6 For examples on physical therapy, see Heap, "Training Women for a New 'Women's Profession,'" 135–58, and Stonehouse, *Moving Together*; on social work, Burke, *Seeking the Highest Good*; and on nursing, McPherson, *Bedside Matters*.

7 Heap, Millar, and Smyth, *Learning to Practise*; Heap, "Training Women for a New 'Women's Profession,'" 135–58; Prentice and Theobald, *Women Who Taught*; and McPherson, *Bedside Matters*.

8 There were just over 13,000 occupational therapists practising in Canada in 2009 according to the Canadian Institute for Health Information (CIHI). Of these, only 8 per cent are "male." http://www.cihi.ca/CIHI-ext-portal/pdf/internet/INFO_09NOV10_PDF_EN.

9 For examples of this very rich literature, see Bourke, *Dismembering the Male*; Koven, "Remembering and Dismemberment," 1167–202; and Reznick, *Healing the Nation*.

10 Lewis, *History*. While the goal for history recovered is to restore material that was actively excluded, in the case of occupational therapy, the material was simply neglected and ignored. Thus, my effort at recovery of this history is directed at collecting it in the first instance. See also Boutilier and Prentice, *Creating Historical Memory*, 3–9, for issues specific to women and written history.

11 Heap and Stuart, "Nurses and Physiotherapists," 179–93. See also McPherson and Stuart, "Writing Nursing History in Canada," 3–22.
12 Dutil and Ferland, *L'histoire de l'ergothérapie au Québec.*

CHAPTER ONE

1   Leacy, *Historical Statistics of Canada*, series A2–14.
2   Ibid., series A125–63.
3   Ibid., series A67–69.
4   In regard to children sent by Dr Barnardo, see Valverde, *The Age of Light, Soap, and Water*, 30.
5   Frager and Patrias, *Discounted Labour*, 17–53.
6   Bosch, "Starr, Ellen Gates," 838–42.
7   The insignia for occupational therapists carried the motto "Per Mentum et Manus ad Sanitatem" [Through mind and hand to health].
8   Prentice, *Canadian Women*, 127.
9   Chief Public Health Officer, *Report on the State of Public Health in Canada*, 2008, 11.
10 Duffin, *History of Medicine.*
11 Bliss, M. *William Osler.*
12 Ibid.
13 Gagan and Gagan, *For Patients of Moderate Means*, 71–97. Prime Minister William Lyon Mackenzie King tried to establish a form of government-funded health care for Canadians during his lengthy period in office but was unsuccessful. It was not until 1957 that the Hospital Insurance and Diagnostic Services Act was approved by Parliament, and not until 1966 that free access to physician services was finally established with the Medical Care Act.
14 See Mitchinson, *The Nature of Their Bodies*, 312–55, for references to Bucke's experiments with women; and Warsh, *Moments of Unreason*, 37–62, in regard to Hobbs's use of alcohol with his patients.
15 Bockoven, *Moral Treatment in American Psychiatry*, 10–19; see also Stevenson, "The Life and Work of Richard Maurice Bucke," 1127–54.
16 Griffin, *In Search of Sanity*, 32–3.
17 Rompkey, "Grenfell, Sir Wilfred Thomason," 270; see also Rompkey, *Grenfell of Labrador*, 125–40.
18 Rompkey, *Jessie Luther at the Grenfell Mission.*
19 Cook, "The Triumph and Trials of Materialism," 377–472.
20 J.S. Woodsworth, the former minister who founded the Co-operative Commonwealth Federation (CCF), had advocated what he called "practical Christianity." Allen has suggested that the social gospel movement was a way to define a new mission for the church's role in society. Allen, *The Social Passion.*
21 Ibid. One of the results of the social gospel movement was the opening of the Fred Victor Mission in 1894 in Toronto to deal with poverty and homelessness.

22 According to the twelfth-century philosopher Maimonides, Leviticus 25:35 translates as "You shall strengthen the stranger and the dweller in your midst and live with him" (i.e., strengthen him until he needs no longer fall [upon the mercy of the community] or be in need). Maimonides spoke of eight degrees of giving, or *Tzedaka*, the highest being to strengthen the person's hand, so that the person will not need to ask for assistance from others.

23 Leiby, *A History of Social Welfare and Social Work in the US*, 122.

24 Mackenzie King, who had spent time at Hull House while a student at the University of Chicago, was elected to Parliament in 1908. He became minister of labour the following year and may have brought some increased understanding to the position from his experience with immigrants at Hull House. However, this experience was apparently of little value in his handling of immigration while prime minister in the 1930s and 1940s, when he actively restricted immigration of particular groups.

25 Morton, *A Short History of Canada*, 141–7.

26 Leiby, *A History of Social Welfare*, 32–3.

27 Cook, "The Triumph and Trials of Materialism," 377–472.

28 Duffin, *History of Medicine*.

29 Dodd, "Eugenics," 205–6. Elizabeth Upham Davis, a prominent American occupational therapist, also spoke of the movement as a sensible means of dealing with society's ills.

30 Dewey, *Experience and Education*, 86–112.

31 For details on Kidner's contributions, see Friedland and Silva, "Evolving Identities," 349–60; and Friedland and Davids-Brumer, "From Education to Occupation" 27–37.

32 Morton, *A Short History of Canada*, 135. See also Ginzberg, *Women and the Work of Benevolence*.

33 Prentice, *Canadian Women*, 82.

34 Griffiths, *The Splendid Vision*, 50.

35 Leacy, *Historical Statistics*, Series D8–55.

36 Prentice, *Canadian Women*, 128.

37 Prentice, "Schoolmistresses," 567–8.

38 Prentice, *Canadian Women*, 132.

39 Errington, "Pioneers and Suffragists," 73.

40 Frager and Patrias, *Discounted Labour*, 75–84.

41 Valverde, *The Age of Light, Soap, and Water*, 30. See also Koven, *Slumming*, for an analysis of this expectation.

42 Cleverdon, *The Woman Suffrage Movement in Canada*, 155.

43 Griffiths, *The Splendid Vision*, 13–46; and Morton, *A Short History*, 134–5. Lady Aberdeen, wife of Governor General Lord Aberdeen, was the first president of the NCWC. She was a strong and very influential woman who believed in the importance of organized philanthropy to the well-being of society. She worked to bring together women of different racial and religious backgrounds, making it

clear that the NCWC would not exclude those considered to be "not acknowledging God and Christ."

44 McLeod, *In Good Hands*.
45 Frager and Patrias, *Discounted Labour*.
46 Prentice, *Canadian Women*, 159.
47 Ibid., 172.
48 Errington, "Pioneers and Suffragists," 64.
49 Richardson, "The Historical Relationship," 20.

CHAPTER TWO

1 Cited in Greenland and Colombo, *The New Consciousness*, 175.
2 Bockoven, *Moral Treatment in American Psychiatry*.
3 Ibid., 12–13. See also Barris, Kielhofner, and Watts, *Psychosocial Occupational Therapy*, 176–7; Pinel, "Medical Philosophical Treatise on Mental Alienation," 19–24; and Tuke, "Reform in the Treatment of the Insane," 46–8.
4 Greenland, "Three Pioneers," 835; and Stogdill, "Joseph Workman," 1–7.
5 Bockoven, *Moral Treatment in American Psychiatry*, 12.
6 Stevenson, "The Life and Work of Richard Maurice Bucke," 1127–54.
7 Greenland, "The Compleat Psychiatrist Dr R.M. Bucke," 75.
8 Greenland and Colombo, *The New Consciousness*, 175.
9 Greenland, "What's New," 80 (for Inspector W.J. O'Reilly's report). It is unclear whether employing women to work with male patients was new only to Bucke or whether it was also unknown elsewhere. It should be noted that many of Bucke's treatments would not be seen as humane today. His writings show, for example, that in the belief that masturbation was related to mental disease, he attempted to discourage the activity by using an experimental treatment involving penile wires. He also carried out gynecological surgeries in the belief that they could cure various mental conditions. See also Mitchinson, *The Nature of Their Bodies*; and Mitchinson, "R.M. Bucke," 239–54.
10 The Canadian film *Beautiful Dreamers*, produced by Michael Maclear in 1990, shows the impact of Whitman on Bucke personally and on his treatment approach.
11 Greenland, "Three Pioneers," 135. Clarke had been the assistant superintendent at Rockwood since 1882, but by 1885, feeling there was too much political interference in asylum affairs, he had decided to leave. However, in 1885, when Superintendent Dr Metcalfe, Clarke's brother-in-law, was killed by a patient, Clarke accepted the position of superintendent.
12 Clarke also had family connections with Workman, as his older sister, Jane, was married to Workman's son.
13 Centre for Addition and Mental Health (hereafter CAMH) Archives, C.K. Clarke, *Statement*, 6.
14 Ibid., 13.

15 Clarke, "The Fourth Maudsley Lecture," 283.

16 Brown, *Dorothea Dix*, 190.

17 Kirkbride, *On the Construction*, 73–80.

18 Greenland, "Three Pioneers," 129–30. Greenland describes earlier treatment facilities in Canada: in Quebec, 1714; in Saint John, NB, 1835; at the Toronto Asylum, 1841; at the Beauport Asylum in Quebec, 1845; and at the Nova Scotia Hospital, 1858.

19 Foucault, *Madness and Civilization*, 158.

20 Charland, "Benevolent Theory," 61–80. See also Sacks, "The Lost Virtues of the Asylum," which expressed support for the idea that a retreat or asylum is a means of removing an individual from his or her stressful environment and providing protection; and Garton, "Seeking Refuge," 25–45.

21 Rush, *Inquiries and Observations upon the Diseases of the Mind*, 224.

22 CAMH Archives, Clarke's Kingston report for 1893 describing Beach Grove, n.p.

23 Moher, "Occupation as a Factor," 62.

24 Reaume, *Remembrances of Patients Past*, 180. Reaume spearheaded a campaign to see the patients' work commemorated in plaques situated on the grounds of the original asylum.

25 Reaume, "Patients at Work," 82.

26 Warsh, *Moments of Unreason*, 117.

27 Herring, "Diversional Occupation," 245.

28 Ibid. The issue of occupying the large number of patients unable to perform work-like activities and thereby left with no occupations speaks to the "Matthew effect" in health care; see Link and Milcarek, "Selection Factor," 280, which discusses how those who most need help are ignored, while those who are easiest to treat receive the most attention: "For to all those who have, more will be given, and they will have an abundance; but from those who have nothing, even what they have will be taken away."

29 Clarke, "The Military Hospital for Mental Cases at Cobourg," 9.

30 Osler, *Aequanimitas*, 356.

31 For the role of volition in teaching, see Ellis, *Outlines of the History and Formation of the Understanding*, 41; and in terms of the psychological development of the child, see Dewey, *Psychology*, 359–73. Kielhofner brought these views into contemporary occupational therapy in his "model of human occupation." Kielhofner, *Conceptual Foundations of Occupational Therapy*, 187–217.

32 Ach, *On Volition*, 13.

33 Ibid.

34 Ibid., 14.

35 Ibid., 13–14.

36 Bandura, "Self-Efficacy," 191–215.

37 See, for example, Burke, "A Clinical Perspective on Motivation," 254–8; Fidler, "From Crafts to Competence," 567–73; and White, "The Urge towards Competence," 271–4.

38 Jarvis, "Mechanical and Other Employments," 129–45.

39 Ibid., 142–3.
40 Bockoven, *Moral Treatment in American Psychiatry*, 75.
41 Meyer, "The Philosophy of Occupation Therapy," 639–42. See also Joseph and Moon, "From Retreat to Health Centre."
42 Time-sharing and multiple processors, serial and parallel processing, and conscious and unconscious processing were among the paradigms explored in neuropsychology. See Gardner, *The Mind's New Science*, for a detailed discussion.
43 Giambra, "A Laboratory Based Method," 2–3.
44 Smallwood and Schooler, "The Restless Mind," 946–58.
45 Ibid.
46 Schneider and Shiffrin, "Controlled and Automatic Processing," 40–4. Of interest, activities that do not require a high degree of concentration allow the mind to wander and are thought to spur spontaneous thought.
47 Csikszentmihalyi, *Flow*, 71–93.
48 Meyer, "The Philosophy of Occupation Therapy," 639–42.
49 Selye, *The Stress of Life*, 417.
50 Ibid.
51 Beck et al., *Cognitive Therapy of Depression*.
52 Friedland, "Diversional Activity," 603. See early reference to this issue in Haas, "Is Diversional Occupation Always Therapeutic," 117–20.
53 The Mental Hygiene Committee was initially called the Mental Hygiene Society.
54 Beers, *A Mind That Found Itself*, 203–7.
55 Addams, *My Friend, Julia Lathrop*, 163. See CAMH Archives, Farrar Papers, for a letter from Meyer (20 July 1943), who conveys his concern about Beers's mental health at the time Beers's book was published and suggests that the book presents a very one-sided view.
56 Addams, *My Friend, Julia Lathrop*, 152.
57 Dunton, *Occupation Therapy*, 16.
58 Newberry Library Archives, Chicago School of Civics and Philanthropy, box 1, file 20, Graham Taylor Papers, Yearbook 1908–1911.
59 Metaxas, "Eleanor Clarke Slagle and Susan Tracy," 39–70. See also Frank, "Opening Feminist Histories of Occupational Therapy," 989–99.
60 Beers, "The Need and Value of Play," 209–15.
61 Clarke, "Fourth Maudsley Lecture," 284.
62 Timothy Eaton was the proprietor of Eaton's, the department store founded in 1869 that at its height had stores in all major cities across Canada.
63 Canadian Medical Association, "The Canadian National Committee for Mental Hygiene," 832–3.
64 Herring thought that the worker "should be brimming over with enthusiasm and energy, and be able to impart the same spirit to his or her pupils." See Herring, "Diversional Occupation," 248.
65 Friedland, "Occupational Therapy and Rehabilitation," 259.
66 Friedland and Renwick, "Psychosocial Occupational Therapy," 467–71.

67 On changes in psychiatric occupational therapy practice, see Friedland and Renwick, "Psychosocial Occupational Therapy," 467–71; and Renwick et al., "Crisis in Psychosocial Occupational Therapy," 279–84.

68 Peloquin, "The 2005 Eleanor Clark Slagle Lecture," 611–25.

CHAPTER THREE

1   Boris, *Art and Labor*, 5.
2   Levine, "The Influence of the Arts-and-Crafts Movement," 248–9.
3   Bloom Hoover, "Diversional Occupational Therapy," 881–5.
4   Friedland, "Why Crafts?" 201–13.
5   Reaume, "Patients at Work," 69–96.
6   Ibid.
7   Cumming and Kaplan, *The Arts and Crafts Movement*, 6–28.
8   Hilton, *The Pre-Raphaelites*, 10.
9   Cate, *Correspondence of Thomas Carlyle and John Ruskin*.
10 Ruskin, *Arrows of the Chace*, 540.
11 Naylor, *The Arts and Crafts Movement*, 25.
12 Carlyle, *Past and Present*, 132.
13 Cumming and Kaplan, *The Arts and Crafts Movement*, 12.
14 Ruskin, *On the Nature of Gothic Architecture*, 12, 13.
15 Davis, "Ruskin and the Art-Workmen," 84.
16 Boris, *Art and Labor*, 83.
17 Ruskin, *Fors Clavigera*, 31.
18 Davis, "Ruskin and the Art-Workmen," 82.
19 Boris, *Art and Labor*, 123.
20 Naylor, *The Arts and Crafts Movement*, 94.
21 Harris, "Ruskin and Social Reform," 17.
22 Morris and Ruskin do not appear to have interacted to any degree, but they did see one another occasionally. While Morris was living in London with his Oxford classmate Edward Burne-Jones, Ruskin would stop by to visit on the nights when he was teaching at the Working Men's College.
23 Thompson, *The Work of William Morris*, 1–55.
24 These factory workers were thought to be the people referred to in William Blake's "dark Satanic mills." Blake, "Milton," 95.
25 Morris, "The Beauty of Life," 53.
26 Ibid., 54.
27 Morris, "Art and the Beauty of the Earth," 80–94.
28 Kelvin, *William Morris on Art and Socialism*.
29 Morris, "An Empty Pocket Is the Worst of Crimes," 123.
30 Morris, "The Worker's Share of Art," 18–19.
31 Cumming and Kaplan, *The Arts and Crafts Movement*, 9–27. See also Morris, *News from Nowhere*, for his utopian world.
32 Morris, "The Lesser Arts," 253.

33 It is apparent that there were male roles and female roles in these artistic ventures: the men created the works, while the women provided the decorative touches. See Barter, *Apostles of Beauty*.

34 Addams and Starr visited Morris; James Mavor, professor of economics at the University of Toronto, was a friend of Morris's; and George Barton, a founder of the National Society for the Promotion of Occupational Therapy (NSPOT), studied with Morris.

35 Kirchhoff, *William Morris*, 167. Morris did not foresee the ability of the machine to function as an extension of the artist's imagination.

36 Boris, *Art and Labor*, 5–123.

37 Ibid., 29.

38 Levine, "The Influence of the Arts-and-Crafts Movement," 248–54.

39 There were several of these retreats in the United States. Roycroft, established by Elbert Hubbard in 1895 in East Acton, NY, was promoted as a social and industrial experiment. See Boris, *Art and Labor*, 146–50.

40 Kahler, "Art and Life," n.p.

41 Stankiewicz, "From the Aesthetic Movement to the Arts and Crafts Movement," 165–73.

42 Wilde, *Extracts from Wilde's Lecture on Art and the Handicraftsman*. http://www.burrows.com/founders/art.html.

43 William Morris Societies exist in Canada and the United States (as well as the United Kingdom and elsewhere) and are very active. Exhibitions of Morris's work continue to be mounted and are very successful (e.g., *The Earthly Paradise*, Art Gallery of Ontario, 1993; *William Morris: Creating the Useful and the Beautiful*, Huntington Library, San Marino, California, 2002; and *Apostles of Beauty*, Art Institute of Chicago, 2009).

44 Panayotidis-Stortz, "Artist, Poet and Socialist," 36–43. See also Thompson, *The Work of William Morris*.

45 Cumming and Kaplan, *The Arts and Crafts Movement*, 7.

46 Canadian Architect and Builder, "Hamilton," 68. Note that an article by Gagen, "History of Art Societies in Ontario," published in *Canada: An Encyclopedia*, states that the association was inaugurated in 1894.

47 Leard-Coolidge, "William Morris and Nineteenth-Century Boston," 164.

48 Pepall, "Under the Spell of Morris," 19–35. Hart House at the University of Toronto was built in the arts and crafts style and in its early years had arts and crafts studios for members (who were all male). See also Russell, "A Mutable Monument," 19–30.

49 Hart House was not fully co-educational until 1972. Indeed women were still barred from attending events there during the time of US presidential candidate Kennedy's visit in 1957. A reporter from the student newspaper, the *Varsity*, and a few of her friends dressed in male attire in order to report on the debate in which Kennedy was to participate. The reporter, Judy Graner Sarick, and her friends were found out and escorted out of the building just before the debate began. Watt, "Rights of Passage," 9.

50 Russell, "The Mutable Monument," 20. The building has many arts and crafts features. See Kilgour, *A Strange Elation*.

51 Licht, "The Founding and Founders," 269–77.

52 University of Toronto Archives and Records Management Services (hereafter UTARMS), James Mavor Papers, box 33, file 17B, and box 10A.

53 Bott, "Re-educational Work," 269–72.

54 Constitution and By-laws of the Society of Arts and Crafts of Canada.

55 Reid, "Applied Art," 55.

56 Cawthra Adamson served as president of the Arts and Crafts Society of Canada, and Reid served as its vice-president. She had studied with Charles Ashbee's Guild of Handicraft in England, and her interior design company, Thornton-Smith, decorated such important buildings as the Senate Chamber in Ottawa and the Royal Alexander Theatre in Toronto. Her work with the Belgian Soldiers' Fund during World War I was noteworthy and especially creative. See Gwyn, *Tapestry of War*; Phipps, *A History of the Cawthra Estate*; and Pringle, "Mrs. Agar Adamson," 1925.

57 Carless, *The Arts and Crafts of Canada*, 18.

58 Panayotidis, "James Mavor," 166–7.

59 McCarthy, *Women's Culture*, 59–79.

60 Peck, "Handicrafts from Coast to Coast," 210.

61 Ibid., 201–16.

62 Canadian Handicrafts Guild (hereafter CHG) Archives, C11.D1, 1912.

63 McLeod, *In Good Hands*, 94.

64 McCord Museum Archives, Women's Art Society of Montreal, drawer 2, folder 2, CHG. See also CHG Archives, C11.D1 074, 1916, for news clippings on the sale of soldiers' work.

65 CHG Archives, Minutes of 13 March 1917, drawer 2, folder 2.

66 Anticipating that many of the toys that had been made in Germany before the war would no longer be purchased, the CHG encouraged soldiers to make toys that could then be said to be "Made in Canada." CHG Archives, C11.D1 072, 1916. According to McLeod (*In Good Hands*, 174), the campaign was launched in 1915 and incorporated in 1916 as a category in annual guild exhibitions. A prize was awarded for the best mechanical, most original, and most saleable cheap toy made by a returned solider. CHG Archives, Obituary for Mrs James H. Peck, *Gazette*, 8 November 1943, C17.D3 012. See also "A Handicraft Display," *Quebec Telegraph*, 22 March 1916.

67 Hall, "Neurasthenia," 47–9.

CHAPTER FOUR

1 The people who ran the centres were often referred to as "settlers." See Barnett and Barnett, *Practicable Socialism*, 105.

2 James, "Reforming Reform," 58.

3 Vicinus, *Independent Women*, 215–16.
4 Greadle, "Hill, Caroline Southwood (1809–1902)."
5 See chapter 5 for Pestalozzi's influence on educational reform and indirectly on the origins of occupational therapy.
6 Wilcock, "Creating Self," 77–8; and Darley, "Hill, Octavia."
7 Darley, "Hill, Octavia."
8 Maurice, *Octavia Hill*, 162. These letters, many of which are between Hill and Ruskin, provide an excellent description of the conditions and the extraordinary work that Hill managed to do. Of interest to occupational therapists is the fact that Hill also took her tenants on "outings."
9 Darley, "Hill, Octavia."
10 McLeod, *In Good Hands*, 203–33.
11 Ibid., 171.
12 In the various tributes following her death, this clinic is referred to as a "nursing home."
13 Casson, "Some Experiences in Occupational Therapy," 265–8.
14 Friedland, "Thomas Bessell Kidner," 292–300.
15 Wilcock, "Creating Self and Shaping the World," 77–88.
16 Wilcock, *An Occupational Perspective of Health*, 381.
17 Burke, *Seeking the Highest Good*, 11.
18 Ibid., 214.
19 Barnett, *Practicable Socialism*, 105.
20 Bosch, "Starr, Ellen Gates," 840.
21 Addams was a founder of the Women's Peace Party in 1915. She received the Nobel Peace Prize in 1931, the first woman so honoured.
22 Muncy, "Lathrop, Julia Clifford," 490–2.
23 Swarthmore College Peace Collection, Jane Addams Papers, series 1, suppl., 10 May 1930.
24 Lovett, "Jane Addams at Hull House," 349–50.
25 Addams, *Twenty Years at Hull-House*, 371–400.
26 James, "Reforming Reform," 65.
27 City of Toronto Archives, Settlement House, series Q, correspondence, file 2, 7 May 1914.
28 University of Illinois at Chicago (UIC) Archives, University Library, Jane Addams Memorial Collection, Addams correspondence, 5 March 1920; and "President Falconer Makes Statement," *Varsity*, 2 March 1920.
29 UIC Archives, University Library, Jane Addams Memorial Collection, reel 16, 0916.
30 Macphail, "Tribute to Jane Addams," 202.
31 University of Michigan, Jane Addams Papers 1860–1960, reel 45, #1325.
32 Rompkey, *Jessie Luther*, 217; and Addams, *Twenty Years at Hull-House*, 371–400.
33 Addams, *Twenty Years at Hull-House*, 371–400.
34 Dobschuetz, "Slagle, Eleanor Clarke," 803.

35 The school joined the University of Chicago and became the School of Social Service Administration in 1920. See Muncy, "Lathrop, Julia Clifford," 491.

36 Breines, "Rabbi Hirsch," 567–8.

37 Loomis and Wade, *Chicago*, n.p. Rabbi Hirsch was also the director of Chicago's Jewish Manual Training School, which opened in 1890 to teach new skills to Russian immigrant Jews. See also Boris, *Art and Labor*, 88.

38 Loomis and Wade, *Chicago*, n.p.

39 Dobschuetz, "Slagle, Eleanor Clarke," 805. The dates given for Slagle's tenure as director of the Favill School are often conflicting. Slagle had many prominent friends, including Eleanor Roosevelt, who spoke at her retirement banquet in 1937.

40 Loomis, "The Henry B. Favill School," 36.

41 Dobschuetz, "Slagle, Eleanor Clarke," 804–5.

42 The term "settlers" was used by Barnett to describe the volunteer work of the university students at Toynbee Hall, the first Settlement House in the United Kingdom. See note 19 above.

43 James, "Practical Diversions and Educational Amusements," 48–66.

44 James, "Reforming Reform," 56.

45 Valverde, *The Age of Light, Soap, and Water.*

46 Ibid., 59.

47 Burke, *Seeking the Highest Good*, 41–60.

48 Wasteneys, "A History of the University Settlement," 304.

49 Ibid., 77.

50 Receiving help without converting to Christianity could be problematic. The Jewish population, which had doubled between 1908 and 1915 with successive waves of emigration primarily from eastern Europe, needed more help than their own community could offer. Three missions (Presbyterian Mission to the Jews; Nathaniel; and the Toronto Jewish Mission) tried to help, but as their goal was to Christianize and Canadianize the Jews, their help was not welcome. See Wasteneys, "A History of the University Settlement," 238–40.

51 Ibid. The settlement house movement appealed to those Christian social reformers who supported cooperation over competition. The Co-operative Commonwealth Federation (CCF) – the precursor of the New Democratic Party (NDP) – took up many of the secular principles of the social gospel movement in the 1930s.

52 University of Toronto Monthly, "The Settlement Movement," 40.

53 Stebner, "The Settlement House Movement," 1067. Although the board of Central Neighbourhood House was intentionally non-sectarian, Elizabeth Neufeld (the Jewish director) and the board were accused of engaging in Jewish propagandism. Neufeld replied to the charges saying, "We don't talk religion at all. We leave that to the ministers and rabbis. Citizenship is our gospel. Jane Addams is our John the Baptist and our Bible is the daily press (when it knows enough to talk sense)."

54 Burke, *Seeking the Highest Good*, 67–72.

55 Wasteneys, "A History of the University Settlement," 65, 284.

56 Vicinus, *Independent Women*, 239.

57 Ibid., 222.

58 UTARMS, Department of Graduate Records, Hastings, Charles, A1973-0026/142(77). The death from typhoid fever of one of Hastings's daughters may have motivated him to work on the implementation of pasteurized milk.

59 UTARMS, James Mavor Papers, *Report on Workmen's Compensation for Injuries in Ontario*, 1900, box 33, file 17B, and box 10A. See also Wasteneys, "A History of the University Settlement," 38.

60 Burke, *Seeking the Highest Good*, 42.

61 In correspondence, Mackenzie King had commented on being a resident at Passmore Edwards as well as at Hull House. See UIC Archives, Jane Addams Memorial Collection, Mackenzie King to Addams, 10 May 1930.

62 Vicinus, *Independent Women*, 211–46.

63 Ibid., 246.

64 The Manitoba Society of Occupational Therapists of Canada considered becoming part of the Department of Public Health and Social Welfare in 1920.

65 Library and Archives Canada (hereafter LAC), Department of Veterans' Affairs (hereafter DVA) fonds, RG 38, Clarke and MacIver correspondence, also Bell and Hincks, v. 205, file NCF, vol. 1. A special course in mental hygiene social training was established in 1920. The curriculum for the eight-week course included one hour a week devoted to the study of occupational therapy, including the application of psychology to occupational therapy, principles and practices of occupational therapy, and home crafts.

CHAPTER FIVE

1 Kidner, *Educational Handwork*, 9.

2 Wollons, *Kindergartens and Cultures*, 2–3. Pestalozzi's ideas informed Caroline Hill's work with children and impressed her daughter, the social reformer Octavia Hill (see chapter 4), who was in turn to influence occupational therapy.

3 After 1887, kindergartens were recognized by the government of Ontario and received a share of the provincial grant.

4 Wollons, *Kindergartens and Cultures*, 19.

5 Murray, *Froebel as a Pioneer in Modern Psychology*, 1130. See also Froebel, Michaelis, and Moore, *Autobiography of Friedrich Froebel*.

6 Wollons, *Kindergartens and Cultures*, 25.

7 Salomon, *The Theory of Educational Sloyd*, 25.

8 Ibid., 1–2.

9 Ibid., 5.

10 Ibid., 73.

11 Gay, "Association and Practice," 375.

12 Foden, *Philip Magnus*, 174–5. See also B. Bailey, "Magnus, Sir Philip."

13 Foden, *Philip Magnus*, 211.

14   Ibid., 222.

15   Dewey, *The School and Society*, 132.

16   Levin, "The Debate over Schooling," 74.

17   Cutchin, "Using Deweyan Philosophy," 304.

18   Dewey, *The School and Society*, 135.

19   Breines, "Pragmatism," 523–4.

20   Bosch, "Starr, Ellen Gates," 840. The argument has been advanced that the idea of imposing values (in this instance regarding art) contradicts the goal of reducing class distinction.

21   Wilson, Stamp, and Audet, *Canadian Education*, 296.

22   Ibid., 320.

23   Panayotidis-Stortz, "Every Artist," 168.

24   Ibid., 170.

25   Robertson also had difficulty determining just where manual training fit. Writing in 1901, he rather ambiguously stated, "It is not technical education, although it gives, during the period of general education, the necessary preparation whereby anyone may derive the full measure of benefit from technical instruction at a later age." Robertson, *Manual Training*, 8.

26   Frost and Michel, "Macdonald, Sir William Christopher."

27   "Macdonald Manual Training School," *Truro Daily News*, 4 October 1900.

28   Robertson reported that girls were often taught domestic science – not manual training – during this time, an idea that had been promoted by the female social activists of the time. Robertson, *Industrial Training and Technical Education*, 1790.

29   Robertson, *Manual Training*, 17.

30   Robertson, *Industrial Training and Technical Education*, 151.

31   In 1910, Kidner told the Royal Commission on Industrial Training and Technical Education that, in England, manual training had been found to be a great preparation for industrial training.

32   Robertson was the general manager of the Macdonald Manual Training Fund and the Macdonald Rural Training Fund.

33   McGill Library Archives, Staff Records, RG 0043, Robertson-Kidner correspondence.

34   LAC, CAOT fonds, Kidner Family Papers. See also Friedland and Davids-Brumer, "From Education to Occupation," 29; and Friedland and Silva, "Evolving Identities," 349.

35   Kidner, "A Cheap Sand-Table," 138.

36   Kidner, "Cardboard Work," 163.

37   Kidner, "The Teacher," 142.

38   Kidner, *Educational Handwork*, 10.

39   Lillard, *Montessori*, 50–90.

40   Bell's mother had been deaf and, like his father, he had become a teacher of people who were deaf. Mabel had received an excellent education both in the US and abroad but at age 16 had been sent to Bell who was considered to be the

best vocal coach in Boston. See Gray, *Reluctant Genius*. See also materials from Alexander Graham Bell Historical Museum, Baddeck, Nova Scotia.

41 Gray, *Reluctant Genius*, 394–5.

42 "Technical Education Classes Will Be Started in October," *Morning Albertan*, 12 September 1911.

43 Calgary Archives, Kidner's reports to Calgary Board of Education, 11 December 1912, 334.

44 "Technical Education," *Morning Albertan*, 28 February 1913.

45 Lanning, "Millar, John."

46 Panayotidis-Stortz, "Artist, Poet, and Socialist," 41.

47 Morton and Wright, *Winning the Second Battle*, 33.

48 "T.B. Kidner Leaving Calgary for Govt. Service," *Morning Albertan*, 3 January 1916; and "T.B. Kidner Takes Post on Dominion's Hospitals Board," *Morning Albertan*, 11 January 1916.

49 It is unclear how much of this idea was Kidner's and how much was developed in collaboration with others, including Ina Matthews (see chapter 8).

CHAPTER SIX

1 The Rooms, Provincial Archives Division, Newfoundland and Labrador, Jessie Luther Papers, manuscript based on diary and letters, 249 (unpublished).

2 McCarthy, *Women's Culture*, 2–19. Female artists lived in a somewhat circumscribed world, as women in the world of art were seen primarily as collectors and fundraisers.

3 These materials have been edited and published in Rompkey, *Jessie Luther at the Grenfell Mission*.

4 Ibid., 10.

5 Hull House was the first settlement house in the United States (see chapter 4). Jessie Luther's work at Hull House preceded that of the legendary American occupational therapist Eleanor Clarke Slagle, who came to Hull House a decade later.

6 University of Illinois at Chicago, *Opening New Worlds*, 41.

7 The Rooms, Provincial Archives Division, Newfoundland and Labrador, Jessie Luther Papers, "Industrial treatment for neurasthenics from a layman's point of view." Compare Jessie's experience to the theory put forward by Ach regarding the role of "the will" in recovery. She adds a temporal aspect to his theory by noting that activities were needed while the will still had the power to act. See Ach, *On Volition*.

8 Rompkey, *Jessie Luther at the Grenfell Mission*, xxix; The Rooms, Provincial Archives Division, Newfoundland and Labrador, Jessie Luther Papers, manuscript based on diary and letters, 2. See also Anthony, "Dr Herbert J Hall."

9 Hall, "Work-Cure," 12.

10 Ibid., 13. Although Hall refers to the Butler Hospital in this article, he does not mention Jessie Luther.

11 Rompkey, *Jessie Luther at the Grenfell Mission*, 10.

12 Ibid., xxi–xxiii.

13 Rompkey, "Grenfell, Wilfred Thomason," 270; see also Rompkey, *Grenfell of Labrador*, 125–40.

14 Ibid., xxx.

15 While she was referred to in the literature on Luther as "director of occupational therapy," her title was likely "director of handicrafts." She would not have had any formal training as an occupational therapist, but would have become registered as such because of her experience in the field.

16 Luther, "Hooked Mats," 78–9, 106. Luther wrote vivid descriptions of her early visits to St Anthony. The mission had two hundred inhabitants and thirty-five houses whose floors were covered in hooked mats, most of which she termed "ugly." The women used their mat frames at any time for leisure, but especially at "matting season" in February, when their duties to help with the fishing had abated. She described the women's attempts to hook into the rugs the words "Don't Spit" in an effort to stop a habit that was not only unpleasant but also dangerous because it might spread tuberculosis. Luther taught the women principles of colour and design, often using dyes that she had made herself. Those who managed a high standard of workmanship were able to establish home industries and sell their mats.

17 There are frequent entries in the Canadian Handicrafts Guild minutes about Grenfell and Luther and the materials that they requested from the guild. For example, in 1907, the guild was to send homespun suitable for clothing in trade for embroidered Indian coats. The minutes state that the CHG agreed to send wool and to begin collecting rags for weaving and note that the "weaving part of their industrial work is in charge of Miss Luther, St Anthony." Grenfell Mats were to become a popular item. See CHG Archives, Minutes, 28 March 1907.

18 American Occupational Therapy Association (hereafter AOTA) Archives, RG 4, Dunton-Hall correspondence, 1 September 1921, series 1, box 2, file 16.

19 Head and Friedland, *Jessie Luther's World of Occupation, circa 1906*, poster for World Federation of Occupational Therapists, Santiago, Chile, 2010.

20 Rompkey, *Jessie Luther*, 197.

21 Luther's involvement at the mission tapered off after what appears to have been disagreements over the management of the Grenfell Industries. However, her decreased involvement may also relate to a subtext in Jessie's story – a romantic relationship between herself and Grenfell. Jessie adored "the doctor," tended to his every whim, and worked hard to help him realize his dreams for the mission. Grenfell paid great attention to Luther, taking her with him on recreational excursions as well as on working visits. He even invited her to join his mother in attending the ceremony at Harvard when he received an honorary degree. One cannot help but imagine Luther's great disappointment when Grenfell not only married another woman, but married someone who became involved in the work at the mission (albeit not that successfully). See also Lynch, *Helping Ourselves*, 5.

22 See the description of Luther's attempts to have her material published in Romp-key, *Jessie Luther*, xi–xiii.

23 McLeod, *In Good Hands*, 11–13; see also Biographical Society of Canada, *Prominent People of the Province of Quebec, 1923–1924*.

24 CHG Archives, Peck, "Things That I Remember," C17.D3 012.

25 "Noted Social Worker Dies," *Gazette*, 8 November 1949.

26 CHG Archives, Peck, "Things That I Remember," C17.D3 012.

27 Peck described winning six pairs of gloves while in Paris, because she could puff smoke through her nose. CHG Archives, Peck, "Things That I Remember," C17. D3 012.

28 McLeod, *In Good Hands*, 20.

29 Peck also helped to found the women's branch of the Antiquarian and Numismatic Society.

30 CHG Archives, *Bulletin*, C11.D1 059.

31 Peck, "The Canadian Handicraft Movement," 8.

32 Ibid., 14.

33 Ibid., 9, 14.

34 CHG Archives, *Bulletin*, C11.D1 059.

35 Ibid.

36 The CHG was at 598A St Catherine Street West, and Holt Renfrew was at 401 St Catherine Street West. CHG Archives, *Bulletin*, C11.D1 059.

37 Forbes was the vice-president of the Great War Veterans' Association and a highly respected paediatric orthopedic surgeon.

38 CHG Archives, "Obituary for Mrs James H Peck," *Gazette*, 8 November 1943, C17.D3 012.

39 Peck took her young daughter, Hester, with her to England. Hester also became involved in the work with soldiers in Canada. Peck refers to the loom in a letter to Marius Barbeau, dated 20 December 1928 (Museum of Canadian Civilization). See also McLeod, *In Good Hands*, 20.

40 UTARMS, Haultain-Primrose correspondence, 10 November 1927; Haultain, "Address by H.E.T. Haultain," 57–9; and Dunlop, "A Brief History of Occupational Therapy," 7. According to Segsworth (in *Retraining Canada's Disabled Soldiers*, 18), Major MacKeen, then district vocational officer for Montreal, asked Peck to organize the work.

41 CHG Archives, Peck, "Things That I Remember," C17.D3 012.

42 CHG Archives, Barbara Carter Collection, C17.D3 012 (reference to letter from Jane Addams).

43 Peck, "From the Canadian Handicrafts Guild," cxxx–cxxxiv.

44 AO, Homewood Sanitarium fonds, Fonds F 1398, minute books of the Board of Directors, 6 July 1912. See also Warsh, *Moments of Unreason*, 118. Pratt regretted his own limited education and wanted an institution where pupils could learn trades through the skilful use of their hands.

45 Jessie Luther was the director of handicrafts at the Butler Hospital.

46 AO, Homewood Sanitarium fonds, Fonds F 1398, annual reports, A.T. Hobbs, 1913.

47 Ibid.

48 Examples of the easy crossing of borders for work and education include Ada Wells Ford, an American, who attended Mount Allison University (program in art) in Sackville, NB, for a course in arts and crafts; Jessie Stewart of Manitoba, who received a bachelor of science degree in fine arts and teachers' college training at Columbia University in New York City prior to attending the ward aides course at the University of Toronto in 1919.

49 AOTA Archives, Register of Occupational Therapists; and LAC, Military Hospitals Commission fonds, acc. 2001-1242, box 4, vol. 1, file 3-28-HX.

50 Root's work experiences reflect the major influences on occupational therapy: the Arts and Crafts movement; educational reform (manual training and sloyd method); the settlement house movement (teaching handicrafts in parish schools and girls' clubs); and mental hygiene (Devereux Mansion in Marblehead, MA, where she worked with Dr Hall, doing weaving and pottery).

51 Moher, "Occupation as a Factor in the Treatment of Insanity," 55–67.

52 Herring, "Diversional Occupation of the Insane," 248.

53 LAC, CAOT fonds, LeVesconte Papers, draft history of occupational therapy in Canada.

54 AO; Windsor Public Library Archives; and LAC, CAOT fonds, LeVesconte Papers.

55 Miss Bathgate went on to attend the ward aides course at U of T in 1918.

CHAPTER SEVEN

1 McMurtrie, *Reconstructing the Crippled Soldier*, 37.

2 Koven, "Remembering and Dismemberment," 1172. See also Bourke, *Dismembering the Male*, 31–75.

3 Morton and Wright, *Winning the Second Battle*, 6–8. See also Macphail, "The General Theme," 1–8.

4 Hospitals were "assembled" in Canada and set up overseas complete with Canadian-trained personnel to treat Canadian soldiers. For example, the Ontario Military Hospital, Orpington, England, came into service on 14 October 1914. Orpington included a needlework room and two wards with verandahs. The Princess Patricia's Canadian Light Infantry was the first contingent of the Canadian Expeditionary Force (CEF) to arrive in England and the first Canadian unit to go to battle. Princess Patricia (who became Lady Patricia Ramsay) taught needlework to the patients at Orpington once a week. She also started the Ladies' Work Association, with the artist Miss Lewis in charge and other ladies to help. They taught people to make lace; do woodcarving, beadwork, basketwork (Indian and other sorts), and old English embroidery; and to knit, sew, paint, and stencil. They also made net bags with the men who had been blinded. See Phillips, "Impressions of the Ontario Military Hospital," 24–6.

5 Sassoon speaks of "getting a Blighty" in his *Memoirs of an Infantry Officer* as does Robert Graves in *Goodbye to All That*. Some "Blighty" wounds were reportedly self-inflicted and often did not achieve the intended return to England. Keshen

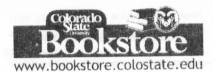

have self-inflicted wounds

during Canada's Great War,

...mmission (hereafter MHC)

...he Somme. By the end of

...had enlisted had died. See

...Commission," 337–9.

...liers' Commission (ISC) by

...ISC was now placed under

...ment Sir James Lougheed.

...anch and establish its own

...Commission, *The Report*

...*ada, May 1918.* All three

...resented the same day (21

...the MHC upon being ap-

...home owned by Mr and

...urpose. Ina Matthews was

...).

...nical College in 1907, Pre-

...plan for re-educating the

...red workers back to work,

...le to return to their former

15 LAC, MHC fonds, "The Provision of Employment for Members of the CEF on Their Return to Canada," Sessional Paper 35a, 6–7.

16 Ibid., 9. Concern for injured soldiers degenerating into unemployables is also highlighted in Reznick's work *John Galsworthy and Disabled Soldiers of the Great War.*

17 LAC, MHC fonds, "Provision of Employment for Members of the CEF on Their Return to Canada," Sessional Paper 35a, 9.

18 Bourillon, "Functional Readaptation," 30. "For instance, an accountant, amputated of a leg, can resume his clerical work and do it as in the past without any reduction of salary, while a pianist deprived of the use of an indispensable finger by paralysis or the cutting of the tendons will be unable to exercise his profession and be reduced to poverty."

19 Canadian ward aides did not serve overseas and were thus protected from the ethical dilemmas faced by health professionals who did. The latter group were obliged to treat wounded soldiers so that they could return as quickly as possible

to the front, where they again risked death. See Cooter, "Malingering in Modernity," 125–48.

20 Bloom Hoover, "Diversional Occupational Therapy in World War I," 881. See also Harris, *The Redemption of the Disabled;* and Friedland, "Diversional Activity," 603–8.

21 Bloom Hoover, "Diversional Occupational Therapy in World War I," 883.

22 Galsworthy, *Another Sheaf*, 8.

23 McLennan, Introduction, 9. See also Koven, "Remembering and Dismemberment," for the new set of obligations that the injured soldier was to accept.

24 Todd, "Returned Soldiers and the Medical Profession," 355.

25 Price, "Lives and Limbs," 1–16.

26 In the August 1918 issue of *Reconstruction*, the article entitled "The Film in England" (p. 8) states that some 6,650 soldiers had viewed the film.

27 "Filmdom Screenings for Picture Patrons," *Toronto Daily News*, 24 August 1918.

28 Keshen, *Propaganda and Censorship*, 59–61.

29 Harris, *The Redemption of the Disabled*, 44–5.

30 LAC, DVA fonds, RG 32, Scammell-Segsworth correspondence. Kidner had come to Calgary after his time in Nova Scotia and New Brunswick as an organizer of manual training in the schools (see chapter 5). He was appointed as vocational secretary in December 1915.

31 LAC, DVA fonds, RG 38, Kidner-Haultain correspondence, vol. 232. Ontario attempted to keep control over its vocational programs and remain independent of Ottawa – except for receiving financial support. Ultimately, its program was seen as inferior and was made to align with that of the other provinces.

32 Morton and Wright, *Winning the Second Battle*, 33.

33 The terms "vocational training" and "occupational therapy" were used interchangeably at this time. See comment for OSOT appeal in Primrose, "Ontario Society of Occupational Therapy," March 1923.

34 "Returned Soldiers Take to Vocational Training," *Toronto Globe*, 4 March 1916.

35 Morton and Wright, *Winning the Second Battle*, 32.

36 Special Committee on Returned Soldiers, *Proceedings*, 102.

37 Kidner, "Vocational Work," 145. There was concern that soldiers who had been trained to do as they were told would find it difficult to think for themselves in their new situation.

38 Trent, "Ward Aides," 2–3.

39 Barton, *Re-education*, 5.

40 Galsworthy, *Another Sheaf*, 6–7.

41 Bourke, *Dismembering the Male*, 31–75.

42 Dobell, "Organization of the Training of the Disabled," 15.

43 Attention was drawn to the fact that in Canada, of some five thousand men who had needed re-education, only about three hundred had refused the opportunity, whereas in England and France, there was great difficulty inducing men to accept the training offered. See Reconstruction, "Explaining Popular Misconceptions," 12.

44 According to Invalided Soldiers' Commission, *Report of the Work of the Invalided Soldiers' Commission* of 1918, "All pensions are determined by the disability of the applicant without reference to his occupation prior to enlistment, *and no reduction can be made from the amount awarded owing to the man having undertaken work or perfected himself in some form of industry*," 49. This applied especially to those disabled men who were granted courses of re-education by the Invalided Soldiers' Commission. In January 1918, J.K.L. Ross, whose wife Ethel Matthews is mentioned in chapter 8, was named chair of the Board of Pension Commissioners after having served for two years in the navy in command of a destroyer on the North Atlantic.

45 Slagle toured Canadian military hospitals in 1917 as a guest of Kidner. They had likely met at the founding meeting of NSPOT. See Dobschuetz, "Slagle, Eleanor Clarke," 804.

46 Black, "Salvaging War's Waste," 472.

47 Kidner, *Occupational Therapy*, 41.

48 AOTA, "President's Report," 290–8. During that visit to Clifton Springs in 1917, Kidner had met occupational therapist Winifred Brainerd when the group visited Clifton Springs Sanitarium. Soon thereafter he invited her to direct the ward aides course at the University of Toronto.

49 Prosser, "War Work in Vocational Education," 263–70.

50 Creighton, "Graded Activity," 745–8.

51 Hayes, "Ward Occupational Therapy for the Military Hospitals," 439–40.

52 Freidson, *Profession of Medicine*, 71.

CHAPTER EIGHT

1 Milwaukee-Downer College (hereafter MDC) Archives, Goodman, "Occupational therapy," *The Kodak*, series 6, box 3, folder 1.

2 Lowe, "Women, Work, and the Office," 253–69. For examples of work taken on by women during the war, see the leaflets from the Department of Public Information at http://pw2oc.mcmaster.ca/node/37689.

3 While women were applauded for their often non-traditional work during the war, they were also criticized. Dr James Burnet, writing in the *Canadian Practitioner and Review* in 1917, commented that these jobs, along with those of amateur nurses, presented a threat to morality, and that the sexual basis of their choices needed to be recognized. He was particularly concerned over the "certain glamour, if nothing more, in the wearing of male attire." Burnet, "Women War-Workers," 418.

4 Socks knit by Marion Simpson of Hamilton, Ontario, were sent along with a note for the soldier and a request for a reply from him, thus making a personal, and much needed, connection. See http://pw2oc.mcmaster.ca/case-study/socks-boys-marion-simpson-and-knitters-first-world-war. See also Blunden, *Undertones of War*, descriptions of life in the trenches.

5 Church, "War Time Experiences of Toronto, Canada," 25. By September 1914, the Ladies Branch of the Centre and South Toronto Conservative Club had begun collecting funds for "the Soldiers Socks and Cap Fund." See letter from Mrs Arthur (Gertrude) Van Koughnet thanking Ina Matthews for her contribution, in Matthews, *The Oslers*, 31.

6 See Friedland and Rais, "Helen Primrose LeVesconte," for reference to Amelia Earhart's work with the VAD in Toronto. LeVesconte, soon to become a prominent occupational therapist, was a member of the VAD at the Spadina Military Hospital in Toronto during the war. Some Canadian VADs worked overseas; for example, Alice Lighthall, the daughter of Cybel (see this chapter) served in France, as did Isabella Mary (Abbott) Plummer, the mother of Canadian actor Christopher Plummer. Plummer, *In Spite of Myself*, 27.

7 Haultain, "Address by H.E.T. Haultain at 25th Anniversary," 58–9.

8 LAC, CAOT fonds, Haultain to Primrose, 10 November 1927, file: copies of correspondence 1918–1920s.

9 Haultain, "Address by H.E.T. Haultain at 25th Anniversary," 59.

10 Marchildon, "Matthews, Wilmot Deloui."

11 Information on Mrs W.D. Matthews's activities is available from a variety of public sources, including a pamphlet on the Curative Work Shop printed in 1927.

12 T.D. Regehr, "Ross, James." The Ross Convalescent Home at 100 King's Road eventually became St Rita's Hospital. The home that J.K.L. and Ethel built in 1905 was adjacent, at 74 King's Road. Now the Martin Arms hotel, it retains the original dining room. See "Sydney Resident Owner of First Triple Crown Winner," *Cape Breton Post*, 26 April 2008. (Some accounts reverse the house numbers on King's Road.)

13 Ibid. J.K.L. was perhaps best known for owning racehorses. See also Ross, *Boots and Saddles*. Ross served in the navy during the war and in 1918 became chair of the Board of Pensions.

14 See NSARM, MG 1, Dr Murdoch D. Morrison Papers, vol. 709, no. 9, for a description of the staffing and renovations carried out under the direction of an officer of the Royal Victoria Hospital in Montreal. J.K.L. Ross had inherited $16 million on his father's death and was very generous with his wealth until he went bankrupt in 1928. An obituary for the first soldier to die at the Ross Military Hospital notes that the matron, "Miss" Ross, provided a wreath for the coffin. It is likely that the matron was Mrs Ross. *Sydney Post*, 17 February 1917.

15 The first indication of Ina's interest in the war effort is of her having sent a contribution to the "Soldiers Socks and Cap Fund." The contribution consisted of her own cheque plus a collection she had organized at Roches Point, in Ontario, which was her summer home. Five young boys, the sons of family and neighbours, had also collected money for the fund (a letter from Mrs Van Koughnet, dated 3 September 1914, thanks Ina for her contribution; see Matthews, *The Oslers*, 31). Family members recalled that Ina always had fine knitting and

needlework on the go. See Morton and Wright, *Winning the Second Battle*, 19–43, for the work done by women at home.

16 The home is now the Newman Centre at the University of Toronto.

17 Personal communication from family member.

18 Ibid.

19 LAC, Military Hospitals Commission fonds, RG 38, Sexton to Robertson, 8 October 1915. Robertson was formerly with the Macdonald Manual Training Fund (see chapter 5), where he had worked closely with Kidner.

20 "Training Disabled Soldiers," *Morning Chronicle* (Halifax), 27 October 1915. See also Hunt, *Nova Scotia's Part in the Great War*, 330, in which he notes that Ina had a pamphlet describing the early efforts of France in rehabilitating "war cripples."

21 Fingard, "Murray, George Henry." Ina and the Rosses likely had personal and business connections to Murray that would have made it easier for them to gain his support. For example, Murray would have known J.K.L. Ross through his dealings with Dominion Coal and Steel. While Murray served as an MP in Halifax, his wife remained in North Sydney, and in such a small community, these families would likely have known one another socially.

22 Hunt, *Nova Scotia's Part in the Great War*, 338.

23 Matthews, *The Oslers*. This edited and annotated collection of letters provides a rare glimpse of the war as seen through the eyes of this large and prominent family. Annabel ("Amo") Matthews was the daughter of E.B. Osler (and niece of Sir William Osler, the internationally known physician), wife of Wilmot L. Matthews, and sister-in-law of Ina Matthews (MacKinnon). Don Matthews, who edited the collection, is Amo's grandson. The letters were found by chance in a trunk in the attic. Arnold writes to his sister-in-law (Amo) of having seen Ina on 28 March 1916 (p. 133).

24 Discussions with family members.

25 Matthews's role is recorded in several reports of the time. See Morton and Wright, *Winning the Second Battle*, 15, 32; Segsworth, *Retraining Canada's Disabled Soldiers*, 10; Hunt, *Nova Scotia's Part in the Great War*; and LAC, Military Hospitals fonds, RG 38, Scammell to Segsworth, 28 April 1919, vol. 203, file 20-189. These references suggest a concern that Ina's name not be omitted, but no information about her or her initial plan has ever been reported despite it being unusual for a woman to have been involved at this level. Of note is the discrepancy in the description of Ina Matthews provided by family members. One source describes her as a quiet person whose husband was the more forceful party. In addition, it was pointed out that Ina was not very attractive, while her sister Ethel was considered a beauty and very social. However, a letter dated 19 May 1916 from Isobel (daughter of Edward Osler) disputes this view: "I saw Ina the other day looking so pretty and in great spirits" (Matthews, *The Oslers*, 141). Of the many great nieces, nephews, cousins, and grandchildren contacted, none could remember anything of note regarding Ina or her ability to have made

such a plan. Her daughter-in-law, Marjorie MacKinnon, was able to contribute the most information, although she married into the family just two years before Ina's death and so her knowledge was limited. Her husband, Peter, who was Ina's son, died very soon thereafter.

26 LAC, Military Hospitals fonds, RG 38, Scammell to Segsworth, 28 April 1919, vol. 203, file 20-189.

27 Edmonton Public School Archives and Museum, Board Minutes (#304), Report No. 19-1914 of Committee on School Management. Goodman was also offered a position in Saskatchewan.

28 Edmonton Public Schools Archives and Museum, Goodman correspondence, acc. 84-1-3173.

29 MDC Archives, OT History File, McNary to Goodman, 3 December 1954, series 6, box 3.

30 Edmonton Public School Archives and Museum, Goodman correspondence, acc. 84.1.3173.

31 MDC Archives, Upham to Board of Administration, 17 September 1918, series 1, box 7. See also Gutman, "Influence of the U.S. Military," 256–62.

32 MDC Archives, Upham Davis to Sabin, undated, series 1, box 7.

33 MDC Archives, President's Informal Report, 22 November 1918, series 1, box 8.

34 MDC Archives, Goodman correspondence, series 6, box 3.

35 Ibid. Sabin, president of MDC, wrote to the American consul in Winnipeg on 12 October 1918 saying that the college was not aware of any law that would prohibit "the entry of Canadians who are of the teaching or nursing profession, among the so-called 'learned professions,'" and asked that he use his authority to secure permission for Goodman to enter into the United States. The American consul general replied: "In going over the list of professions admissible to the United States, no mention is made of what is known as 'occupational therapy.' If you are in touch with any person of influence in Washington, they may be able to go into the subject with the Secretary of Labor, who would doubtless instruct the immigration officials to admit Miss Goodman" (15 October 1918).

36 MDC Archives, Goodman to Upham, 2 September 1918, series 1, box 7.

37 The first fieldwork site was at Muirdale Tuberculosis Sanitarium.

38 MDC Archives, newspaper advertisements for occupational therapy program at MDC, 29 September 1918 (*Milwaukee Sentinel*), 6 October 1918 (*Milwaukee Journal*), series 9, box 2.

39 See MDC Archives, application signed by Dunton and endorsed by Slagle, series 1, box 1.

40 AOTA Archives, Dunton-Hall correspondence regarding a meeting with American Hospital Association, 27 March 1922, series 1, box 2, file 16.

41 See Goodman, "The Industrial Case," 193–203; and Goodman, "Corrective Work for Children," 181–8.

42 MDC Archives, series 6, boxes 2, 3, and 9; series 1, boxes 7 and 8. See also http://www.caot.ca/default.asp?pageID=2115.

43 McGill University Archives, Lighthall Family Papers, MS 216 C23/4. Cybel and W.D.'s correspondence was prohibited but occurred nonetheless.

44 Wollons, *Kindergartens and Cultures*; and Murray, *Froebel as a Pioneer*.

45 McGill Archives, Lighthall Family Papers.

46 Ibid.

47 Ibid.

48 Westmount Historical Association Archives, Lighthall Papers; and McLeod, *In Good Hands*, 220.

49 McLeod, *In Good Hands*, 231, 322.

50 LAC, Military Hospitals Commission fonds, Kidner to Warters regarding Wiltshire, 25 February 1918, acc. 2001-1242, box 4, vol. 1, file 3-28-WI. In the United States in 1919, some 125 of 1,200 aides in service were men. See *Report of the In*

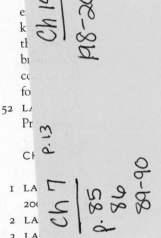

51 S   Military Convalescent

    H   year. Haines had wide

    e   for four years. Kidner

    k   tire state and reported

    th   oke of her as "the real

    b   rected to say that the

    c   that rate. LAC, DVA

    fo   4, file 3-28-HX.

52 L   Census Classification

    Pr

    Ch

1 LA   n, 15 May 1918, acc.

   200

2 LA   e History."

3 LA   series 1-495, acc. 1995/0002, box A-13, file: Copies of Correspondence 1918–1920s. The university was to provide some accommodation, some equipment, and some teaching staff, while the MHC would provide the balance. Haultain noted that the classes were expected to grow very rapidly.

4 UTARMS, "President's Report," 30 June 1918, 15.

5 Burke, *Seeking the Highest Good*, 51–60.

6 Haultain was known for developing the Iron Ring Ceremony for graduating engineers, which persists to this day. For many years "the rings were made by returned crippled soldiers, originally under the guidance of the occupational therapy girls." See Jones, *Delineations of Destiny*, 28.

7 UTARMS, Haultain to Primrose, 10 November 1927.

8 Bott, "Re-educational Work for Soldiers," 270.

9 Bott, "Mechanotherapy," 441; and "Re-educational Work for Soldiers," 269–72. See also Heap, "Training Women for a New 'Women's Profession'"; and Stone-

house, *Moving Together*. Adapted – or remedial (a later term) – exercises likely began with mechanotherapy.

10 Bott, "Functional Re-education," 13.

11 Treatment was given between four and five each afternoon, and a regular "motor service" (i.e., volunteer drivers) transported the patients between the hospitals and the university. Bott, "Re-educational Work for Soldiers," 271.

12 Stonehouse, *Moving Together*, 1–12.

13 UTARMS, Senate Minutes, 13 January 1928, vol. 15, 255–6. Dean Primrose stated that he had, at the October meeting of the senate, inadvertently referred to the late Colonel Wilson and Professor Bott as the originators of training in occupational therapy in Hart House during the later stages of the war, whereas the work had its inception in the engineering department under the direction of Professors Haultain and C.H.C. Wright.

14 United States Army Medical Department, "On the Subject of Reconstruction," 104–7.

15 Creighton, "Graded Activity," 745–8.

16 CAMH Archives, C.K. Clarke Papers, "Statement on Occupational Therapy"; Hall, "Work-Cure," 12–14; and Stevenson, "The Life and Work of Richard Maurice Bucke," 1128–54. This psychological approach to treatment continues today as soldiers returning from the war in Afghanistan learn to deal with the residual effects of their physical injuries as well as with post-traumatic stress disorder, operational stress injuries, or combat-induced stress. Building self-esteem, confidence, and skills is still seen as a key starting point for decreasing dependency. See English, "Leadership and Operational Stress in the Canadian Forces," for a discussion on recent approaches to prevention and treatment of operational stress disorders.

17 UTARMS, Haultain files, CV, 21 September 1961; and Young, *Engineering Education at Toronto*, 142. Haultain appears to have done an excellent job, and he was kept at his position in an ever-expanding unit longer than he wished. By June 1919, exhausted, he informed President Falconer that he had found a worthy successor in Major George Drew. UTARMS, Haultain files, A67-007, 375. According to Jones in *Delineations of Destiny*, Haultain "[o]riginated and carried through, without any remuneration, an extensive program of occupational therapy." But see also Haultain's letter of 2 October 1918 to U of T president Falconer in which he agreed to accept a salary of $5,000 from the Military Hospitals Commission. UTARMS, Haultain correspondence, A67-007.

18 LAC, CAOT fonds, Haultain-Primrose correspondence, 10 November 1927, series I-495, acc. 1995/0002, box A-13. Haultain's wife, Frances Muriel Cronyn, whom he married in 1909, enrolled in the ward aides course in 1919 at age thirty-eight.

19 Haultain, "Address by H.E.T. Haultain," 59.

20 Brainerd, "OT and Me," 280. Kidner asked Brainerd, "Are you tied down here, young woman?" She replied, "Not that I know of." Mr Kidner said, "We'll send for you to come to Canada some day."

21 Ibid., 278–9.
22 Brainerd, "The Beginning of the Training School," 54–6. According to LeVes-conte's draft history, Brainerd was replaced by Jessie Scott, whereas other records name Burnette as the replacement (to be discussed later in this chapter). It is likely that Burnette was in charge, while Scott was an instructor.
23 Ibid., 54.
24 LAC, DVA fonds, Waters and Segsworth correspondence, 15 May 1918, acc. 2001-1242, box 4, p. 128, file 3-28-W1, vol. 1.
25 LAC, DVA fonds, Warters and Kidner correspondence, box 4, file 3-28-W1, vol. 1. The salary issue was set out by W.J. Warters, district vocational officer for Winnipeg, in a letter to Kidner on 9 May 1918. The scale differentiated between teachers in shops (starting at $100), teachers in classrooms (at $120), and men in charge of departments with assistants under them ($150). All had increments set out and ceilings that were to remain no matter how long individuals were in employment.
26 AOTA Archives, Dunton correspondence. Dunton wrote to Brainerd on 12 September 1918 telling her he was glad to have her back in the United States. A year later (16 December 1919), he wrote asking her to share her expertise on using painting as an activity for soldiers, saying that her knowledge would help others and should be passed on.
27 "Assistant Vice-President N.L. Burnette Retires," *Northern Star*, January–February 1951, 26, 29; and personal communication with Burnette's daughter.
28 Construction of a new provincial psychiatric facility at Whitby had been started in 1912; plans were set aside by the war and the subsequent need for more convalescent beds. From 1916 to 1919, Whitby Hospital's buildings were under the control of the MHC.
29 LAC, "Military Hospitals Report," 14 November 1917.
30 Segsworth, *Retraining Canada's Disabled Soldiers*, 37. See also AOTA Archives, Dunton to Slagle, 7 September 1918.
31 In 1932, Burnette was awarded an honorary degree by L'école d'hygiène sociale appliqué, Université de Montreal. The citation noted his contributions to public health and his work to bring about a betterment of general social conditions in the Canadian community.
32 Burnette, *Invalid Occupation in War Hospitals*, 29.
33 Burnette, "Invalid Occupation as a Guide," 230.
34 LAC, CAOT fonds, Ward Aides Courses. Others listed as teaching the course included Messrs Chester, Banks, Paton, Harrod, and Jeffreys; Misses Scott, Harris, Patterson, and Stewart; and Professors Price, Guess, and Arkley.
35 Burnette, *Invalid Occupation in War Hospitals*.
36 For discussion of these issues, see Koven, "Remembering and Dismemberment"; and Bourke, *Dismembering the Male*. These works examine society's attempts to mitigate the plight of the injured soldier without ascribing to him the characteristics typically applied to the crippled child. When so-called effeminate crafts

(e.g., weaving, basketry) were taught, it was made clear that the crafts were but the medium for the first mental stimulus – "the agency by which a patient is induced to forget himself and take an interest again in other people and other things." See Canada, *Canada's Work for Disabled Soldiers*, 58.

37   Burnette, *Invalid Occupation in War Hospitals* (foreword). Burnette set out ten principles for occupational therapy; these were based on the fifteen principles of occupational therapy that Burnette helped Dunton formulate for a 1918 publication.

38   Ibid., 24.

39   Burnette, "Invalid Occupation as a Guide," 231. This idea foreshadows the well-known statement by American occupational therapist Mary Reilly that "man, through the use of his hands as they are energized by mind and will, can influence the state of his own health." Reilly, "Occupational Therapy Can Be One of the Great Ideas," 87.

40   Burnette, "Invalid Occupation as a Guide," 231.

41   Ibid. See Rigby and Letts, "Environment and Occupational Performance," 17–29, for a contemporary perspective.

42   Ibid., 229.

43   Ibid., 231. Burnette writes "useful and beautiful things," reversing the phrase made famous by William Morris. In his manual (*Invalid Occupations in War Hospitals*), he acknowledges that he is not championing a return to the age of handi-work but reminds readers that "no machine produces except what the mind of man desires and conceives" (p. 21). And while he also discusses technique and the finished product in terms of their psychological value, Burnette sees occupations as providing an opportunity to educate the soldier on the "beauty of design [to] ... develop his good taste" (p. 21).

44   Burnette, "Occupational Therapy and Mental Hygiene," 18–29.

45   Ibid., 23.

46   Burnette, "Invalid Occupation as a Guide," 228.

47   Burnette, "Occupational Therapy and Mental Hygiene," 21.

48   LAC, DVA fonds, Arnold-Parkinson correspondence, 20 September 1920; and Nettleton to Arnold, 17 September 1920, acc. 2001-01151-2, box 604.

49   Griffin, *In Search of Sanity*, 32–3.

50   See Burnette, "Occupational Therapy in Canadian War Hospitals," 402; and Haultain, "News Notes: H.E.T. Haultain," 58, for descriptions of the uniform. There is some discrepancy regarding the colour. A grad of 1944 recalled that the uniforms of the original ward aides with whom she worked were olive green. Veils appear to have been worn more commonly than hats at this time. Some-time over the next four decades, the insignia moved from the hat to the buckle of the belt. It remained there until the 1960s when therapists began to come out of uniform.

51   See Brintnell and Goldenberg, "Occupational Therapy," for a discussion of the holistic concepts fundamental to the profession. Mind, body, and spirit were

seen as the interacting elements in the therapeutic activities provided to the soldiers. These elements were represented by the triangular form of the insignia as put forth in Trent, "Ward Aides," 2–4.

52 Stead, "The Ontario Society of Occupational Therapy," 8.

53 LAC, CAOT fonds, DSCR Ward Occupations Series, *Note-Books for the Use of Ward Aides Only.* See also Trent, "Ward Aides," 2–3. At a later time, the Latin words *Per Mentum et Manus ad Sanitatum* (through mind and hand to health) were added to the insignia.

54 Haultain, "Address by H.E.T. Haultain," 58.

55 Pringle, "God Bless the 'Girls in Green'!," 48.

56 A play, *The Green Goddess,* starring George Arliss, was presented as a fundraiser for OSOT on 15 January 1923 at the Royal Alexandra Theatre in Toronto. Dr Primrose, as chairman of the advisory board, provided an address on the work of the society and its plans for the future. See OSOT Archives, Annual Meetings, box 1, folder 1920.

57 Burnette, "The Status of Occupational Therapy in Canada," 6–8.

58 LAC, CAOT fonds, Haultain-Kidner correspondence, 19 March 1918 and 26 March 1918.

59 A similar debate occurred in relation to the name of the professional society, a concern being that "occupational therapy" was too cumbersome. Suggested alternatives included "ergotherapy." See Dunton, editorial, 267–8. Interestingly, he had used the term "work therapy" (the literal translation of ergotherapy) almost two decades earlier in an item entitled "Invitation: Occupation and Amusement," 4.

60 George Barton, who organized the founding of the National Society for the Promotion of Occupational Therapy in the United States, was concerned about the meanings conveyed by the various titles being proposed. He said, "One thing I cannot and will not stand for is the use of 'occupational workers.' It means nothing … it does not even suggest the hospital to the casual reader, and it is bad English. We cannot, I think, lose a single opportunity to rub in the word 'therapeutics.' I will insist always that this be the matter of prime importance, both from my interest in the development of a new line of medicine, and from my horrid vision as a sociologist [sic] of what may occur if therapeutics is forgotten." Quoted in Licht, "The Founding and Founders," 269–70.

61 Burnette, "Invalid Occupation as Guide," 230.

62 Segsworth, *Retraining Canada's Disabled Soldiers,* 18.

63 CHG Archives, address given by May Phillips, 13 March 1917, drawer 2, folder 2.

64 Peck's work was also known in other jurisdictions where similar work was being planned. For example, Sir James Lougheed, the president of the MHC, provided a letter of introduction for Mrs Van Koughnet (of Toronto) to visit Peck and discuss the work she was doing.

65 Peck's early experiences in England and with using crafts to treat one of Dr Alexander Mackenzie Forbes's patients had prepared her for this work (see chapter 6).

66 The street numbering has since been changed. The site is occupied by a new building, le Pavillion Birks.

67 There is a story that Gault promised his bishop, William Bennett Bond of the Diocese of Montreal, that if God would give him a son, he would provide a building for the Theological College. By that time, Gault's wife had given birth to eight children, with only a daughter surviving beyond infancy. Gault must have decided to reverse the order of his offer, for he gave the building in 1881, a year before the birth of his son Andrew Hamilton. Andrew Hamilton Gault went on to found the Princess Patricia's Canadian Light Infantry, which was to play such a strong role in the war. Hinton, "Andrew Frederick Gault"; see also Tolmatch, "The Extraordinary Bequest of Brigadier A. Hamilton Gault," 20–1.

68 LAC, Military Hospitals Commission, interdepartmental correspondence, Sexton to Kidner, 6 February 1918.

69 LAC, Kidner to MacKeen, acc. 2001-1242, box 4, file 3-28-HX.

70 LAC, DVA fonds, Brennan-Rexford correspondence, 27 October 1919.

71 While it is clear that the course was held on the McGill premises, there is as yet no information to indicate that it was given under the auspices of the university.

72 "McGill Gives Building to Help Soldiers," Herald, 31 January 1918.

73 See the discussion of Cybel Lighthall in chapter 8.

74 The district vocational officer of Unit "G" complained that aides attending the U of T course had "practically no Hospital Training while in Toronto." He noted that such training was needed not only to better equip the ward aide but also to give the hospitals the assurance that the ward aides were capable of carrying on. LAC, DVA fonds, acc. 2001-1242, box 4, file 3-28-WI, vol. 1.

75 Hall, "The Nurse and the O.T. Aide," 562.

76 Howland, "Occupational Therapy," 411.

77 National Conference of Social Work, "Report of International Conference on the Rehabilitation of the Disabled," 88–95.

78 Susan Tracy (the nurse who published Invalid Occupations in 1910) thought that nurses were needed because of their medical background, which also helped them gain the confidence of doctors and patients, something that might not occur with non-medically oriented teachers or craftworkers.

79 LAC, DVA fonds, letter from Sexton, 23 January 1919, acc. 2001-1242, box 4, file 3-28-VA. See also exchange of letters regarding seven students (Millar, Little, Scott, Merritt, Sutherland, Holmes, and Twigg) from British Columbia who were to attend the ward aides course. All were said to have skills in handiwork, some had relatives who had been killed or were at the front. The course at Columbia University, Teachers College School of Practical Arts, was given by the Department of Nursing and Health and was to appeal to "teachers, supervising nurses and social workers but others, particularly those with a knowledge of craft work, will be admitted." It stressed art subjects (design, drawing), teaching methods, and psychology.

80 LAC, DVA fonds, acc. 2001-1242, box 4, file 3-28-SJ. There is an exchange of some eight letters regarding the application of Miss Annie L. Brock of Saint

John, NB, who was thirty-eight years old and considered outside the acceptable age range.

81 Gilligan, *In a Different Voice*, 4–23. See also Hamlin, "Embracing Our Past," 1028–35; and Frank, "Opening Feminist Histories of Occupational Therapy," 989–99.

82 This special course was likely instituted in response to feelings that the West was being ignored. Andrews wrote to Sir James Lougheed on 4 September 1919 stating that "there is a feeling in the West that Eastern ladies are being given preference in these jobs." LAC, DVA fonds, acc. 2001-1242, box 4, file 3-28-WI, vol. I.

83 Neither Mrs Haultain nor Miss Lash Miller (both of whom were students) was considered "in a position to agree to remain with the Commission for a period of 12 months." LAC, CAOT fonds, Haultain-Arkley correspondence, acc. 1995/0002, box A-13, file: copies of correspondence 1918–1920s. Mrs Haultain became the vice-president of the newly formed OSOT in 1921 but appears gradually to have withdrawn from the profession. The couple later divorced and Professor Haultain spent the last years of his life living at the National Club in Toronto.

84 Colman, "Recruitment Standards and Practices in Occupational Therapy, 1900–1930," 742–8.

85 LAC, CAOT fonds, Haultain correspondence, 12 March 1918.

86 Segsworth, *Retraining Canada's Disabled Soldiers*, 24.

87 LAC, DVA fonds, correspondence between the director of vocational training and Dr G.H. Graham, 3 January 1919. For example, one letter asks that Dorothy (the daughter of Sir James A. Lougheed, then president of the MHC), who graduated from the "Calgary District" class in December 1918, should be sent to British Columbia; and Major T.W. Anderson, a stockbroker, writes to request that his sister be sent back to Toronto from Ste Anne de Bellevue and that she should not lose any holidays in the process.

88 McGill Archives, Lighthall Family Papers, Rexford to Lighthall, 10 September 1918.

89 LAC, Segsworth-Sexton correspondence, acc. 2001-1242, box 4, file 3-28-HX.

CHAPTER TEN

1 LAC, DVA fonds, Stupart's "Report on Ward Aides to Dr W.C. Arnold," acc. 2001-1424, box 3, vol. 5, file 3-28-TO.

2 There is a listing of twenty-two women who had taken the course and since resigned as ward aides. Of the group who had resigned, 40 per cent were married.

3 The records that do exist (which are inconsistent) refer to the graduates in terms of where they had been placed following graduation. Thus, the actual numbers of students in the courses are likely higher.

4 Middleton, *The Municipality of Toronto*, 73.

5 I met with Doris Stupart's daughter Elizabeth in 2003 to discuss her mother's career.

6 LAC, correspondence, acc. 2001-1242, box 4, file 3-28-TO, vol. 1, p. 146. The motto of Roycroft was "Life without industry is guilt; industry without art is brutality." Roycroft's goal was to combine art with utility – just as William Morris had recommended. The original request from Stupart was to send Misses Mowat and Leask. The two aides who were eventually sent were Misses Pickford and Lasby. Leatherwork and metal craft were thought especially suited to the men who were working in their own homes.

7 LAC, DSCR fonds, Stewart to DeLaporte, 20 June 1923.

8 Eaton's was a large department store with branches across Canada.

9 LAC, acc. 2001-1242, box 3, file 3-28-TO, vol. 5. The facilities featured in Stupart's report were Westminster Hospital, Byron Sanatorium, and the Vetcraft Shop, all in London; Pearson Hall, Euclid Hall Hospital, Davisville Hospital, and Dominion Orthopaedic Hospital, in Toronto; the Brant Hospital in Burlington; the Mountain Sanatorium in Hamilton; the Cottage Sanatorium in Gravenhurst; and the Sydenham Hospital and the Mowat Sanatorium in Kingston. The report was submitted to Dr W.C. Arnold on 7 December 1920.

10 Pringle, "God Bless the 'Girls in Green'!," 48–50.

11 OSOT Archives, box 1, folder 1920s. The motion to award life membership to Stupart also included the phrase "and whereas Miss Stupart has recently been married and this Society should show recognition of her outstanding ability and assistance." Presumably the reference to her marriage was to indicate that she would now be leaving the profession.

12 Helen Primrose LeVesconte was a graduate of the first diploma class at U of T and the director of occupational therapy at the university for over thirty years. She worked on a history of the profession and requested information from graduates of the ward aides course.

13 LAC, CAOT fonds, Hudson Edwards and LeVesconte correspondence, 20 March 1970.

14 Ibid.

15 Segsworth, the vocational secretary, had issued a directive (26 December 1919) sanctioning the practice of working with civilians where it seemed especially desirable to do so, but Rexford, then the acting vocational secretary, criticized the practice and asked the ward aides to account for their actions in detail (e.g., how many patients, how much time spent, who paid for the materials, etc.). Eventually, Riches, the district vocational officer, provided this information to Rexford for Hudson (23 January 1920). See LAC, DVA fonds, box 4, file 3-28-RE.

16 Ibid., Riches-Parkinson correspondence, 28 November 1918.

17 LAC, CAOT fonds, Hudson Edwards to LeVesconte, 14 September 1969.

18 Ibid., 20 March 1970.

19 Ibid., 21 October 1968.

20 Ibid., 20 March 1970.

21 Ibid.

22 Ibid.

23 LAC, CAOT fonds, Ward Aides files. Griffin was not in the first class but was in a course within the first year.

24 Hall and Buck, *Handicrafts for the Handicapped*, 115.

25 LAC, DVA fonds, Griffin to Drew, 4 September 1920, acc. 2001-1242, box 4, file 3-28-WI. George Drew was later to become the premier of Ontario (1943–48).

26 LAC, DVA fonds, acc. 2001-1242, box 4, file 3-28-VA. A letter dated 9 November 1918 stated that there would be no more courses after the one beginning 15 October 1918 because there were enough graduates to meet the need. However, the course continued to be offered through to the summer of 1919. For this special western course, a request was made to accept three over-age aides from Winnipeg. Two students were sent from British Columbia, one of whom was a widow (Mrs Partington), whose husband had been killed in France. Partington was accepted and worked at Shaughnessy Hospital in British Columbia after graduating.

27 LAC, DVA fonds, Major Drew (as vocational officer for Ontario) to Mr Parkinson, 3 September 1919, acc. 2001-1242, box 4, file 3-28-WI, vol. 1. In an earlier exchange of letters, Segsworth (who was then the administrator of the Vocational Branch in Ottawa) tells Riches (vocational officer in Regina) that he is "probably a little bit sensitive as most Westerners are." He defends their interaction, saying, "There is nothing in any of my letters which gives you the right to gather that I consider Western people less patriotic than those in the East." LAC, DVA fonds, Segsworth to Riches, 15 March 1918, acc. 2001-1242, box 4, file 3-28-RE. This sentiment was also common in the United States, where there was criticism that everything was being run by a set of easterners.

28 Handwritten four-page letter, 8 January 1920, complaining about the state of the ward aides' uniforms. LAC, DVA fonds, acc. 2001-1242, box 4, file 3-28-WI.

29 LAC, DVA fonds, Rexford to Griffin, 12 January 1920, acc. 2001-1242, box 4, file 3-28-WI, vol. 1.

30 LAC, DVA fonds, Rexford to Hannibal, 17 December 1920, acc. 2001-1242, box 4, file 3-28-TO.

31 Winnipeg General Hospital, *Winnipeg General Hospital Reports and Accounts*, 1920–1922.

32 AOTA Archives, RG 4, application for approval as active member, approved by Dunton, box 2, file 14.

33 LAC, DVA fonds, Sexton to Segsworth, 13 September 1918, acc. 2001-1242, box 4, file 3-28-HX.

34 Information about Jean Blanchard was provided by her daughter, Ann Kerr-Linden, who had tape-recorded an oral history with her mother when Blanchard was seventy-eight. She also presented the information in a class at the Joint Centre for Bioethics at the University of Toronto.

35 Between 9 October and 2 November 1918, 1,682 people died in Toronto from the Spanish influenza. Wilton, "Spanish Flu Outdid WWI in Number of Lives Claimed," 2036–7.

36 It was common at the time for a woman about to give birth to be with her own mother, who would then assist with the birth and early care of the newborn.

37 Lotz, *Head, Heart and Hands*, 17, 20.

38 Ibid., 19–20. Mary Black's papers form part of her family's archives, which are housed at the Nova Scotia Archives and Records Management (NSARM) primarily in MG 1, vol. 2876. Additional information is found in other files within MG 1 as well as in MG 20 and NSARM micro reel #9493.

39 LAC, Sexton to Black, 23 January 1919, acc. 2001-1242, box 4, file 3–28, p. 128.

40 Ibid.

41 LAC, CAOT fonds, Black to Bignell, 3 August 1986. Black remembered the names of the girls in her group as Alice Stairs, Anna McGregor, Jean Hardy, Dorothy Yuill, Gertrude Creelman, and Ethel Harrison.

42 NSARM, MG 1, Mary Black, Item #9 of the agreement between the DSCR and the applicant for training as a ward aide, 1919, vol. 2876. It was often the case that soldiers who had not yet gone overseas were injured or became ill and required occupational therapy services.

43 Nova Scotia Hospital, *Sixty-Fourth Report of the Nova Scotia Hospital*, 10. The classes likely centred on four different activities in occupational therapy.

44 Twohig notes that it was common for residents of Atlantic Canada, and women in particular, to travel to the northeastern states in search of better work opportunities. Twohig, "Once a Therapist," 110.

45 NSARM, MG 1, Houston to Robeson, 9 June 1922, vol. 2876.

46 This hospital eventually housed five thousand patients and had between twenty-five and thirty trained occupational therapists.

47 The Junior League must have withdrawn an offer to Mary Black and then made it again. In its letter dated 3 July 1930, the league stated that Helen LeVesconte was to have come to run the department in the Winnipeg General Hospital. However, LeVesconte's family "was much opposed to her leaving her home at present." The league was therefore seeking Black's services (again).

48 NSARM, MG 1, Black to Slagle, n.d., vol. 2876.

49 Lotz, *Head, Heart, and Hands*, 20. Lotz dedicates his book on the crafts people of Nova Scotia to Mary Black.

50 McKay, *Quest of the Folk*, 152–213. McKay argues that Black was part of tourism's bid to sell folk art and rewrite Nova Scotia's cultural history. He singles out Black for her role in reviving crafts, but notes that she thought little of the weaving produced in Nova Scotia, comparing it unfavourably to the refinement and beauty of weaving in the United States. To correct the situation, Black recommended providing good designs to rural craftworkers for them to copy. Black thought that the economic and cultural motivations for the handicrafts movement had to be indissolubly linked.

51 Brackley, "Mary E. Black." Black also received a number of honours, including the Queen Elizabeth II Silver Jubilee Medal, prizes for her weaving, and many honorary positions.

CHAPTER ELEVEN

1   Griffin, "Some Results of Occupational Therapy," 289.
2   Margaret Harris, a Canadian-trained ward aide from Pictou, NS, and a graduate
    of Mount Allison and the ward aides' class at the U of T, became the head in-
    structor at the St Louis School of Occupational Therapy. See Gibbon, "History
    of Occupational Therapy in the Maritimes," 73–4. Concerns about the "brain
    drain" continue in Canada, as a number of graduates go to the United States to
    earn enough money to pay back student loans.
3   Hayes, "Ward Occupational Therapy for the Military Hospitals," 438–41. See
    also Fagile Low, "The Reconstruction Aides," 38–42.
4   UTARMS, "President's Report," 16 April 1921.
5   Farrar, "Rehabilitation in Nervous and Mental Cases among Ex-Soldiers," 17–25.
6   Many vocational officers became members of NSPOT, including F.M. Riches
    from Saskatchewan, H.W. Hewett of Alberta, and F.H. Sexton of Nova Scotia.
    Others involved in the war effort, such as Dr J.S. Hogg and Norman Burnette of
    Ontario, J.G. Miller of Alberta, and John Kyle of British Columbia, also became
    members. Dr E.A. Bott, who had run the educational program for physiotherapy
    at Hart House in Toronto, was an associate member, and Sir James Lougheed,
    the president of the Military Hospitals Commission, was an honorary member.
    Edith Griffin, then supervisor of occupations at the Tuxedo Hospital in Win-
    nipeg, had been invited to speak at NSPOT's annual meeting in 1920, although
    she was not a registered member. See AOTA Archives, proceedings of annual
    meetings of NSPOT from 1917 to 1919.
7   Stewart, "Occupational Therapy in Canada," 382. In 1922, Jessie Stewart spoke
    to the Maryland Occupational Therapy Society about the work done in Canada
    prior to and after the war. There is some confusion about when the Manitoba
    society was established (1920 or 1922) and whether it was called the Manitoba
    Society of Occupational Therapists of Canada or the Canadian Society of Oc-
    cupational Therapists of Manitoba.
8   OSOT Archives, letters from 1920, box 4, folder 1920.
9   Hall, "The Roll Call," 162–4.
10 Griffin, "Some Results of Occupational Therapy," 281–9. Some injured soldiers
    would likely not have a job if no accommodations were made for their condi-
    tion. The term "curative workshop" was replaced in later years by "sheltered
    workshop."
11 "Occupational Therapeutists: War Experiment Now Ranks as Profession," *Win-
    nipeg Evening Tribune,* 14 July 1923.
12 OSOT Archives, Charter of 1968.
13 Committee members were Misses M. Bickell, M. Orr, H. De Laporte, E. Jackes, P.
    Wallis, and Mrs M. Graham.
14 OSOT Archives. The notice that the letters patent had been granted for the
    purpose of incorporating OSOT (dated 3 February 1921) was sent directly to Sir

Frederick Stupart, the director of the Meteorological Service of Canada at that time.

15 UTARMS, "President's Report," 1921.

16 OSOT Archives, "President's Report," Drawing Room Meeting, Government House, 16 April 1921. The physicians were Drs C.K. Clarke, J.H. Elliott, Glasscoe, D. Graham, W.H. Hill, J.H. Holbrook, G. Howland, J.S. McCullogh, A. Primrose, and C.D. Parfitt. The other prominent citizens were: Mr C.W. Bishop, N.L. Burnette, Prof. J.A. Dale, C.J. Decker, Col. Gartshore, Prof. H.E.T. Haultain, the Hon. Mr Rollo, and Sir Frederick Stupart.

17 OSOT Archives, Primrose to Dr G.E. Wilson, 2 December 1921. The physicians were Wilson, Cunningham, Howland, Elliott, Fleming, and Smith. Minutes of the first meeting of the committee of physicians appointed by Dr Primrose for the Advisory Board, December 1921 (n.d.).

18 OSOT Archives, Minutes of the first meeting of the Committee of Physicians, December 1921. The committee consisted of Drs Wilson, Howland, Cunningham, Fleming, along with Misses Stupart, Graham, and Marks.

19 Heap, "Training Women for a New 'Women's Profession,'" 135–58. See also Gritzer and Arluke, *The Making of Rehabilitation*, for discussion of the medicalizing of occupational therapy in the name of rehabilitation; and Friedland, "Occupational Therapy and Rehabilitation," 373–80.

20 Primrose, "Ontario Society of Occupational Therapy," 292–3.

21 "'Is Practical Christianity' Occupational Therapy Praised," *Toronto Evening Telegram*, 2 May 1925. A second article appeared in "The Woman about Town" section of the same newspaper two days later. Underscoring its intended female audience, the article ended with a description of the dress Mrs Cockshutt had worn (one of the new flowered chiffons in pinkish mauve tones). See "Most Successful Annual Therapy Meeting," *Toronto Evening Telegram*, 4 May 1925.

22 In 1932, the Junior League sponsored a full-time position in occupational therapy at the Hospital for Sick Children and received thirty applications.

23 OSOT Archives, Nagle, "Draft for Article." Volunteering was also an issue in physical therapy in Canada (see Heap, "Training Women") and in occupational therapy in the United States (see Gutman, "Occupational Therapy's Link to Vocational Reeducation," 907–15).

24 Reznick, *Healing the Nation*, 116–37. The first workshops, at Shepherds Bush, were opened on 1 October 1916. The British Red Cross Society and the Order of St John of Jerusalem financed the equipping of the workshops. Such workshops had been connected with the treatment of "cripples" in the past. Of interest is the claim that Nova Scotia opened the first curative workshop for injured soldiers in Sydney six months earlier (see chapter 8).

25 Jones, "The Problem of the Disabled," 281. Jones described having the power to compel soldiers to attend the workshop, but noted that power was not needed.

26 Myers, "Pioneer Occupational Therapists in World War I," 208–15; and Schwab, "The Experiment in Occupational Therapy at Base Hospital 117," 580–93. These

parallel accounts provide fascinating descriptions of the workshops. Of interest is the idea of using the workshop to help sensitize the soldier to the noise that he would be hearing upon returning to the battlefield. See also Reznick, *Healing the Nation*, 123–7.

27 Bourke, *Dismembering the Male*, 31–75.

28 Reed and Sanderson, *Concepts of Occupational Therapy*, 177–8.

29 OSOT Archives, letter from OSOT Executive to the Executive of the IODE in Ontario, 29 April 1922. The IODE certainly supported OSOT in many of its endeavours, but this particular plan put forward by Stupart was never realized.

30 OSOT Archives, Stupart to the IODE, 29 April 1922. The wording of this communication suggests that the workshop may have been seen as the major site for occupational therapy – that is, as a community service on its own and not as an extension of hospital services.

31 Stewart, "Convalescent Workshops," 381–3.

32 The booklet, which is undated, was reprinted in the *U of T Monthly* of 1923 but likely appeared before that date. The officers of the society and board of management are listed. The honorary president remained the lieutenant-governor of Ontario, and Falconer was the vice-president. The president of OSOT was now E. Muriel Bickell; the vice-president, C. Helen Mowat; the secretary, Aileene Marks; and the treasurer, Miss M. Boyd. Dr Primrose was the chairman of the board of management, with Dr Howland the vice-chairman. There were thirty-six board members, seventeen of whom were physicians. Other members included Mrs W.D. Matthews (mother of Ina Matthews, who helped develop the scheme for re-educating injured soldiers; see chapter 8), Sir Frederick Stupart, Prof. Haultain, Mr Chester (an instructor in the ward aides course), and Mrs D.A. Dunlap (of the Dunlap Observatory).

33 Primrose, "Ontario Society for Occupational Therapy," 412–14. The *Toronto Evening Telegram* reported that the curative workshop under the direction of Kathleen de Courcy O'Grady housed 77 patients in 1928; 41 were supported by bursaries, 21 were financed through the Workmen's Compensation Board, and 15 were patients who paid privately. "Occupational Therapy Grows in Canada: Toronto Branch Cleared $6500 at Street Fair," *Toronto Evening Telegram*, 26 September 1928. See also Mowat, "Bursaries in Field Service Work," 41–3.

34 The work at Toronto General Hospital is described as having been carried out as a special branch of the Social Service Department. See Cosbie, *The Toronto General Hospital*.

35 Primrose, "Ontario Society for Occupational Therapy," 412–14.

36 A similar approach was implemented in the 1990s in Ontario. Funds from the Ontario Ministry of Health supported the development of new student fieldwork opportunities in settings that did not employ occupational therapists. Some of these venues opted to establish occupational therapy services after the project ended and the value of the service had been demonstrated (see Friedland, Polatajko, and Gage, "Expanding the Boundaries," 301–9).

37 McDonald, "Curative Workshops," http://www.caot.ca/default.asp?pageid=1487. The Toronto Junior League also gave $250 to OSOT to provide a bursary at the Hospital for Sick Children. "What Women Are Doing," *Toronto Evening Telegram*, 9 May 1925.

38 B.K. Sandwell, text of radio broadcast, in *Street Fair Extra*, 6 June 1936. Sandwell was editor of *Saturday Night Magazine*. Gordon Sinclair (a popular radio commentator and journalist) and various lords and ladies were also involved. The fairs included a variety of events, such as a dog show, horse racing, boxing, bingo, kissing booths, and refreshments. See "Therapy Street Fair Is Opened," *Globe and Mail*, 30 May 1930. See also Trentham, "Occupational Therapy Street Fair."

39 Canadian Association of Occupational Therapy, editorial, 99–100. Dr Ruth Franks, who wrote this editorial, exhorted therapists to develop a body of volunteers to help in settlement houses and other social service agencies as a means of educating the public about occupational therapy.

40 Occupational Therapy and Rehabilitation, "Meeting of the Quebec Occupational Therapy Society," 313.

41 Reid, "Ergotherapy," cited in S. Licht, *Occupational Therapy Source Book*, 81–7.

42 Court, "Canada's First Women Postgraduates in Psychiatry." Franks, a member of Central Neighbourhood Settlement House, was especially concerned about the welfare of children.

43 LAC, CAOT fonds, Minutes, 20 November 1930 (W.J. Dunlop, secretary).

44 LAC, CAOT fonds, Robinson Papers. The patrons who followed Viscountess Willingdon were the Countess of Bessborough, Lady Tweedsmuir, the Countess of Athlone, the Viscountess Alexander of Tunis, and Governors General Vincent Massey, Georges Vanier, Roland Michener, Jules Leger, Edward Schreyer, and Jeanne Sauvé. Of interest is the fact that Her Excellency Sharon Johnston, the wife of the current governor general of Canada (His Excellency David Johnston), graduated from Physical and Occupational Therapy at the University of Toronto in 1966.

45 Dunton, editorial, 267–8. Dunton mentions the quaintness and beauty of Canada.

46 American Occupational Therapy Association, "Fifteenth Annual Meeting of the AOTA," 397–402. Many dignitaries attended, including the lieutenant-governor of Ontario and the chairman of the board of governors of U of T. Lists of distinguished guests included some familiar names: T.B. Kidner (see chapters 5, 7, and 13), Eleanor Clarke Slagle, Dr W.R. Dunton, Winifred Brainerd (the first director of the ward aides course at U of T; see chapter 9), and Dr Doane (the newly elected president of AOTA). Presentations were made at the conference by several Canadians, including Drs Jackson, Hincks, Stevenson, and McGie, and Maude Richardson (from the Whitby Hospital), and C. Helen Mowat (from the Toronto Curative Workshop). A tea was given by the Toronto Association of Occupational Therapy at the workshop, and a banquet was held at the Royal York Hotel. Speakers at the banquet included Dr Hincks, Dr Primrose, Mr Kidner, Mr Dunlop, Mrs Slagle, and the Hon. W.G. Martin.

47 Son of George Gooderham of the Gooderham and Worts Distillery family.
48 LAC, CAOT fonds, LeVesconte Papers, draft history of occupational therapy in Canada.
49 Ibid.
50 Canadian Association of Occupational Therapy, "The Canadian Journal of Occupational Therapy," 3.
51 The run for CJOT in October 2009 was 5,750, with an additional 986 readers viewing the online version only.
52 Howland, "President's Address," 4–6.
53 Howland, editorial, 4.
54 Ibid.
55 Ibid.
56 R. Franks, editorial, 99–100.
57 Goode, "Encroachment," 903. See also Hamilton, "News Notes," 60–3.

CHAPTER TWELVE

1   LeVesconte, "Our Basic Tools," 52.
2   OSOT Archives, "President's Report," 1921.
3   "Therapy Course Will Be Given by University," Varsity, 30 January 1922. The lectures were held from 5 to 6 PM. The first two, on the meaning of intelligence, were given by Dr Peter Sandford of the Ontario College of Education. Dr Goldwin Howland was to discuss nervous diseases in the next three, and the content of the remaining lectures was yet to be determined.
4   Pringle, "God Bless the 'Girls in Green'!," 48–52.
5   LAC, CAOT fonds, LeVesconte Papers, draft history of occupational therapy in Canada.
6   Friedland, University of Toronto: A History, 282–3.
7   UTARMS, Senate Minutes, 8 January 1926, A1968-0012, roll 7, vol. 14, 576–7.
8   Friedland, Robinson, and Cardwell, "In the Beginning," 16.
9   According to LeVesconte's oral history, the final notice was given just ten weeks before the start date.
10 UTARMS, "Occupational Therapy," University of Toronto commencement booklet, 1926.
11 Gillett, "The Four Phases of Academe," 36–47.
12 AOTA Archives, Registry. Wright had experience in military hospitals (Wolsey Barracks Hospital and Davisville Hospital) as well as at the Toronto Hospital for Consumptives in Weston, Ontario. She continued as supervisor of the program until 1933 when LeVesconte took over; in 1936, Wright was an instructor of the Institutes Branch of the Department of Agriculture in Ontario.
13 Gauvreau, "Presbyterianism, Liberal Education, and the Research Ideal," 54.
14 Ibid., 51. The significance of a liberal arts foundation for the education of health professionals in general and occupational therapists in particular has continued to be of interest. Yerxa and Sharrott, "Liberal Arts: The Foundation for Oc-

cupational Therapy," 153–9, make a strong case for a liberal arts education as preparation for occupational therapy – in sharp contrast to those who support no prerequisite courses, or allow other professional courses such as kinesiology.

15 UTARMS, Senate Minutes, 8 January 1926, A1968-0012, p. 576.

16 After Toronto, the programs were added in the following order: 1950, McGill; 1954, Université de Montréal; 1959, Kingston (special course); 1960, University of Alberta and University of Manitoba; 1961, University of British Columbia; 1968, Laval; 1967, Queen's; 1970, University of Western Ontario; 1980, Dalhousie University; 1984, Mohawk College (OT assistants); 1986, University of Ottawa; 2007, Université de Sherbrooke; and, in 2008, the Université du Québec à Trois Rivières. In the 1960s, the University of Saskatchewan was preparing to offer a program, but an apparent lack of available OT faculty caused the plans to collapse. There are now plans to open a program in 2012.

17 "Unique Function Seen in University Halls," *Globe and Mail*, 11 June 1928.

18 Bruce, "An Address," 8. Mabel (McNeill) McRae was something of an exception to the rule described by Bruce. A graduate of Havergal College and the occupational therapy class of 1930, she was working in a Toronto hospital and already married to a newly graduated physician when Dr Howland asked her to go to Scotland, to the Astley Ainslie Hospital, to help develop its occupational therapy service. Her husband followed her overseas; she lived in residence at the hospital and he found an internship in another town; and they were together on weekends. Mabel had an adventurous spirit; she loved occupational therapy and the opportunities it gave her to be independent and to flourish. At age ninety, she still spoke with great delight about her work (personal communications, 1995 and 1996; and student video interview, 1996).

19 American Occupational Therapy Association, "Status of Training Schools," 426–7.

20 LeVesconte, "School Section: University of Toronto, 49–51.

21 Dunlop, "Occupational Therapy – A Career for Young Women," 271–2.

22 UTARMS, Department of OS&OT, Elizabeth Spaulding Sime Papers. There were questions on family social work, community resources, the history of the English Poor Law, the problem of relief, and the characteristics of a good boarding home.

23 University of Toronto Student's Administrative Council, *Torontonensis*, 1928, 124–5.

24 LAC, DVA fonds, RG 38, Clarke to MacIver, vol. 205, file NCF, vol. 1.

25 "Defenders Rally to Refute Varsity 'Trade School' Dig," *Mail and Empire*, 20 November 1929.

26 "Therapy Course Not Discontinued," *Varsity*, 21 January 1930.

27 "Too Many Graduates for Available Openings," *Toronto Evening Telegram*, 2 May 1930.

28 *University of Toronto Monthly*, "Occupational Therapy Course Lengthened," 192.

29 Ibid. The heavy course load continued, but it did not stop students from participating in university life. Even with thirty-five hours of classes each week, oc-

cupational therapy students had proportionately the highest membership in the Women's Training Corp during World War II. Students enjoyed themselves and were popular members on campus. They had a reputation for not taking their craft courses too seriously; for example, in their woodworking course during the 1940s, they reportedly said, "Give us the job and we'll finish the tools"!

30 LAC, CAOT fonds, "Isobel Robinson Oral History."

31 The idea of combining occupational therapy and physical therapy had been considered as early as 1929; see Howland, "The Value of Occupational Therapy in Nervous Diseases," 319. Howland presented his case for a four-year course with a degree. He argued that the Workmen's Compensation Board workers were trained in that way and that in a country like Canada, with its population spread so thinly, the combined worker could be supported where separate services could not. When the U of T committee was considering the course in physiotherapy in 1929, it recommended that the "required academic subjects" be taken together with occupational therapy. It went on to state that arrangements would later be made to enable a student wishing to take both courses to do so by taking one of the courses for two years and then taking an additional year of practical work in the other field. See also LAC, CAOT fonds, LeVesconte Papers, draft history of occupational therapy in Canada. I graduated as a physical and occupational therapist from the University of Toronto in 1960. As a product of the "experiment" with combined training, I could practise as an occupational therapist and/or a physical therapist. Physical therapy, then as now, was more circumscribed; it focused on the science of movement and its interventions were aimed at improving movement. As a discipline, it was, and remains, larger and better understood. Indeed, that was often given as the reason why most graduates of the combined-training program chose to practise as physical therapists; in that capacity, they could more readily understand and explain to others what they were doing and why.

32 Rochon Ford, A Path Not Strewn with Roses, 46–57.

33 There is as yet no information regarding the name "Primrose" and whether it might have had a connection with the family of Dean Primrose or was simply a female first name.

34 Friedland and Rais, "Helen Primrose LeVesconte," 132–3.

35 LeVesconte recalled the arrival of the "people in green uniforms" (i.e., the ward aides) and how effective their work was. When asked about the activities the ward aides used, she replied, "I hate to mention what they did, but then they did the only thing that was sensible to do, something that ... they could measure, that ... a man couldn't say, 'I can't do that because' ... [It was] basketry." UTARMS, "LeVesconte Oral History," 25.

36 Ibid., 4, 12. Earhart had come to Toronto to visit with her sister Muriel, who was attending Saint Margaret's School for teachers. Wanting to be useful to the war effort, she decided to stay on and do volunteer work with the VAD at Spadina Military. See also "Amelia Earhart Once V.A.D. in Toronto," Toronto Star Weekly, 16 June 1928.

37 UTARMS, "LeVesconte Oral History," 38–45. A striking characteristic reported by women who had been in that first course was the stellar quality of the people who lectured to them. LeVesconte recalled (fifty years later) that Professor Wallace had been such a popular lecturer in English that no one ever missed a class. Dr Cates (of the Cates and Basmajian text) lectured in anatomy, and Dr Best (of Banting and Best insulin fame) lectured in physiology. A great favourite was Dr Blatz, who taught psychology and was just then forming the Institute of Child Study. His students reported being dazzled by his words and his charismatic nature. See Friedland and Rais, "Helen Primrose LeVesconte," 134, for a discussion of "The Green Goddesses," which referred to the students' famous green uniforms and, of course, their beauty.

38 Ibid., 134–5.

39 "Occupational Therapy Society," *Toronto Telegram*, 1 May 1925.

40 LeVesconte, *Guideposts of Occupational Therapy*, 54.

41 Ibid., 18.

42 LeVesconte, "Expanding Fields," 12.

43 Friedland and Rais, "Helen Primrose Levesconte," 131–41.

44 LeVesconte, "Expanding Fields," 7.

45 LeVesconte, "Some Aspects of Rehabilitation in Canada," 47–53. She showed a grasp of demographic issues by including comparative statistics, historical facts, and current policy concerns.

46 The material for her book, still in draft form and without references, is broad in scope yet detailed in its examination of ideas and events. She describes a profession with deep and strong roots, one that is destined to grow and become a significant part of the health care landscape. LAC, CAOT fonds, LeVesconte Papers. However, for all her devotion and passion, she was unable to complete the work for publication.

47 LeVesconte wanted to move out of the army "Huts" that had served as temporary housing for the program in 1949. A temporary move into the School of Practical Science was made in 1961. The next temporary move, to 256 McCaul Street in 1966, was followed by a permanent move into the Rehabilitation Sciences Building at 500 University Avenue in 2002. That move brought occupational therapy, physical therapy, speech-language pathology, and the new Graduate Department of Rehabilitation Science under one roof and into a space with good classrooms and study areas, faculty offices with proper walls, and research space.

CHAPTER THIRTEEN

1 Cardwell, "President's Address," 139–40.

2 Dunlop, as director of extension at U of T, was in charge of the course. When the program came into the Faculty of Medicine as part of the Department of Rehabilitation Medicine in 1950, Dr Zinovieff was brought from England to lead it. He was succeeded by Drs Jousse, Crawford, and Milner (a rehabilitation engineer and the first – and only – non-physician to lead the department. A series of as-

sociate deans, all of them male physicians, followed as head of the department until 1994 when occupational therapy became a separate department within the Faculty of Medicine with its own chair. This change put the department on an equal footing (theoretically) with all of the other departments in the faculty.

3 Young, "Obituaries," 389–92. Discussions with relatives of Dr Primrose provided additional details.

4 Smith, "Roll of Honour," 115. Howard Primrose was killed on 26 May 1916.

5 UTARMS, Primrose diary, vol. 2.

6 Primrose was known to direct morning prayers on Sundays on the front porch of his cottage in Muskoka; all would be assembled and anyone who missed the event would be made to sit on a stool. However, Primrose was generally in a hurry to end the prayers and get on with his fishing or other outdoor activities.

7 UTARMS, letter from Mary Louise Gaby.

8 Primrose was president of the Toronto Medical Society in 1900 and of the Academy of Medicine in 1918. In 1931, he became president of the American Surgical Association and in 1932 president of the Canadian Medical Association. See Young, "Obituaries," 389–92.

9 The name of the building (Medical Arts) was considered appropriate for its time, when medicine was still considered more of an art than a science. Situated on the southwest corner of St George and Bloor Streets in Toronto, it was the first purpose-built medical office building in Toronto and was celebrated for its Georgian proportions and craftsmanship.

10 "'Is Practical Christianity' Occupational Therapy Praised," *Toronto Evening Telegram*, 2 May 1925.

11 LAC, Primrose to director of Christie Street Hospital, acc. 2001-1242, box 3, file 3-28, vol. 5.

12 British Medical Journal, "Obituary: Alexander Primrose," 257.

13 Falconer, "Inaugural Address," 10.

14 Gauvreau, "Presbyterianism, Liberal Education and the Research Ideal," 59.

15 Ibid., 39.

16 Hamilton [Stupart], "News Notes," 60–3.

17 Greenlee, *Sir Robert Falconer*, 337–9.

18 Gauvreau, "Presbyterians, Liberal Education and the Research Ideal," 52.

19 Heap, "Training Women for a New 'Women's Profession,'" 147.

20 Friedland and Davids-Brumer, "From Education to Occupation," 27–37; and Friedland and Silva, "Evolving Identities," 349–60.

21 Larsson, "Restoring the Spirit," 45–59.

22 AOTA Archives, RG 4, Dunton-Barton correspondence, 28 February 1917, box 1, file 12.

23 Ibid., 19 and 28 February and 6 March 1917, box 1, file 12.

24 NSPOT, the organization Kidner had helped to found, changed its name to the American Occupational Therapy Association in 1921.

25 Kidner was the head of the Advisory Service on Institutional Construction for the NTBA.

26 Kidner, "Accommodation for Occupational Therapy in Federal Tuberculosis Sanatoriums," 292–4.

27 Kidner served as acting president in 1930 after the sudden death of both the president and the vice-president, Havilland and Carr respectively.

28 Friedland and Silva, "Evolving Identities," 349–60.

29 Friedland, "From Education to Occupation," 33. Mrs Kidner took her daughter, Lilian, and Lilian's three daughters with her. Lilian had already separated from her (Canadian) husband by this time. Kidner's two sons remained in the United States.

30 AOTA Archives, Dunton-Slagle correspondence, 8 April 1929.

31 Barton had distanced himself from the organization early on, and Hall died in 1923 just after completing his term in office. Hall's life and work are captured in a two-part article by his granddaughter in 2005. See Anthony, "Dr Herbert J Hall," 3–19, 21–32.

32 Dunton, "Addresses Made at the Memorial Meeting for Thomas Bessell Kidner," 443–5.

33 AOTA Archives, RG 4, Dunton-Hall correspondence, series 1, box 2, file 16.

34 Friedland and Silva, "Evolving Identities," 349–60. Members were warned to "make certain that the back door is very carefully fastened against pretenders, that others do not crawl in under the fence, and that those who are permitted to enter the front door have the proper credentials of admission." Elwood, "The National Board," 341–2.

35 AOTA Archives, text of Kidner's radio talk broadcast, 5 February 1924, box 1, file 11.

36 AOTA, "Presidents," 290–8. For an analysis of Kidner's contributions in Canada, the United States, and England, respectively, see also Friedland and Davids-Brumer, "From Education to Occupation"; Friedland and Silva, "Evolving Identities"; and Friedland, "Thomas Bessell Kidner and the Development of Occupational Therapy."

37 Friedland and Davids-Brumer, "From Education to Occupation," 27–37.

38 Occupational Therapy and Rehabilitation, "Addresses at the Memorial Meeting for Thomas Bessell Kidner," 435–45.

39 "Thomas B. Kidner Dies; Therapy Group Head," New York Times, 16 June 1932, 21.

40 Howland, "Presidential Address," 7.

41 LeVesconte, "Dr. Goldwin W. Howland," 70.

42 His mother was Laura Chipman, whose sister had married Leonard Tilley, also a father of Confederation. See Osgoode Hall Archives, Oral History, Mr Justice William Howland interview by Kates for the Osgoode Society, book 1, C-81-1-0-126, container Q367.

43 University of Toronto Students' Administrative Council, Torontonensis 1900.

44 LeVesconte, "Dr. Goldwin W. Howland," 70.

45 Osgoode Hall Archives, Oral History, Mr Justice William Howland interview by Kates for the Osgoode Society, C-81-1-0-126, container Q367. Mrs Howland's

son, Mr Justice William Howland, recalls her driving around poor areas of the city leaving food baskets and presents at the homes of those less fortunate at Christmas.

46 Ibid.

47 Bott, "Re-educational Work for Soldiers," 269–72.

48 LeVesconte, "Dr. Goldwin W. Howland" 67–70.

49 Osgoode Hall Archives, Oral History, Mr Justice William Howland interview by Kates for the Osgoode Society, C-81-1-0-126, container Q367. Mr Justice Howland remarked that besides his work in neurology, occupational therapy was a great interest in his father's life.

50 The physician's gatekeeper role was acknowledged in the United States as well. In deciding on a presenter for a paper on occupational therapy at a conference of the AMA, Eleanor Clarke Slagle wrote to Dunton, 3 March 1930, as follows: "[T]he paper on occupational therapy should be presented by a physician [i.e., not by Kidner] because knowing as I do the temper and temperament of doctors in general, and of the AMA in particular … If we could get a big man to speak for us we could get a big audience." Not even Kidner, past president of AOTA, former advisor to the US government, and then a successful consultant, was considered a "big man."

51 Howland, "President's Address," 8.

52 Worthington and Moynihan, "What Is Occupational Therapy?," 10.

53 Osgood Hall Archives, Oral History, Mr Justice William Howland interview by Kates for the Osgoode Society, C-81-1-0-126, container Q367. Mr Justice Wm Howland's oral history talks about his father's hobbies and his fondness for the summer property in Muskoka. Howland was at a fishing camp in Algonquin Park when Tom Thomson's body was found floating on Canoe Lake. Howland was the first to examine the body and to pronounce his death from drowning.

54 Farrar, "Historical Notes," 368–70.

55 Knowles, "Memories of Dr Dunton."

56 AOTA Archives, Hall, Dunton-Hall correspondence, 2 June 1922, series 1, box 2, folder 16.

57 Mill, On the Subjection of Women, 28.

58 Miller, Toward a New Psychology of Women, 4–11.

59 Maxwell and Maxwell, "Inner Fraternity and Outer Sorority," 330–58.

60 "The Renowned Professor Higgins" was created by G.B. Shaw in the play Pygmallion and later in the musical My Fair Lady.

61 Cardwell, "President's address," 139–40.

62 LAC, CAOT fonds, "Isobel Robinson Oral History."

CHAPTER FOURTEEN

1 Burnette, "The Status of Occupational Therapy in Canada," 182.

2 Leacy, Historical Statistics of Canada, series A125–63.

3 Johnson, "The Teacher in Occupational Therapy," 45–51.

4   Howland, "Occupational Therapy," 407–17.

5   Ibid., 415.

6   McGill Archives, Lighthall Family Papers.

7   AOTA Archives, Slagle to Dunton, 28 April 1931. Slagle writes that "It is a little bit refreshing to go to another country and find that they also have difficulties and that personalities seem to stand out even more strongly than in this country." When I started my course in physical and occupational therapy in 1957, we were given a brief component on nursing practices (including instruction in bed-making) and were given to understand that the hospital was the nurses' domain.

8   See Heap and Stuart, "Nurses and Physiotherapists," 179–93.

9   LeVesconte, "Expanding Fields of Occupational Therapy," 11.

10   Burnette, "Invalid Occupation as a Guide," 227.

11   Ibid., 229.

12   Dunlop, "Occupational Therapy – A Career for Young Women," 271–2.

13   Burnette, "Invalid Occupation as a Guide," 228.

14   See comments in Punnett, "Occupational Therapy North of 53," 291–4, regarding work at the Grenfell Mission not being "therapeutic." The definition of what was and was not therapeutic was often in flux.

15   Kidner, "President's Address," 431.

16   Gutman, "Occupational Therapy's Link to Vocational Reeducation," 907–15; and J. Ross, Occupational Therapy and Vocational Rehabilitaion.

17   Meyer, "The Philosophy of Occupation Therapy," 639–42.

18   Hooper and Wood, "Pragmatism and Structuralism in Occupational Therapy," 40–50.

19   Friedland, "Occupational Therapy and Rehabilitation," 373–80.

20   LeVesconte, "An Experiment in Pre-industrial Work," 323.

21   American Occupational Therapy Association, "Annual Meeting of the American Occupational Therapy Association," 745.

22   Kidner, "Reconstruction Schemes in Hospitals," 119. See also Colman, "Maintaining Autonomy," 63–70.

23   Prud'Homme, "What Is a Health Professional?"

24   Howland, "The Value of Occupational Therapy," 317–20; and LeVesconte, "Expanding Fields of Occupational Therapy," 4–12.

25   Blom-Cooper, Occupational Therapy, 49–51.

26   Byers, "Vocational Training in the Treatment of Pulmonary Tuberculosis," 1–7.

27   Creighton, "Graded Activity," 745–8.

28   Bott, "Mechanotherapy," 441–6.

29   LAC, CAOT fonds. See correspondence between Haultain and Primrose regarding the origins of the ward aides program and occupational therapy (chapter 9).

30   Hampson, "Occupational Treatment at Crippled Children's School, Toronto," 57.

31   Gutman, "Occupational Therapy's Link to Vocational Reeducation," 907–15. See also Barris, Cordero, and Christiaansen, "Occupational Therapists' Use of

Media," 679–84, for a discussion of the changing image of occupational therapy that could be seen from their 1986 study, one that resembled physical therapy practice and was less true to the heritage of occupational therapy.

32 Burnette, "The Status of Occupational Therapy in Canada," 8.

33 MacFarlane, "Occupational Therapy and Physiotherapy Combine," 99. When LeVesconte, the newly appointed director of the occupational therapy program at U of T, had spoken of the desirability of combining occupational therapy and physical therapy in 1935, she had envisioned a four-year degree course that would offer courses common to physiotherapy and occupational therapy for the first three years and courses specializing in a particular field in the final year. The combined course that came about in 1950 was not a degree course, and it entailed having all the students take all the courses with the intent that graduates should practise in both fields.

34 Gritzer and Arluke, *The Making of Rehabilitation*, 151–6.

35 A committee of ten physicians and the directors of the two departments (Helen LeVesconte and Lillian Pollard) held its first meeting on 20 October 1949 to discuss the courses that could be combined into one, to choose a name for the combined course, and to draw up a calendar. Minutes of meetings that followed show that a variety of topics caused concern, including the notion raised at the first meeting that perhaps not enough thought had gone into the change. In discussions about specific courses, the dean of medicine raised the concern that the university was not the medium for the teaching of diversional crafts. When it came to choosing specific crafts, Dr Mary Jackson, a psychiatrist and strong member of CAOT's advisory body, recommended that weaving be retained, as it had already been proven to be of great value. In the end, 150 hours were to be devoted to a selected group of crafts. Another interesting discussion centred on a course in public speaking. Lillian Pollard, the head of physiotherapy, said that she had found that most students were inarticulate and unable to direct groups effectively. The course, called "Diction," was approved and thirty hours were allotted to it.

36 For a discussion of the accepted scope of rehabilitation and the ramifications for occupational therapy, see Friedland, "Occupational Therapy and Rehabilitation," 373–80. See also Brintnell et al., "The Rehabilitation Era," 27–8.

37 The latest iteration of occupational therapy education at U of T is a two-year professional master's degree that requires a four-year undergraduate degree for entry. Effective in 2008, CAOT granted academic accreditation only to educational programs that led to a professional master's degree, which was seen as the entry credential. In the United States, there is a growing consensus that the entry-level designation should be a doctoral degree.

38 For a discussion on general systems theory in medical care, see Kielhofner, *Model of Human Occupation*, 24–31. See also Engel, "The Need for a New Medical Model," 37–53; and Guirguis, "Unemployment and Health," s10–s13.

39 LAC, CAOT fonds, LeVesconte Papers, draft history of occupational therapy in Canada; and Friedland, "Occupational Therapy and Rehabilitation," 373–80.

40 In 1983, the question of moving into a community college was raised when Dr Fred Lowy, then dean of the Faculty of Medicine, explained to the Department of Physical Medicine and Rehabilitation that the dearth of research coming from the department raised questions about its continued existence in the university. As there was a program at Mohawk College in Hamilton, his comment was in keeping with a direction that had already been taken elsewhere. The department moved quickly to disarm the dean of his views, and as more faculty members gained doctoral degrees, a greatly increased level of research activity followed.

CHAPTER FIFTEEN

1 G. Frank, "Opening Feminist Histories of Occupational Therapy," 996.
2 Townsend and Polatajko, *Enabling Occupation II*.
3 Townsend and Wilcock, "Occupational Justice and Client-Centred Practice," 75–87.
4 Metaxas, "Eleanor Clarke Slagle and Susan E. Tracy," 39–70.
5 Townsend and Polatajko, *Enabling Occupation II*, 153–72.
6 G. Frank, "Opening Feminist Histories of Occupational Therapy," 996–7.
7 Sands, "When Is Occupation Curative?," 118. Society's interest in spiritualism (including séances) may also have influenced the work of early occupational therapists; making a connection with the past (and the people in it) was seen as a means of gaining guidance and moving forward.
8 McColl, "Spirit, Occupation and Disability," 217–28.
9 Canadian Association of Occupational Therapists, *Occupational Therapy Guidelines for Client-Centred Practice*. These first guidelines, produced in 1983, recognized the contribution of ward aides who had included the concept of the spirit as an essential component of restoring health. See also Brintnell and Goldenberg, "Occupational Therapy," 43.
10 Kirsh, "A Narrative Approach to Addressing Spirituality in Occupational Therapy," 55–61.
11 Egan and Delaat, "The Implicit Spirituality of Occupational Therapy Practice," 115–21.
12 The Daughters of the American Revolution supported an occupational therapy program on Ellis Island in the early 1900s so that new immigrants could engage in occupational therapy during their time in the detention centre. One chaplain recalled telling a woman from an Eastern European country of the various things she could do in the occupational therapy workshop. His advice was followed by a dead silence until she said, "Do you mean I can choose what I can do?" Colonial Homes, "Our Threshold of Liberty," 38.
13 Breines, "Media Education Based on the Philosophy of Pragmatism," 461–4. See also Reynolds, "Textile Art Promoting Well-Being," 58–67.

14 Isabel Fryzberg's *Creative Works Studio* in Toronto helps people with mental illnesses who live in the community. It is located away from the hospital and views
   the illness as an everyday part of life.

15 "Arts for Life," *Baycrest Breakthroughs*, 5–6.

16 See conference on "The Art of Public Health," Dalla Lana School of Public
   Health, University of Toronto, 2010.

17 Education departments in art galleries such as the Art Gallery of Ontario offer
   workshops in creativity and innovation to businesses and corporations.

18 Rather like a kaleidoscope, the various pieces (reflecting the components of
   holism) remain, but with each turn, the pattern (and the intervention) changes.
   This analogy comes from discussions with my colleague Professor Sharon
   Friefeld.

19 For a discussion of current implications of the concept of holism, see McColl,
   "Holistic Occupational Therapy," 72–8.

20 Punnett, "Occupational Therapy North of 53," 291.

21 Macdonald, "Helping Them to Help Themselves," 16.

22 Wood, "Weaving the Warp and Weft of Occupational Therapy," 44–52.

23 Whalley Hammell, "Sacred Texts," 6–13. Hammell bases much of her concern
   about basic assumptions in occupational therapy on whether they are culturally
   specific (ableist, class-bound, etc.).

24 Townsend and Polatajko, *Enabling Occupation II*, 9–61.

25 LeVesconte wrote about her views on the role of the therapist in several publications. See LeVesconte, "Our Basic Tools of Treatments," 52; *Guideposts to Occupational Therapy*, 54; and "The 4th Therapist," 61–4.

26 Fine, "Resilience and Human Adaptability," 493–503.

27 Townsend and Polatajko, *Enabling Occupation II*.

28 Ibid.

29 For recent studies on the current interest in this area, see Palmadottir, "Client-
   Therapist Relationships," 394–401; and Taylor et al., "Therapeutic Use of Self,"
   198–207.

30 Some models take into account the need for long-term relationships to facilitate
   developmental transitions and transitions in care levels. See, for example, Provincial Rehabilitation Reference Group, *Managing the Seams*; and Jacobsen and
   Greenley, "What Is Recovery?"

31 Peloquin, "The Fullness of Empathy," 26.

32 J.D. Frank, "The Therapeutic Use of Self," 92–102.

33 Kirsh and Tate, "Developing a Comprehensive Understanding," 1054–74.

34 Rollnick and Miller, "What Is Motivational Interviewing," 325–34.

35 Mee and Sumsion, "Mental Health Clients," 121–8.

36 Rollnick and Miller, *Motivational Interviewing*, 38.

37 LeVesconte went so far as to say that without a therapeutic relationship there
   could be no expectation of change. Current work recognizes the effects of context (e.g., institutional policies and practices, health care resources) on the op-

portunity to form these relationships. See Mortenson and Dyck, "Power and Client-Centered Practice," 261–7.

38 Gagan and Gagan, "Hospitals."

39 Blom-Cooper, *Occupational Therapy.*

40 Putnam, "The Prosperous Community," 61–74.

41 Bowlby-Sifton, "The Dementia Story," 3–6.

42 "To Teach People to Work Their Own Cure," *Toronto Star Weekly,* 3 June 1922.

43 The Manitoba Society for Occupational Therapy has provided a useful booklet (*Occupational Therapists and Primary Health Care*) outlining evidence for various potential roles for occupational therapy in primary health care. These roles deal with seniors' health promotion, chronic disease management, rural practice, injury prevention and return to work, assistive technology, homelessness, mental health and wellness, transitions from correctional-based settings to the community, health promotion in the schools, and child and youth health promotion. Similarly, successful advocacy by OSOT has prompted Ontario's Ministry of Health and Long-Term Care to expand the list of interdisciplinary health providers to include occupational therapists

44 Friedland and Silva, "Evolving Identities," 349–60.

45 Yerxa, "Health and the Human Spirit for Occupation," 412–18; and Kielhofner, *Model of Human Occupation: Theory and Application.* See also Wright, *Physical Disability,* for a classic work in this field.

46 Pentland and McColl, "Occupational Integrity," 135–7. The attraction of this approach was promoted by an American occupational therapy group a number of years ago when it designed a T-shirt that read, "The doctor saved my life but the OT made it worth living."

47 "Occupational Therapeutists – War Experiment Now Ranks as Profession," *Winnipeg Evening Tribune,* 14 July 1923.

48 See also Harris, "Toward a Restorative Medicine," 1710–12; and Guirguis, "Unemployment and Health," S10–S13.

49 Engel, "The Need for a New Medical Model," 37–53. See also Davidson and Strauss, "Beyond the Biopsychosocial Model," 44–55.

50 Yerxa, "Some Implications of Occupational Therapy's History," 79–83. Doble and Santha, "Occupational Well-Being," 184–90, would consider that the opportunity to enhance well-being could be had through meeting more psychological occupational needs such as the need for affirmation, agency, renewal, etc.

51 Kidner, Editorial, 501.

BIBLIOGRAPHY

ARCHIVES

American Occupational Therapy Association (AOTA) Archive, Baltimore
Archives of Ontario (AO), Toronto
Art Gallery of Ontario Archives, Toronto
Canadian Association of Occupational Therapy (CAOT), Ottawa
Canadian Handicrafts Guild (CHG) Archives, Montreal
Centre for Addictions and Mental Health (CAMH) Archives, Toronto
City of Toronto Archives, Toronto
Edmonton Public Schools Archives and Museum, Edmonton
Glenbow Archives, Calgary
Library and Archives Canada (LAC), Ottawa
Manitoba Society of Occupational Therapy (MSOT) Archives, Winnipeg
McCord Museum Archives, Montreal
McGill University Archives, Montreal
Milwaukee-Downer College (MDC) Archives, University of Wisconsin-Milwaukee
Newberry Library Archives, Chicago
Nova Scotia Archives and Records Management (NSARM), Halifax
Ontario Society of Occupational Therapy (OSOT) Archives, Toronto
Osgoode Hall Archives, Toronto
Provincial Archives of Newfoundland and Labrador (The Rooms), St John's
Swarthmore College Archives, Swarthmore, Pennsylvania
University of British Columbia Archives, Vancouver
University of Illinois at Chicago (UIC), Chicago
University of Toronto Archives and Records Management (UTARMS), Toronto
Westmount Historical Society Archives, Montreal
Whitby Hospital Archives, Whitby, Ontario
Women's Art Association of Canada (WAAC) Archives, Toronto
Windsor Public Library Archives, Windsor, Ontario

NEWSPAPERS

Cape Breton Post
Chronicle Herald (Halifax) and predecessor papers
Chronicle-Telegraph (Quebec) and predecessor papers

Globe and Mail (Toronto) and predecessor papers
Milwaukee Journal
Milwaukee Sentinel
Morning Albertan
Morning Chronicle (Halifax)
New York Times
Toronto Evening Telegram
Sydney Post (Nova Scotia)
Toronto Daily News
Toronto Star
Toronto Star Weekly
Truro Daily News
Varsity (Toronto)
Winnipeg Evening Tribune

WORKS CITED AND CONSULTED

Ach, N. "On Volition." http://www.uni-konstanz.de/kogpsych/ach.atm.

Addams, J. *My Friend, Julia Lathrop*. 3rd edn. New York: Macmillan, 2005.

– *Twenty Years at Hull-House*. 15th edn. New York: Macmillan Company, 1951.

Allen, R. *The Social Passion: Religion and Social Reform in Canada 1914–1928*. Toronto: University of Toronto Press, 1990.

American Occupational Therapy Association. "Fifteenth Annual Meeting of the American Occupational Therapy Association." *Occupational Therapy and Rehabilitation* 10, no. 6 (1931): 397–402.

– "Presidents of the American Occupational Therapy Association (1917–1967)." *American Journal of Occupational Therapy* 21, no. 5 (1967): 290–8.

– "Sixteenth Annual Meeting of the American Occupational Therapy Association." *Occupational Therapy and Rehabilitation* 11, no. 5 (1932): 387–92.

– "Status of Training Schools." *Occupational Therapy and Rehabilitation* 6 (1938): 426–7.

Anderson, B. *Occupational Therapy: Its Place in Australia's History*. Camperdown, NSW: NSW Association of Occupational Therapists, 1988.

Anthony, S.H. "Dr Herbert J Hall: Originator of Honest Work for Occupational Therapy 1904–1923." *Occupational Therapy in Health Care* 19, no. 3 (2005): Part 1, 3–19; Part 2, 21–32.

Bailey, B. "Magnus, Sir Philip, First Baronet (1842–1933)." *Oxford Dictionary of National Biography*. Oxford University Press. http://www.oxforddnb.com/view/printable/40870.

Bain, K. *What the Best College Teachers Do*. Boston: Harvard University Press, 2004.

Bandura, A. "Self-Efficacy: Toward a Unifying Theory of Behavioral Change." *Psychological Review* 84, no. 2 (1977): 191–215.

Barker, P. *Regeneration*. New York: Plume Books, 1991.

Barker-Schwartz, K. "Reclaiming Our Heritage: Connecting the Founding Vision to the Centennial Vision." *American Journal of Occupational Therapy* 63, no. 6 (2009): 681–90.

Barnett, S.A., and H.O. Barnett. *Practicable Socialism*. 3rd edn. London: Longman's Green, 1915.

Barris, R., G. Kielhofner, and J.H. Watts. *Psychosocial Occupational Therapy: Practice in a Pluralistic Arena*. Thorofare, NJ: Slack, 1988.

Barter, J. *Apostles of Beauty: Arts and Crafts from Britain to Chicago*. Exhibition catalogue. Chicago: Art Institute of Chicago, 2009.

Barton, G.E. *Re-Education: An Analysis of the Institutional System of the United States*. Chicago: Houghton Mifflin Company, 1917.

Beck, A.T., A.J. Rush, B.F. Shaw, and G. Emery. *Cognitive Therapy of Depression*. New York: Guilford Press, 1979.

Beers, C.W. *A Mind That Found Itself*. Nutley, NJ: National Association for Mental Health, 1908.

– "The Need and Value of Play, Recreation, and Diversional Occupation among the Insane." *Playground* 7 (1913): 209–15.

Biographical Society of Canada. *Prominent People of the Province of Quebec, 1923–1924*. Montreal: Biographical Society of Canada, 1924.

Black, A. "Salvaging War's Waste." *Red Cross Magazine*, October 1917, 465–72.

Blake, W. "Milton." In *The Complete Poetry and Prose of William Blake*, edited by D.V. Erdman, 95. Berkeley: University of California Press, 2008.

Bliss, M. *William Osler: A Life in Medicine*. Toronto: University of Toronto Press, 1999.

Blom-Cooper, L. *Occupational Therapy: An Emerging Profession in Health Care*. London, UK: College of Occupational Therapists, 1989.

Bloom Hoover, J. "Diversional Occupational Therapy in World War I: A Need for Purpose in Occupations." *American Journal of Occupational Therapy* 50, no. 10 (1996): 881–5.

Blunden, E. *Undertones of War*. London, UK: Penguin Books, 1928.

Bockoven, J.S. *Moral Treatment in American Psychiatry*. New York: Springer Publishing Company, 1972.

Boris, E. *Art and Labor: Ruskin, Morris, and the Craftsman Ideal in America, 1876–1915*. Philadelphia: Temple University Press, 1986.

Bosch, J.L. "Starr, Ellen Gates." In *Women Building Chicago 1790–1990: A Biographical Dictionary*, edited by R.L. Schultz and A. Hast, 838–42. Bloomington: Indiana University Press, 2001.

Bott, E.A. "Functional Re-education." In *Reconstruction Bulletin*, 13. Toronto: J. de Labroquerie Tache, 1918.

– "Mechanotherapy." *American Journal of Orthopedic Surgery* 16, no. 7 (1918): 441–6.

– "Re-educational Work for Soldiers," *U of T Monthly* 17, no. 7 (1917): 269–72.

Bourillon, M. "Functional Readaptation and Professional Re-education of the Disabled Victims of the War." *American Journal of Care for Cripples* 3 (1916): 23–8.

Bourke, J. *Dismembering the Male: Men's Bodies, Britain and the Great War.* Chicago: University of Chicago Press, 1996.

Boutilier, B., and A. Prentice. *Creating Historical Memory: English-Canadian Women and the Work of History.* Vancouver: University of British Columbia Press, 1997.

Bowlby-Sifton, S. "The Dementia Story: Challenging the Art of Occupational Therapy." *Canadian Journal of Occupational Therapy* 64, no. 1 (1997): 3–6.

Brackley, C. "Mary E. Black." OT *Now* (Canadian Association of Occupational Therapists). http://www.caot.ca/default.asp?pageid=1463.

Brainerd, W. "The Beginning of the Training School for Teachers of Occupation Therapy at the University of Toronto." *Proceedings of the Second Annual Meeting of the National Society for the Promotion of Occupational Therapy.* New York: 1918.

– "OT and Me: Early Days at the Sanitarium, Clifton Springs, New York." *American Journal of Occupational Therapy* 21, no. 5 (1967): 278–80.

Breines, E. "Media Education Based on the Philosophy of Pragmatism." *American Journal of Occupational Therapy* 43, no. 7 (1989): 461–4.

– "Pragmatism as a Foundation for Occupational Therapy Curricula." *American Journal of Occupational Therapy* 41, no. 8 (1987): 522–5.

– "Rabbi Hirsch Influenced the Chicago School of Civics and Philanthropy." *American Journal of Occupational Therapy* 46, no. 6 (1992): 567–8.

Brintnell, E.S., M.T. Cardwell, H.M. Madill, and I.M. Robinson. "The Fifties and Sixties. The Rehabilitation Era: Friend or Foe." *Canadian Journal of Occupational Therapy* 53 (1986): 27–8.

Brintnell, E.S, and K. Goldenberg. "Occupational Therapy." In *Rehabilitation Teams: Action and Interaction,* edited by E. Boberg and E. Kassirer, 43–53. Ottawa: Minister of National Health and Welfare, 1983.

British Medical Journal. "Obituary: Alexander Primrose." *British Medical Journal* 2, no. 4363 (1944): 257.

Brown, R.C., and R. Cook. *Canada 1896–1921: A Nation Transformed.* Toronto: McClelland & Stewart, 1981.

Brown, T.J. *Dorothea Dix: New England Reformer.* Cambridge, MA: Harvard University Press, 1998.

Bruce, H. "An Address." *Canadian Journal of Occupational Therapy* 1, no. 2 (1933): 6–9.

Burke, J.P. "A Clinical Perspective on Motivation: Pawn versus Origin." *American Journal of Occupational Therapy* 31, no. 4 (1977): 254–8.

Burke, S.Z. *Seeking the Highest Good: Social Service and Gender at the University of Toronto, 1888–1937.* Toronto: University of Toronto Press, 1996.

Burnet, J. "Women War-Workers and the Sexual Element." *Canadian Practitioner and Review* 42, no. 10 (1917): 417–19.

Burnette, N. "Invalid Occupation as a Guide to the Vocational Fitness of the Handicapped." *Canadian Journal of Mental Hygiene* 1 (1919): 227–31.

– *Invalid Occupation in War Hospitals*. Toronto, 1919.

– "Occupational Therapy and Mental Hygiene." *Mental Hygiene Bulletin* 1, no. 3 (1921): 18–29.

– "Occupational Therapy in Canadian War Hospitals." *Modern Hospital* 11, no. 5 (1918): 401–2.

– "The Status of Occupational Therapy in Canada." *Canadian Journal of Occupational Therapy* 2 (1923): 179–82.

Byers, J.R. "Vocational Training in the Treatment of Pulmonary Tuberculosis." *Canadian Medical Association Journal* 8, no. 1 (1918): 1–7.

– "Original Communications: Vocational Training." *Canadian Practitioner and Review* 63, no. 4 (1918): 115–19.

Canada. Department of Soldiers' Civil Re-establishment. *Canada's Work for Disabled Soldiers*. Ottawa: Canadian Board of Pension Commissioners, 1919.

– *Canada's Work for Disabled Soldiers*. Ottawa: Head Office of the Department of Soldiers' Re-establishment, 1920.

Canadian Architect and Builder. "Hamilton: The Arts & Crafts Association." *Canadian Architect and Builder* 8, no. 5 (1895): 68.

Canadian Association of Occupational Therapists. "The Canadian Journal of Occupational Therapy." *Canadian Journal of Occupational Therapy* 1, no. 1 (1933): 3.

– *Occupational Therapy Guidelines for Client-Centred Practice*. Ottawa: Department of National Health and Welfare, 1991.

Canadian Medical Association. "Canadian National Committee for Mental Hygiene." *Canadian Medical Association Journal* 23, no. 6 (1930): 832–3.

– Editorial: "The Invalided Soldiers' Commission and the New Department of Soldiers Reestablishment." *Canadian Medical Association Journal* 8, no. 5 (1918): 429–35.

– "The Military Hospitals Commission." *Canadian Medical Association Journal* 6, no. 4 (1916): 337–9.

Cardwell, T. "President's Address." *Canadian Journal of Occupational Therapy* 33, no. 4 (1966): 139–40.

Carless, W. *The Arts and Crafts of Canada*. Montreal: McGill University Publishing, 1925.

Carlyle, C. *Past and Present*. London, UK: Chapman and Hall, 1843.

Casson, E. "Some Experiences in Occupational Therapy." *Medical Press and Circular* 197, no. 5185 (1938): 265–8.

Cate, G. *The Correspondence of Thomas Carlyle and John Ruskin*. Stanford, CA: Stanford University Press, 1982.

Charland, L.C. "Benevolent Theory: Moral Treatment at the York Retreat." *History of Psychiatry* 18, no. 1 (2007): 61–80.

Chief Public Health Officer. *Report on the State of Public Health in Canada, 2008.* Ottawa: Public Health Agency Canada, 2008.

Christie, N. *Engendering the State: Family, Work, and Welfare in Canada.* Toronto: University of Toronto Press, 2000.

Church, T.L. "War Time Experiences of Toronto, Canada." *National Municipal Review* 7, no. 1 (1918): 23–7.

Clarke, C.K. "The Fourth Maudsley Lecture." *Journal of Mental Science* 69, no. 286 (1923): 279–96.

– "The Military Hospital for Mental Cases at Cobourg." *Saturday Night,* 23 February 1919.

Cleverdon, C.L. *The Woman Suffrage Movement in Canada.* Toronto: University of Toronto Press, 1974.

Code, L. "Feminist Theory." In *Changing Patterns: Women in Canada,* 2nd edn, edited by S. Burt, L. Code, and L. Dorney, 19–57. Toronto: McClelland & Stewart, 1993.

Colman, W. "Maintaining Autonomy: The Struggle between Occupational Therapy and Physical Medicine." *American Journal of Occupational Therapy* 46, no. 1 (1992): 63–70.

– "Recruitment Standards and Practices in Occupational Therapy, 1900–1930." *American Journal of Occupational Therapy* 44, no. 8 (1990): 742–8.

Colonial Homes. "Our Threshold of Liberty." *Colonial Homes* 16 (October 1990): 36–40.

Constitution and By-laws of the Society of Arts and Crafts of Canada. Edward P. Taylor Research Library and Archives, Art Gallery of Ontario, Toronto. Ottawa: Canadian Institute for Microreproductions, 1998.

Cook, R. "The Triumph and Trials of Materialism (1900–1945)." In *The Illustrated History of Canada,* edited by C. Brown, 377–472. Toronto: Lester & Orpen Dennys, 1987.

Cooter, R. "Malingering in Modernity: Psychological Scripts and Adversarial Encounters During the First World War." In *War, Medicine and Modernity,* edited by M. Cooter, M. Harrison, and S. Sturdy, 125–36. Sutton: Stroud, 1998.

Cosbie, W.G. *The Toronto General Hospital: A Chronicle 1819–1965.* Toronto: Macmillan of Canada, 1975.

Court, J. "Canada's First Women Postgraduates in Psychiatry." http://www.utpsychiatry.ca/centenary/vignette/ Nov07-Vig5-FirstWomenPG.pdf.

Creighton, C. "Graded Activity: Legacy of the Sanatorium." *American Journal of Occupational Therapy* 47, no. 8 (1993): 745–8.

Csikszentmihalyi, M. *Flow: The Psychology of Optimal Experience.* New York: Harper and Row, 1991.

Cumming, E., and W. Kaplan. *The Arts and Crafts Movement*. London: Thames and Hudson, 1991.

Cutchin, M. "Using Deweyan Philosophy to Rename and Reframe Adaptation-to-Environment." *American Journal of Occupational Therapy* 58, no. 3 (2004): 303–12.

Darley, G. "Hill, Octavia (1838–1912)." *Oxford Dictionary of National Biography*. Oxford University Press. http://www.oxforddnb.com/view/article/33873.

Davidson, L., and J.S. Strauss. "Beyond the Biopsychosocial Model: Integrating Disorder, Health, and Recovery." *Psychiatry* 58, no. 1 (1995): 44–55.

Davis, A.E. "Ruskin and the Art-Workmen: Frederick Brigden, Sr., Engraver." *Journal of Pre-Raphaelite Studies* 6/7 (1997): 78–88.

Dewey, J. *Experience and Education*. New York: Macmillan Publishing Co., 1974.

– *Psychology*. New York: Harper and Brothers, 1887.

– *The School and Society*. Delhi, India: Aakar Books, 2008.

Dobell, W. "Organization of the Training of the Disabled in the War." *Special Bulletin*, 1916, 12–28.

Doble, S.E., and J.C. Santha. "Occupational Well-Being: Rethinking Occupational Therapy Outcomes." *Canadian Journal of Occupational Therapy* 75, no. 3 (2008): 184–90.

Dobschuetz, B. "Slagle, Eleanor Clarke." In *Women Building Chicago 1790–1990: A Biographical Dictionary*, edited by R.L. Schultz and A. Hast, 803–5. Bloomington: Indiana University Press, 2001.

Dodd, D. "Eugenics." In *The Oxford Companion to Canadian History*, edited by G. Hallowell, 205–6. Don Mills, ON: Oxford University Press, 2004.

Driver, M. "A Philosophic View of the History of Occupational Therapy in Canada." *Canadian Journal of Occupational Therapy* 35, no. 2 (1968): 52–60.

Duffin, J. *History of Medicine: A Scandalously Short Introduction*. Toronto: University of Toronto Press, 1999.

Dunlop, W.J. "Occupational Therapy – A Career for Young Women." *Social Welfare* 10, no. 12 (1928): 271–2.

– "A Brief History of Occupational Therapy," *Canadian Journal of Occupational Therapy*, 1 (1933): 6–10.

Dunton, W.R. Addresses made at the memorial meeting for Thomas Bessell Kidner. *Occupational Therapy and Rehabilitation* 11, no. 6 (1932): 443–5.

– Editorial. *Occupational Therapy and Rehabilitation* 10 (1931): 267–8.

– "Invitation: Occupation and Amusement." *Maryland Psychiatric Quarterly* 2 (1912): 4.

– *Occupation Therapy: A Manual for Nurses*. Philadelphia and London: W.B. Saunders Company, 1918.

Dutil, E., and F. Ferland. *L'histoire de l'ergothérapie au Québec*. Montreal: Presses de l'Université de Montréal, forthcoming.

Egan, M., and D. Delaat. "Considering Spirituality in Occupational Therapy Practice." *Canadian Journal of Occupational Therapy* 61, no. 2 (1994): 95–102.

Ellis, W. *Outlines of the History and Formation of the Understanding.* London, UK: Smith, Elder and Cornhill, 1847.

Elwood, E. "The National Board of Medical Examiners and Medical Education, and the Possible Effect of the Board's Program on the Spread of Occupational Therapy." *Occupational Therapy and Rehabilitation* 6, no. 5 (1927): 341–8.

Engel, G. "The Need for a New Medical Model: A Challenge for Biomedicine." *Holistic Medicine* 4 (1989): 37–53 (first published in *Science* 196 (1977): 129–36).

English, A. "Leadership and Operational Stress in the Canadian Forces." *Canadian Military Journal,* autumn 2000, 33–8.

Errington, E.J. "Pioneers and Suffragists." In *Changing Patterns: Women in Canada,* 2nd edn, edited by S. Burt, L. Code, and L. Dorney, 59–91. Toronto: McClelland & Stewart, 1993.

Fagile Low, J. "The Reconstruction Aides." *American Journal of Occupational Therapy* 46, no. 1 (1992): 38–42.

Falconer, R. "Inaugural Address." *University of Toronto Monthly* 8 (1907): 6–14.

Farrar, C.B. "Historical Notes: I Remember C.K. Clarke." *American Journal of Psychiatry* 114 (1957): 368–70. .

– "Rehabilitation in Nervous and Mental Cases among Ex-Soldiers." *Canadian Journal of Occupational Therapy* 7, no. 1 (1940): 17–25.

Fidler, G., and J. Fidler. "From Crafts to Competence." *American Journal of Occupational Therapy* 35, no. 9 (1981): 567–73.

Fine, S. "Resilience and Human Adaptability: Who Rises above Adversity? 1990 Eleanor Clarke Slagle Lecture." *American Journal of Occupational Therapy* 45, no. 6 (1991): 493–503.

Fingard, J. "Murray, George Henry." *Dictionary of Canadian Biography.* University of Toronto Press. http://www.biographi.ca/EN/ShowBio.asp?BioId-41977.

Foden, F. *Philip Magnus: Victorian Educational Pioneer.* London, UK: Vallentine, Mitchell, 1970.

Foucault, M. *Madness and Civilization: A History of Insanity in an Age of Reason.* Abingdon, UK: Routledge, 2005.

Frager, R.A., and C.K. Patrias. *Discounted Labour: Women Workers in Canada, 1870–1839.* Toronto: University of Toronto Press, 2005.

Frank, G. "Opening Feminist Histories of Occupational Therapy." *American Journal of Occupational Therapy* 46, no. 11 (1992): 989–99.

Frank, J.D. "The Therapeutic Use of Self." *American Journal of Occupational Therapy* 12, no. 4 (1958): 92–102.

Franks, R. Editorial. *Canadian Journal of Occupational Therapy* 2, no. 4 (1935): 101.

– Editorial. *Canadian Journal of Occupational Therapy* 3, no. 4 (1936): 99–100.

Freidson, E. "Professions and the Occupational Principle." In *The Professions and Their Prospects,* 19–38. Chicago: University of Chicago Press, 1971.

– *Profession of Medicine: A Study of the Sociology of Applied Knowledge.* Chicago: University of Chicago Press, 1988.

Friedland, J. "Diversional Activity: Does It Deserve Its Bad Name?" *American Journal of Occupational Therapy* 42, no. 9 (1988): 603–8.

– "Hilda Goodman." *Occupational Therapy Now*, 2007. http://www.caot.ca/default.asp?pageid=2115.

– "Knowing from Whence We Came: Reflecting on Return-to-Work and Interpersonal Relationships." *Canadian Journal of Occupational Therapy* 68, no. 5 (2001): 266–71.

– "Occupational Therapy." In *TPH: History and Memories of the Toronto Psychiatric Hospital*, edited by E. Shorter, 259–70. Toronto: Wall and Emerson, 1996.

– "Occupational Therapy and Rehabilitation: An Awkward Alliance." *American Journal of Occupational Therapy* 52, no. 5 (1998): 373–80.

– "Thomas Bessell Kidner and the Development of Occupational Therapy in the United Kingdom: Establishing the Links." *British Journal of Occupational Therapy* 70, no. 7 (2007): 292–300.

– "Why Crafts? Influences on the Development of Occupational Therapy in Canada: 1890–1930." Muriel Driver Memorial Lecture. *Canadian Journal of Occupational Therapy* 70, no. 4 (2003): 204–13.

Friedland, J., and N. Davids-Brumer. "From Education to Occupation: The Story of Thomas Bessell Kidner." *Canadian Journal of Occupational Therapy* 74, no. 1 (2007): 27–37.

Friedland, J., H. Polatajko, and M. Gage. "Expanding the Boundaries of Occupational Therapy Practice through Student Fieldwork Experiences: Description of a Provincially-Funded Community Development Project." *Canadian Journal of Occupational Therapy* 68 (2001): 301–9.

Friedland, J., and H. Rais. "Helen Primrose LeVesconte: Clinician, Educator, Visionary." *Canadian Journal of Occupational Therapy* 72 (2005): 131–41.

Friedland, J., and R. Renwick. "Psychosocial Occupational Therapy: Time to Cast Off the Gloom and Doom." *American Journal of Occupational Therapy* 47, no. 5 (1993): 467–71.

Friedland, J., I. Robinson, and T. Cardwell. "In the Beginning: CAOT from 1926–1939." *OT Now* 3, no. 1 (2001): 15–18.

Friedland, J., and J. Silva. "Evolving Identities: Thomas Bessell Kidner and Occupational Therapy in the United States." *American Journal of Occupational Therapy* 62, no. 3 (2008): 349–60.

Friedland, M. *The University of Toronto: A History.* Toronto: University of Toronto Press, 2002.

Froebel, F., E. Michaelis, and H.K. Moore. *Autobiography of Friedrich Froebel.* London, UK: Swan Sonnenschein & Co., 1906.

Frost, S.B., and R.H. Michel. "Macdonald, Sir William Christopher." *Dictionary of Canadian Biography.* University of Toronto Press. http://www.biographi.ca/009004-119.01-e.php?&id_nbr=7550.

Gagan, D., and R. Gagan. *For Patients of Moderate Means: A Social History of the Voluntary Public General Hospital in Canada 1890–1950.* Montreal & Kingston: McGill-Queen's University Press, 2002.

– "Hospitals." In *The Oxford Companion to Canadian History,* edited by G. Hallowell. Oxford University Press.
http://www.oxfordreference.com.myaccess.library.utoronto.ca/views/
ENTRY.html?entry=t148.e751&srn=1&ssid=131383429#FIRSTHIT.

Gagen, R.F. "History of Art Societies in Ontario." In *Canada: An Encyclopaedia of the Country,* edited by J.C. Hopkins, 360–5. Toronto: Linscott, 1898.

Galsworthy, J. *Another Sheaf.* New York: C. Scribner's Sons, 1919.

Gardner, G.H. *The Mind's New Science: History of the Cognitive Revolution.* New York: Basic Books, 1985.

Garton, S. "Seeking Refuge: Why Asylum Facilities Might Still Be Relevant for Mental Health Care Services Today." *Health & History* 11, no. 1 (2009): 25–45.

Gauvreau, M. "Presbyterianism, Liberal Education and the Research Ideal: Sir Robert Falconer and the University of Toronto." In *The Burning Bush and a Few Acres of Snow,* edited by W. Klempa, 39–60. Ottawa: Carleton University Press, 1994.

Gay, H. "Association and Practice: The City and Guilds of London Institute for the Advancement of Technical Education." *Annals of Science* 57 (2000): 369–98.

Giambra, L.M. "A Laboratory Based Method for Investigating Influences on Switching Attention to Task Unrelated Imagery and Thought." *Consciousness and Cognition* 4, no. 1 (1995): 1–21.

Gibbon, M. "History of Occupational Therapy in the Maritimes." *Canadian Journal of Occupational Therapy* 7, no. 2 (1940): 73–4.

Gillett, M. "The Four Phases of Academe: Women in the University." In *The Illusion of Inclusion: Women in Post-Secondary Education,* edited by J. Stalker and S. Prentice, 36–47. Halifax: Fernwood Publishing, 1998.

Gilligan, C. *In a Different Voice: Psychological Theory and Women's Development.* Cambridge, MA: Harvard University Press, 1993.

Ginzberg, L.D. *Women and the Work of Benevolence: Morality, Politics, and Class in the Nineteenth-Century United States.* New Haven: Yale University Press, 1990.

Glazebrook, G.P. *The Story of Toronto.* Toronto: University of Toronto Press, 1971.

Goode, W. "Encroachment, Charlatanism, and the Emerging Profession: Psychology, Sociology and Medicine." *American Sociological Review* 25, no. 6 (1960): 902–14.

Goodman, H. "Corrective Work for Children." *Occupational Therapy and Rehabilitation* 2, no. 3 (1928): 181–8.

– "The Industrial Case from the Accident back to the Job." *Archives of Occupational Therapy* 1, no. 3 (1922): 193–203.

Graves, R. *Goodbye to All That.* London, UK: Penguin Books, 2000.

Gray, C. *Reluctant Genius: The Passionate Life and Inventive Mind of Alexander Graham Bell.* Toronto: HarperCollins, 2006.

Grayson, R. "Footprints on the Sands of Time – Reflecting on the Impact of Attitude." *Australian Occupational Therapy Journal* 40, no. 2 (1993): 55–66.

Gleadle, Kathryn. "Hill, Caroline Southwood (1809–1902)." *Oxford Dictionary of National Biography*. Oxford University Press. http://www.oxforddnb.com/view/article/60328.

Greenland, C. "The Compleat Psychiatrist, Dr. R.M. Bucke's Twenty-Five Years as Medical Superintendent Asylum for the Insane, London, Ontario, 1877–1902." *Canadian Psychiatric Association Journal* 17, no. 1 (1972): 71–7.

– "Three Pioneers of Canadian Psychiatry." *Journal of the American Medical Association* 200, no. 10 (1967): 833–41.

– "What's New? Occupational Therapy in 1883." *Canadian Journal of Occupational Therapy* 29, no. 3 (1962): 79–80.

Greenland, C., and J.R. Colombo. *The New Consciousness: Selected Papers of Richard Maurice Bucke*. Toronto: Colombo & Company, 2007.

Greenlee, J.G. *Sir Robert Falconer: A Biography*. Toronto: University of Toronto Press, 1987.

Griffin, E. "Some Results of Occupational Therapy with Regard to Health, Economics and General Welfare of a Community." *Archives of Occupational Therapy* 1, no. 4 (1922): 281–9.

Griffin, J.D. *In Search of Sanity: A Chronicle of the Canadian Mental Health Association, 1918–1988*. London, ON: Third Eye Publications, 1989.

Griffiths, N.E.S. *The Splendid Vision*. Ottawa: Carleton University Press, 1993.

Gritzer, G., and A. Arluke. *The Making of Rehabilitation: A Political Economy of Medical Specialization, 1890–1980*. Los Angeles: University of California Press, 1985.

Guirguis, S. "Unemployment and Health: Physicians' Role." *International Archives of Occupational and Environmental Health* 72, suppl. issue (1999): S10–S13.

Gutman, S.A. "Influence of the U.S. Military and Occupational Therapy Reconstruction Aides in World War I on the Development of Occupational Therapy." *American Journal of Occupational Therapy* 49, no. 3 (1995): 256–62.

– "Occupational Therapy's Link to Vocational Reeducation, 1910–1925." *American Journal of Occupational Therapy* 51, no. 10 (1997): 907–15.

Gwyn, S. *Tapestry of War: A Private View of Canadians in the Great War*. Toronto: HarperCollins Canada, 2004.

Haas, L.J. "Is Diversional Occupation Always Therapeutic." *American Journal of Occupational Therapy* 1, no. 2 (1922): 117–20.

Hall, H.J. "Neurasthenia. A Study of Etiology, Treatment by Occupation." *Boston Medical and Surgical Journal* 153 (1905): 47–9.

– "The Nurse and the O.T. Aide." *Public Health Nurse*, November 1921, 562.

– "The Roll Call." *Modern Hospital* 19, no. 2 (1922): 162–4.

– "Work-Cure: A Report of Five Years' Experience at an Institution Devoted to the Therapeutic Application of Manual Work." *Journal of the American Medical Association* 54, no. 1 (1910): 12–14.

Hall, H.J., and M. Buck. *Handicrafts for the Handicapped*. New York: Moffat, Yard & Company, 1917.

Hamilton [Stupart], D. "News Notes." *Canadian Journal of Occupational Therapy* 12 (1945): 60–3.

Hamlin, R. "Embracing Our Past, Informing Our Future: A Feminist Re-Vision of Health." *American Journal of Occupational Therapy* 46, no. 11 (1992): 1028–35.

Hampson, J. "Occupational Treatment at Crippled Children's School, Toronto." *Occupational Therapy and Rehabilitation* 12, no. 1 (1933): 55–72.

Harris, G. *The Redemption of the Disabled: A Study of Programmes of Rehabilitation for the Disabled of War and Industry*. New York: D. Appleton and Company, 1919.

Harris, J. "Ruskin and Social Reform." In *Ruskin and the Dawn of the Modern*, edited by D. Birch, 7–55. London: Oxford University Press, 1999.

Harris, J.C. "Toward a Restorative Medicine: The Science of Care." *Journal of the American Medical Association* 301, no. 16 (2009): 1710–12.

Haultain, H.E.T. "News Notes: Address by H.E.T. Haultain at 25th Anniversary of the Ontario Society of Occupational Therapists." *Canadian Journal of Occupational Therapy* 11 (1945): 57–9.

– "Industrial Rehabilitation." *Canadian Medical Association Journal* 8, no. 8 (1918): 703–5.

Hayes, Henry. "Ward Occupational Therapy for the Military Hospitals." *American Journal of Orthopedic Surgery* 16 (1918): 438–41.

Head, B., and J. Friedland. "Jessie Luther." *Occupational Therapy Now*, 2006. http://www.caot.ca/default.asp?pageid=1524.

Heap, R. "From the Science of Housekeeping to the Science of Nutrition and Dietetics at the University of Toronto's Faculty of Household Science, 1900–1950." In *Challenging Professions: Historical and Contemporary Perspectives on Women's Professional Work*, edited by E. Smyth, S. Acker, P. Bourne, and A. Prentice, 141–70. Toronto: University of Toronto Press, 1999.

– "Training Women for a New 'Women's Profession': Physiotherapy Education at the University of Toronto, 1917–40." *History of Education Quarterly* 35, no. 2 (1995): 135–58.

Heap, R., W. Millar, and E. Smyth. *Learning to Practise: Professional Education in Historical and Contemporary Perspective*. Ottawa: University of Ottawa Press, 2005.

Heap, R., and M. Stuart. "Nurses and Physiotherapists: Issues in the Professionalization of Health Care Occupations during and after World War I." *Health and Canadian Society* 3, nos 1–2 (1995): 179–93.

Herring, A.P. "Diversional Occupation of the Insane." *Proceedings of the American Medical-Psychological Association*, 1912, 245–8.

Hilton, T. *The Pre-Raphaelites*. London: Thames and Hudson, 1997.

Hinton, M. "Gault, Andrew Frederick." In *Dictionary of Canadian Biography*. University of Toronto Press. http://www.biographi.ca/009004-119.01-e.php?BioId=40853&query=.

Hooper, B., and W. Wood. "Pragmatism and Structuralism in Occupational Therapy: The Long Conversation." *American Journal of Occupational Therapy* 56, no. 1 (2002): 40–50.

Howland, G. Editorial. *Canadian Journal of Occupational Therapy* 1, no. 1 (1933): 4–5.

– "Occupational Therapy." *Occupational Therapy and Rehabilitation* 5, no. 6 (1926): 407–17.

– "Presidential Address, Annual Convention Canadian Association of Occupational Therapy, 1948." *Canadian Journal of Occupational Therapy* 16, no. 1 (1949): 7.

– "The President's Address at the Annual Convention Canadian Association of Occupational Therapy, 1933." *Canadian Journal of Occupational Therapy* 1, no. 2 (1933): 4–6.

– "The Value of Occupational Therapy in Nervous Diseases." *Occupational Therapy and Rehabilitation* 8 (1929): 317–20.

Hunt, M.S. *Nova Scotia's Part in the Great War.* Halifax: Nova Scotia Publishing Co., 1920.

Invalided Soldiers' Commission. *Report of the Work of the Invalided Soldiers' Commission, Canada, May, 1918.* Ottawa: J. de Labroquerie Taché, 1918.

Jacobson, N., and D. Greenley. "What Is Recovery? A Conceptual Model and Explication." *Psychiatric Services* 52, no. 4 (2001): 482–5.

James, C. "Practical Diversions and Educational Amusements: Evangelia House and the Advent of Canada's Settlement Movement, 1902–09." *Historical Studies in Education* 10, no. 1 (1998): 48–66.

– "Reforming Reform: Toronto's Settlement House Movement, 1900–20." *Canadian Historical Review* 82, no. 1 (2001): 55–90.

Jarvis, E. "Mechanical and Other Employments for Patients in the British Lunatic Asylums." *American Journal of Insanity* 19, no. 2 (1862): 129–45.

Johnson, S.C. "The Teacher in Occupational Therapy." In *Proceedings of the First Annual Meeting of the National Society for the Promotion of Occupational Therapy*, 45–51. Towson, MD: National Society for the Promotion of Occupational Therapy, 1917.

Jones, L.E. *Delineations of Destiny: Biographical Sketches of Some Famous Canadian Professional Engineers.* Toronto: University of Toronto Press, 1985.

Jones, R. "The Problem of the Disabled." *American Journal of Orthopedic Surgery* 16, no. 5 (1918): 273–90.

Jongbloed, L. "Substitutability of Work and the Profession of Occupational Therapists." *Canadian Journal of Occupational Therapy* 51, no. 3 (1984): 131–3.

Joseph, A.E., and G. Moon. "From Retreat to Health Centre: Legislation, Commercial Opportunity and the Repositioning of a Victorian Private Asylum." *Social Science and Medicine* 55, no. 12 (2002): 2193–200.

Kahler, B.R. "Art and Life: The Arts and Crafts Movement in Chicago, 1897–1910." PhD diss., Purdue University, 1986.

Kates, C.J. *Chief Justice W.C.G. Howland: Interviews for the Osgoode Society* [transcript notes]. Toronto: Osgoode Society, 1992.

Kellogg, P.U. "A Canadian City in War Time." *Survey* 38 (1917): 1–14.

Kelvin, N. Introduction to *William Morris on Art and Socialism*, edited by N. Kelvin, xiii–xvi. Mineola, NY: Dover Publications, 1999.

Keshen, Jeffrey. *Propaganda and Censorship during Canada's Great War.* Edmonton: University of Alberta Press, 1996.

Kidner, T.B. "Accommodation for Occupational Therapy in Federal Tuberculosis Sanatoriums." *Modern Hospital* 18 (1922): 292–4.

– "Cardboard Work." *Educational Review* 15 (1902): 164.

– "A Cheap Sand-Table." *Educational Review* 18 (1904): 138.

– Editorial. *Archives of Occupational Therapy* 1 (1922): 449–502.

– *Educational Handwork.* Toronto: Educational Book Co., 1910.

– *Occupational Therapy: The Science of Prescribed Work for Invalids.* New York: W. Kohlhammer/Stugart, 1930.

– "President's Address." *Archives of Occupational Therapy* 3 (1924): 423–31.

– "Reconstruction Schemes in Hospitals for Mental and Nervous Diseases." *Archives of Occupational Therapy* 3, no. 2 (1924): 117–20.

– "The Teacher of Manual Training." *Educational Review* 14 (1900): 142–3.

– "Vocational Work of the Invalided Soldiers' Commission of Canada." *Annals of the American Academy of Political and Social Science* 80 (1918): 141–9.

Kielhofner, G. *Conceptual Foundations of Occupational Therapy.* Philadelphia: F.A. Davis Company, 2004.

– *Model of Human Occupation: Theory and Application.* Philadelphia: Lippincott, Williams, and Wilkins, 2008.

Kilgour, D., ed. *A Strange Elation: Hart House, the First Eighty Years.* Toronto: University of Toronto, 1999.

Kirchhoff, F. *William Morris.* London and Boston: Twayne Publishers, 1978.

Kirkbride, T. *On the Construction, Organization, and General Arrangements of Hospitals for the Insane.* London: Lippincott and Co., 1880.

Kirsh, B. "A Narrative Approach to Addressing Spirituality in Occupational Therapy: Exploring Personal Meaning and Purpose." *Canadian Journal of Occupational Therapy* 63, no. 1 (1996): 55–61.

Kirsh, B., and E. Tate. "Developing a Comprehensive Understanding of the Working Alliance in Community Mental Health." *Qualitative Health Research* 16, no. 8 (2006): 1054–74.

Knowles, F.E. "Memories of Dr Dunton." *Maryland Psychiatrist Newsletter* 22, no 3 (1995): http://www.dunton.org/archive/biographies/William_Rush_Dunton_Jr.htm.

Koven, S. "Remembering and Dismemberment." *American Historical Review* 99 (1994): 1167–202.

– *Slumming: Sexual and Social Politics in Victorian London.* Princeton, NJ: Princeton University Press, 2004.

Lanning, R. "Millar, John." *Dictionary of Canadian Biography*. University of Toronto Press. http://www.biographi.ca/009004-119.01-e.php?&id_nbr=6932&&PHPSESSID=l1ih6dh7lonpvg68qrv4dnqr45.

Larsson, M. "Restoring the Spirit: The Rehabilitation of Disabled Soldiers in Australia after the Great War." *Health & History* 6, no. 2 (2004): 45–59.

Leacy, F.H. *Historical Statistics of Canada*. Ottawa: Statistics Canada, Ministry of Supplies and Services, 1983.

Leard-Coolidge, L. "William Morris and Nineteenth-Century Boston." In *William Morris Centenary Essays*, edited by P. .Faulkner and P. Preston, 156–64. Exeter, UK: University of Exeter Press, 1999.

Leiby, J. *A History of Social Welfare and Social Work in the US*. New York: Columbia University, 1978.

LeVesconte, H. "Dr. Goldwin W. Howland." *Canadian Journal of Occupational Therapy* 17, no. 3 (1950): 67–70.

– "Expanding Fields of Occupational Therapy." *Canadian Journal of Occupational Therapy* 3, no. 1 (1935): 4–12.

– "An Experiment in Pre-Industrial Work for Chronic Women Patients." *Occupational Therapy and Rehabilitation* 13, no. 5 (1934): 317–23.

– "The 4th Therapist." *Canadian Journal of Occupational Therapy* 21, no. 2 (1954): 61–4.

– *Guideposts of Occupational Therapy*. Toronto: University of Toronto Press, 1959.

– "Our Basic Tools of Treatment." *Canadian Journal of Occupational Therapy* 15 (1948): 52–4.

– "The Place of Occupational Therapy in Social Work Planning." *Canadian Journal of Occupational Therapy* 2, no. 1 (1934): 13–16.

– "School Section: University of Toronto." *American Journal of Occupational Therapy* 1, no. 1 (1947): 49–51.

– "Some Aspects of Rehabilitation in Canada." *Canadian Journal of Occupational Therapy* 22 (1955): 47–53.

Levin, R.A. "The Debate over Schooling: Influences of Dewey and Thorndike." *Childhood Education* 68, no. 2 (1991): 71–5.

Levine, R.E. "A Historical Perspective on Professional Values." *Journal of Allied Health* 12, no. 3 (1983): 183–91.

– "The Influence of the Arts-and-Crafts Movement on the Professional Status of Occupational Therapy." *American Journal of Occupational Therapy* 41, no. 4 (1987): 248–54.

Lewis, B. *History: Remembered, Recovered, Invented*. Princeton, NJ: Princeton University Press, 1974.

Licht, S. *Occupational Therapy Source Book*. Baltimore, MD: Williams & Wilkins, 1948.

– "The Founding and Founders of the American Occupational Therapy Association." *American Journal of Occupational Therapy* 21, no. 5 (1967): 269–77.

Lillard, P.P. *Montessori: A Modern Approach*. New York: Schocken Books, 1972.

Link, B., and B. Milcarek. "Selection Factors in the Dispensation of Therapy: The Matthew Effect in the Allocation of Mental Health Resources." *Journal of Health and Social Behaviour* 21, no. 3 (1980): 279–90.

Lochnan, K., D. Schoenherr, and C. Silver. *The Earthly Paradise: Arts and Crafts by William Morris and His Circle from Canadian Collections*. Toronto: Key Porter, 1993.

Loomis, B., and B.D. Wade. *Chicago – Occupational Therapy Beginnings: Hull House, the Henry B. Favill School of Occupations and Eleanor Clarke Slagle*. Chicago: University of Illinois at Chicago, 1973.

– "The Henry B. Favill School of Occupations and Eleanor Clark Slagle." *American Journal of Occupational Therapy* 46, no. 1 (1992): 34–7.

Lotz, J. *Head, Heart, and Hands: Craftspeople in Nova Scotia*, Halifax: Braemer Publishing, 1986.

Lougheed, J.A. *Military Hospitals Commission Canada: Special Bulletin April 1916*. Ottawa: Military Hospitals Commission of Canada, 1916.

Lovett, R.M. "Jane Addams at Hull House." *New Republic*, 14 May 1930, 349–50.

Lowe, G.S. "Women, Work, and the Office: The Feminization of Clerical Occupations in Canada, 1901–1931." In *Rethinking Canada: The Promise of Women's History*, 3rd edn, edited by Veronica Strong-Boag and Anita Clair Fellman, 253–69. Toronto: Oxford University Press, 1997.

Luther, J. "Hooked Mats: How a Native Handicraft of the Women of Newfoundland and Labrador Was Placed on a Paying Basis." *House Beautiful* 40 (1916): 78–106.

Lynch, C. *Helping Ourselves: Crafts of the Grenfell Mission*. Exhibition catalogue. Newfoundland Museum, 1985.

McCarthy, K.D. *Women's Culture: American Philanthropy and Art, 1830–1930*. Chicago: University of Chicago Press, 1991.

McColl, M.A. "Holistic Occupational Therapy: Historical Meaning and Contemporary Implications." *Canadian Journal of Occupational Therapy* 61, no. 2 (1994): 72–8.

– "Spirit, Occupation and Disability." Muriel Driver Memorial Lecture. *Canadian Journal of Occupational Therapy* 67, no. 4 (2000): 217–28.

Macdonald, E.S. "Helping Them to Help Themselves." *House Beautiful* 41 (December 1916): 16–19.

McDonald, H. "Curative Workshops." Canadian Association of Occupational Therapy. http://www.caot.ca/default.asp?pageid=1487.

MacFarlane, J.A. "Occupational Therapy and Physiotherapy Combine at the University of Toronto." *Canadian Journal of Occupational Therapy* 17, no. 3 (1950): 98–9.

McKay, I. *The Quest of the Folk: Antimodernism and Cultural Selection in Twentieth-Century Nova Scotia*. Montreal & Kingston: McGill-Queen's University Press, 1994.

Mackenzie, D. *Canada and the First World War: Essays in Honour of Robert Craig Brown*. Toronto: University of Toronto Press, 2005.

McLennan, J.S. Introduction. *Special Bulletin*, Military Hospitals Commission, April 1916, 9.

McLeod, E.M. *In Good Hands: The Women of the Canadian Handicrafts Guild*. Montreal & Kingston: McGill-Queen's University Press, 1999.

McMurtrie, D.C. *Reconstructing the Crippled Soldier*. New York: Red Cross Institute for Crippled and Disabled Men, 1918.

– "Returning the Disabled Soldier to Economic Independence." *Annals of the American Academy of Political and Social Science* 80 (1918): 62–9.

Macphail, A. "The General Theme." In *The Medical Services (Official History of the Canadian Forces in the Great War 1914–1919)*, 1–8. Ottawa: F.A. Acland, 1925.

Macphail, Agnes. "Tribute to Jane Addams." *Unity*, 1935, 202.

McPherson, K. *Bedside Matters: The Transformation of Canadian Nursing, 1900–1990*. Toronto: Oxford University Press, 1996.

McPherson, K., and M. Stuart. "Writing Nursing History in Canada: Issues and Approaches." *Canadian Bulletin of Medical History* 11 (1994): 3–22.

McQuay, E. "Dr. Goldwin Howland." Canadian Association of Occupational Therapy. http://www.caot.ca/default.asp?pageid=2096.

Manitoba Society of Occupational Therapists. *Occupational Therapists and Primary Health Care*. Winnipeg: Manitoba Society of Occupational Therapists, 2005.

Mansell, D.J. *Forging the Future – A History of Nursing in Canada*. Ann Arbor, MI: Thomas Press, 2004.

Marchildon, G. "Matthews, Wilmot Deloui." *Dictionary of Canadian Biography*. University of Toronto Press. http://www.biographi.ca/009004-119.01-e.php?&id_nbr=7574&interval=25&&PHPSESSID=ggvd5mpm8vfi72ml575rj76u15.

Matthews, D.L. *The Oslers during World War One: Being Letters Chiefly to AMO Matthews from Her Brothers, Cousins, Other Relatives and Friends*. Paiana, Greece: author, 1999.

Maurice, E.S. *Octavia Hill: Early Ideals*. London: George Allen and Unwin, 1928.

Mavor, J. *My Windows on the Street of the World*. Vol. 1. New York: J.M. Dent & Sons, 1923.

– *Report on Workmen's Compensation for Injuries*. Toronto: Warwick Bro's & Rutter, 1900.

Maxwell, J.D., and M.P. Maxwell. "Inner Fraternity and Outer Sorority." In *Work, the Sociology of Work in Canada*, edited by Audrey Wipper, 330–58. Ottawa: Carleton University Press, 1994.

Mee, J., and T. Sumsion. "Mental Health Clients Confirm the Motivating Power of Occupation." *British Journal of Occupational Therapy* 64, no. 3 (2001): 121–8.

Metaxas, V. "Eleanor Clarke Slagle and Susan E. Tracy: Personal and Professional Identity and the Development of Occupational Therapy in Progressive Era America." *Nursing History Review* 8 (2000): 39–70.

Meyer, A. "The Philosophy of Occupation Therapy." *American Journal of Occupational Therapy* 31 (1977): 639–42.

Middleton, J.E. *The Municipality of Toronto: A History.* Vol. 3. Toronto: Dominion Publishing Co., 1923.

Mill, J.S. *On the Subjection of Women.* Greenwich, CT: Fawcett Publications, 1971.

Millar, J. *The School System in the State of New York (As Viewed by a Canadian).* Toronto: Warwick Bro's & Rutter, 1898.

Miller, R. *Toward a New Psychology of Women.* Boston: Beacon Press, 1976.

Mitchinson, W. *The Nature of Their Bodies: Women and Their Doctors in Victorian Canada.* Toronto: University of Toronto Press, 1991.

– "R.M. Bucke: A Victorian Asylum Superintendent." *Journal of Ontario History* 73, no. 4 (1981): 239–54.

Mitchinson, W., P. Bourne, A. Prentice, G. Cuthbert Brandt, B. Light, and N. Black. *Canadian Women – A Reader.* Toronto: Harcourt Brace & Company, 1996.

Moher, T.J. "Occupation as a Factor in the Treatment of Insanity." *Bulletin of the Ontario Hospitals for the Insane* 4, no. 1 (1911): 55–67.

Moran, J. "Medicine, Moral Therapy, and Motives." In *Committed to the State Asylum: Insanity and Society in Nineteenth-Century Quebec and Ontario,* 82–97. Montreal & Kingston: McGill-Queen's University Press, 2000.

Moran, J., and D. Wright. *Mental Health and Canadian Society.* Montreal & Kingston: McGill-Queen's University Press, 2006.

Morris, W. "Art and Beauty of the Earth." In *William Morris on Art and Socialism,* edited by N. Kelvin, 80–94. Mineola, NY: Dover Publications, 1999.

– "The Beauty of Life." In *William Morris on Art and Socialism,* edited by N. Kelvin, 35–55. Mineola, NY: Dover Publications, 1999.

– "An Empty Pocket Is the Worst of Crimes." *Commonweal,* 1886, 123.

– "The Lesser Arts." In *William Morris on Art and Socialism,* edited by N. Kelvin, 1–18. Mineola, NY: Dover Publications, 1999.

– *News from Nowhere.* Toronto: Penguin, 1993.

– "The Worker's Share of Art." *Commonweal,* 1889, 18–19.

Mortenson, W., and I. Dyck. "Power and Client-Centered Practice: An Insider Exploration of Occupational Therapists' Experiences." *Canadian Journal of Occupational Therapy* 73, no. 5 (2006): 261–7.

Morton, D. *A Short History of Canada.* Edmonton: Hurtig Publishers, 1987.

Morton, D., and G. Wright. *Winning the Second Battle: Canadian Veterans and the Return to Civilian Life, 1915–1930.* Toronto: University of Toronto Press, 1987.

Mowat, H. "Bursaries in Field Service Work." *Occupational Therapy and Rehabilitation* 11, no. 1 (1932): 41–3.

Muncy, R. "Lathrop, Julia Clifford." In *Women Building Chicago 1790–1990: A Biographical Dictionary,* edited by R.L. Schultz and A. Hast, 490–2. Bloomington: Indiana University Press, 2001.

Murray, E.R. *Froebel as a Pioneer in Modern Psychology*. Baltimore, MD: Warwich & York, 1914.

Myers, C. "Pioneer Occupational Therapists in World War I." *American Journal of Occupational Therapy* 2, no. 4 (1948): 208–15.

National Conference of Social Work. "Report of International Conference on the Rehabilitation of the Disabled." *Maryland Psychiatric Quarterly* 3, no. 4 (1917): 88–95.

Naylor, G. *The Arts and Crafts Movement: A Study of Its Sources, Ideals, and Influence on Design Theory*. Cambridge, MA: MIT Press, 1971.

Nova Scotia Hospital. *Sixty-Fourth Report of the Nova Scotia Hospital for the Year 1920–1921*. Halifax: Commissioner of Public Works and Mines, 1922.

Occupational Therapy and Rehabilitation. "Addresses at the Memorial Meeting for Thomas Bessell Kidner." *Occupational Therapy and Rehabilitation* 6, no. 6 (1932): 435–45.

– "Meeting of the Quebec Occupational Therapy Society." *Occupational Therapy and Rehabilitation* 8, no. 5 (1929): 313.

Ontario Society of Occupational Therapists. "Occupational Therapy & Family Health Teams in Ontario." http://www.osot.on.ca/eng/otinont/familyHealthTeams.asp.

– "Welcoming Interdisciplinary Primary Health Care." *Link*, no. 78 (April/May 2006): 1–3.

Osler, W. *Aequanimitas, with Other Addresses to Medical Students, Nurses and Practitioners of Medicine*. 3rd edn. New York: McGraw-Hill, 1932.

Oswald, S.G. *University of Toronto Roll of Service 1914–1918*. Toronto: University of Toronto Press, 1921.

Palmadottir, G. "Client-Therapist Relationships: Experiences of Occupational Therapy Clients in Rehabilitation." *British Journal of Occupational Therapy* 69, no. 9 (2006): 394–401.

Panayotidis, E.L. "James Mavor: Cultural Ambassador and Aesthetic Educator to Toronto's Elite." *Journal of Pre-Raphaelite Studies* 8 (Fall/Spring 1997): 163–73.

Panayotidis-Stortz, E. "Artist, Poet, and Socialist: Academic Deliberations on William Morris at the University of Toronto, 1896–1925." *Journal of William Morris Studies* 12, no. 1 (1998): 36–43.

– "'Every Artist Would Be a Workman, and Every Workman an Artist': Morrisian and Arts and Crafts Ideas and Ideals at the Ontario Educational Association 1900–1920." In *William Morris: Centenary Essays*, edited by P. Faulkner and P. Preston, 165–71. Exeter, UK: Exeter University Press, 1999.

Paterson, C. "Rationale for the Use of Occupation in the 19th Century Asylums." *British Journal of Occupational Therapy* 60, no. 4 (1997): 179–83.

Peck, A. "From the Canadian Handicrafts Guild, through Mrs. James H. Peck." *Royal Society of Canada Proceedings and Transactions*, series 2, 11 (1905): cxxx–cxxxiv.

Peck, M.A. "The Canadian Handicraft Movement." In *National Council of Women of Canada Yearbook 1904*, 6–14, 1904.

– "Handicrafts from Coast to Coast." *Canadian Geographical Journal* 9, no. 4 (1934): 201–16.

Peloquin, S. "The Fullness of Empathy: Reflections and Illustrations." *American Journal of Occupational Therapy* 49, no. 1 (1995): 24–31.

– "The 2005 Eleanor Clark Slagle Lecture: Embracing Our Ethos, Reclaiming Our Heart." *American Journal of Occupational Therapy* 59, no. 6 (2005): 611–25.

Pentland, W., and M.A. McColl. "Occupational Integrity: Another Perspective on 'Life Balance.'" *Canadian Journal of Occupational Therapy* 75, no. 3 (2008): 135–7.

Pepall, R. "Under the Spell of Morris: A Canadian Perspective." In *Earthly Paradise*, edited by K. Lochnan, D. Schoenherr, and C. Silver, 19–35. Toronto: Key Porter, 1993.

Phillips, C.J. "Impressions of the Ontario Military Hospital." In *Kentish Homes Visited by the Staff and Nurses of the Ontario Military Hospital, Orpington, Kent, in 1916*, edited by C.J. Phillips, 24–6. Privately published, 1917.

Phipps, K. *A History of the Cawthra-Elliott Estate.* 1989. http://cawthra-bush.org/HISTORICAL/his5.htm.

Pinel, P. "Medical Philosophical Treatise on Mental Alienation." In *Occupational Therapy Source Book*, edited by S. Licht, 19–24. Baltimore, MD: Williams & Wilkins, 1948.

Plummer, C. *In Spite of Myself: A Memoir.* Toronto: Alfred A. Knopf, 2008.

Prentice, A. *Canadian Women: A History.* Toronto: Harcourt Brace Jovanovich, 1988.

– "Schoolmistresses." In *The Oxford Companion to Canadian History*, edited by G. Hallowell, 467–8. Don Mills, ON: Oxford University Press, 2004.

Price, M. "Lives and Limbs." http://www.standford.edu/group/SHR/5-supp/text/price.html.

Primrose, A. "Ontario Society of Occupational Therapy." *University of Toronto Monthly* 24 (1924): 292–3.

– "Ontario Society of Occupational Therapy: How a Lesson from the War Is Being Applied in Times of Peace." *University of Toronto Monthly* 25 (1925): 412–14.

Pringle, G. "God Bless the 'Girls In Green'!: Story of a New Vocation for Women – Occupational Therapy – in Which Dominion of Canada Leads the World." *MacLean's Magazine*, 22 February 1922, 48–52.

– "Mrs. Agar Adamson: Versatile Canadian Artist Who Has Done Much for Art in Toronto." *Saturday Night* 40 (1925): 25.

Prosser, C.A. "War Work in Vocational Education." *Annals of the American Academy of Political and Social Science* 79 (1919): 236–70.

Provincial Rehabilitation Reference Group. *Managing the Seams: Making the Rehabilitation System Work for People.* Report. Ontario: Ontario Ministry of Health and Long-Term Care, 2000.

Prud'Homme, J. "What Is a Health Professional? The Changing Relationship of Occupational Therapists and Social Workers to Therapy and Heathcare in Quebec, 1940–1985." *Canadian Bulletin of Medical History* 28, no. 1 (2011): 71–94.

Punnett, H.R. "Occupational Therapy North of 53." *Occupational Therapy and Rehabilitation* 8 (1929): 291–4.

Putnam, R. "The Prosperous Community: Social Capital and Public Life." *American Prospect* 13 (1993): 36–42.

Quiroga, V.A.M. *Occupational Therapy: The First 30 Years 1900 to 1930.* Bethesda, MD: American Occupational Therapy Association, 1995.

Reaume, G. "Patients at Work: Insane Asylum Inmates' Labour in Ontario, 1841–1900." In *Mental Health and Canadian Society: Historical Perspectives*, edited by J.E. Moran and D. Wright, 69–96. Montreal & Kingston: McGill-Queen's University Press, 2006.

– *Remembrances of Patients Past.* Don Mills, ON: Oxford University Press, 2000.

Reconstruction. "Explaining Popular Misconceptions in Reference to Vocational Training." *Reconstruction*, November 1917–December 1918, 12.

– "The Film in England." *Reconstruction*, August 1918, 7.

Reed, K., and S.N. Sanderson. *Concepts of Occupational Therapy.* 4th edn. Baltimore, MD: Lippincott Williams & Wilkins, 1999.

– "Occupational Therapy Values and Beliefs: The Formative Years: 1904–1929." *OT Practise* 2, no. 7 (2006): 21–5.

Regehr, T.D. "Ross, James." *Dictionary of Canadian Biography.* University of Toronto Press. http://www.biographi.ca/009004-119.01-e.php?&id_nbr=7681&& PHPSESSID=5g8t4fvjomel2vg5ako9hmitr3.

Reid, E.C. "Ergotherapy in the Treatment of Mental Disorders." In *Occupational Therapy Source Book*, edited by S. Licht, 81–7. Baltimore, MD: Williams & Wilkins, 1948.

Reid, G.A. "Applied Art." *Canadian Architect and Builder* 13, no. 3 (1900): 55.

Reilly, M. "Occupational Therapy Can Be One of the Great Ideas of the 20th Century." *American Journal of Occupational Therapy* 16, no. 1 (1962): 87–105.

Reitz, S.M. "A Historical Review of Occupational Therapy's Role in Preventive Health and Wellness." *American Journal of Occupational Therapy* 46, no. 1 (1992): 50–4.

Renwick, R., J. Friedland, V. Sernas, and K. Raybould. "Crisis in Psychosocial Occupational Therapy: A Closer Look." *Canadian Journal of Occupational Therapy* 57 (1990): 279–84.

Reynolds, F. "Textile Art Promoting Well-Being. *Journal of Occupational Science* 11, no. 2 (2004): 58–67.

Reznick, J. *Healing the Nation: Soldiers and the Culture of Caregiving in Britain during the Great War.* Manchester, UK: Manchester University Press, 2004.

– *John Galsworthy and Disabled Soldiers of the Great War.* Manchester, UK: Manchester University Press, 2009.

– "Work Therapy and the Disabled British Soldier in Great Britain in the First World War: The Case of Shepherd's Bush Military Hospital, London." In *Disabled Veterans in History*, edited by D. Gerber, 185–203. Ann Arbor: University of Michigan Press, 2000.

Richardson, S. "The Historical Relationship of Nursing Program Accreditation and Public Policy in Canada." *Nursing History Review* 4 (1996): 19–42.

Rigby, P., and L. Letts. "Environment and Occupational Performance: Theoretical Considerations." In *Using Environments to Enable Occupational Performance*, edited by L.P. Letts, P. Rigby, and D. Stewart, 17–29. Thorofare, NJ: Slack Incorporated, 2003.

Roberts, C.G.D., and A.L. Tunnell. *The Canadian Who's Who, 1936–1937: A Handbook of Canadian Biography of Living Characters*. Vol. 2. Toronto: Murray Printing Co., 1937.

– *The Canadian Who's Who, 1938–1939*. Vol. 3. Toronto: Trans-Canada Press, 2010.

Robertson, J.W. *Industrial Training and Technical Education*. 4th edn. Ottawa: C.H. Parmelee, 1913.

– *Manual Training: The Macdonald Manual Training Schools*. Toronto, 1901.

– *Royal Commission on Industrial Training and Technical Education: Report of the Commissioners, Part IV*. Ottawa, C.H. Parmelee, Printer to the King's Most Excellent Majesty, 1913.

Robinson, I. "The Mists of Time." Muriel Driver Lecture 1981. *Canadian Journal of Occupational Therapy* 48, no. 4 (1981): 145–52.

Rochon Ford, A. *A Path Not Strewn with Roses: One Hundred Years of Women at the University of Toronto 1884–1984*. Toronto: University of Toronto Press, 1985.

Rodgers, D.T. "Idle Womanhood: Feminist Versions of the Work Ethic." In *The Work Ethic in Industrial America, 1850–1920*, 182–209. Chicago: University of Chicago Press, 1974.

Roland, C. *Clarence Hinks: Mental Health Crusader*. Edited by T.P. Morley. Toronto: Dundurn Press, 1990.

Rollnick, S., and W.R. Miller. *Motivational Interviewing: Preparing People for Change*. 2nd edn. New York: Guilford Press, 2002.

– "What Is Motivational Interviewing?" *Behavioural and Cognitive Psychotherapy* 23, no. 4 (1995): 325–34.

Rompkey, R. "Grenfell, Sir Wilfred Thomason." In *The Oxford Companion to Canadian History*, edited by G. Hallowell, 270. Don Mills, ON: Oxford University Press, 2004.

– *Grenfell of Labrador: A Biography*. Toronto: University of Toronto Press, 1991.

– *Jessie Luther at the Grenfell Mission*. Montreal & Kingston: McGill-Queen's University Press, 2001.

Ross, J. *Occupational Therapy and Vocational Rehabilitation*. Chichester, UK: Wiley and Sons, 2007.

Ross, J.K.M. *Boots and Saddles: The Story of the Fabulous Ross Stable in the Golden Days of Racing.* New York: E.P. Dutton & Co., 1956.

Rush, B. *Medical Inquiries and Observations upon the Diseases of the Mind.* 5th edn. Philadelphia: Grigg and Elliot, 1835.

Ruskin, J. *Arrows of the Chace: A Collection of Scattered Letters Published in the Daily Newspapers.* New York: John Wiley & Sons, 1881.

– *Fors Clavigera. Letters to the Workmen and Labourers of Great Britain.* Vol. 5. New York: John Wiley & Sons, 1886.

– *On the Nature of Gothic Architecture.* London: Smith, Elder, 1854.

Russell, P.G. "The Mutable Monument: The Architecture of Hart House." In *A Strange Elation: Hart House, the First Eighty Years,* edited by David Kilgour, 19–25. Toronto: Hart House and University of Toronto Press, 1999.

Salomon, O. *The Theory of Educational Sloyd: The Lectures of Otto Salomon.* Boston: Silver, Burdett, and Co., 1907.

Sands, J.F. "When Is Occupational Therapy Curative?" *Occupational Therapy and Rehabilitation* 7, no. 2 (1928): 115–22.

Sassoon, S. *Memoirs of an Infantry Officer.* Chatham, UK: Mackays of Chatham, 1965.

Schneider, W., and R.M. Shiffrin. "Controlled and Automatic Processing: Detection, Search and Attention." *Psychological Review* 84, no. 1 (1977): 1–66.

Schwab, S.I. "The Experiment in Occupational Therapy at Base Hospital 117." *Mental Hygiene,* no. 3 (1919): 580–96.

Schwartz, K.B. "Occupational Therapy and Education: A Shared Vision." *American Journal of Occupational Therapy* 46, no. 1 (1992): 12–18.

Sedgwick, A., L. Cockburn, and B. Trentham. "Exploring the Mental Health Roots of Occupational Therapy in Canada: A Historical Review of Primary Texts from 1925–1950." *Canadian Journal of Occupational Therapy* 74, no. 5 (2007): 407–17.

Segsworth, W. *Retraining Canada's Disabled Soldiers.* Ottawa: Department of Soldiers' Civil Re-establishment, 1920.

Selye, H. *The Stress of Everyday Life.* New York: McGraw-Hill, 1976.

Serrett, K.D. *Philosophical and Historical Roots of Occupational Therapy.* New York: Haworth Press, 1985.

Shortt, S.E.D. *Victorian Lunacy: Richard M. Bucke and the Practice of Late Nineteenth-Century Psychiatry.* Vol. 2. Cambridge: Cambridge University Press, 1986.

Smallwood, J., and J. Schooler. "The Restless Mind." *Psychological Bulletin* 132, no. 6 (2006): 946–58.

Smith, E. "The Crest Says – 'Per Mentem Et Manus Ad Sanitatem.'" *Canadian Journal of Occupational Therapy* 31, no. 1 (1964): 3–4.

Smith, G.O. "Roll of Honour." In *University of Toronto Roll of Service, 1914–1918.* Toronto: University of Toronto Press, 1921.

Smyth, E., A. Acker, P. Bourne, and A. Prentice. *Challenging Professions: Historical and Contemporary Perspectives on Women's Professional Work.* Toronto: University of Toronto Press, 1999.

Special Committee on Returned Soldiers. *Proceedings.* Ottawa: J. de Labroquerie Taché, 1917.

Stalker, J., and S. Prentice. *The Illusion of Inclusion: Women in Post Secondary Education.* Toronto: Fernwood Books, 1998.

Stankiewicz, M.A. "From the Aesthetic Movement to the Arts and Crafts Movement." *Studies in Art Education* 33 (1992): 165–73.

Stead, Ada. "The Ontario Society of Occupational Therapy." *Wisconsin Journal of Occupational Therapy* 2, no. 2 (1925): 2–9.

Stebner, E. "The Settlement House Movement." In *Encyclopedia of Women and Religion in North America,* edited by R. Skinner Keller, Radford Ruether, and M. Cantlon, 1067. Indiana: Indiana University Press, 2006.

Stevenson, G.H. "The Life and Work of Richard Maurice Bucke: An Appraisal." *American Journal of Psychiatry* 93, no. 5 (1937): 1127–54.

Stewart, I. "James Wilson Robertson." *Dictionary of Canadian Biography.* University of Toronto Press. http://www.biographi.ca/009004-119.01-e.php?&id_nbr=7962&interval=20&&PHPSESSID=j5ctsgkclqegs7902hom403m52.

Stewart, J. "Occupational Therapy in Canada." *Archives of Occupational Therapy* 2 (1923): 381–3.

Stogdill, C.G. "Joseph Workman, MD, 1805–1894, Alienist and Medical Teacher." *Canadian Medical Association Journal* 95, no. 18 (1966): 1–7.

Stonehouse, H. *Moving Together: Physical Therapy and the University of Toronto.* Toronto: University of Toronto Press, 2007.

Strong-Boag, V. "'Ever a Crusader': Nellie McClung, First-Wave Feminist." In *Rethinking Canada: The Promise of Women's History,* 3rd edn, edited by Veronica Strong-Boag and Anita Clair Fellman, 271–83. Toronto: Oxford University Press, 1997.

Taylor, R.R., S.W. Lee, G. Kielhofner, and M. Ketkar. "Therapeutic Use of Self: A Nationwide Survey of Practitioners' Attitudes and Experiences. *American Journal of Occupational Therapy* 63, no. 2 (2009): 198–207.

Thompson, P. *The Work of William Morris.* 3rd edn. Oxford, UK: Oxford University Press, 1993.

Todd, J.L. "Returned Soldiers and the Medical Profession." *Canadian Medical Association Journal* 7, no. 4 (1917): 343–55.

Tolmatch, E. "The Extraordinary Bequest of Brigadier A. Hamilton Gault." *Collage,* 1997, 20–1.

Toronto Association of Occupational Therapy. "Toronto Association of Occupational Therapy Curative Workshop Pamphlet Circa 1926." 1926.

Townsend, E., and H. Polatajko. *Enabling Occupation II: Advancing an Occupational Therapy Vision for Health, Well-Being & Justice through Occupation.* Ottawa: CAOT Publications ACE, 2007.

Townsend, E., and A.A. Wilcock. "Occupational Justice and Client-Centred Practice: A Dialogue in Progress." *Canadian Journal of Occupational Therapy* 71, no. 2 (2004): 75–87.

Tracy, S.E. *Studies in Invalid Occupation: A Manual for Nurses and Attendants.* Boston: Whitcomb & Barrows, 1910.

Trent, M.E. "Ward Aides." *Vocational Bulletin,* June 1919, 2–5.

Trentham, B. "Occupational Therapy Street Fair." Canadian Association of Occupational Therapists. http://www.caot.ca/default.asp?pageid=1462.

Tuke, D.H. "Reform in the Treatment of the Insane." *American Journal of Insanity* 50 (1893): 46–8.

Twohig, P.L. "'Once a Therapist, Always a Therapist': The Early Career of Mary Black, Occupational Therapist." *Atlantis* 28, no. 1 (2003): 106–17.

United States Army Medical Department. "Hart House, Toronto, a Functional Re-Education Center." *Reconstruction and Reeducation of the Disabled Soldier,* 1918, 104–7.

University of Illinois at Chicago. *Opening New Worlds: Jane Addams' Hull-House.* Chicago: University of Illinois at Chicago, 1989.

University of Toronto Faculty of Medicine. "Canada's First Women Postgraduates in Psychiatry." http://www.utpsychiatry.ca/centenary/vignette/Nov07-Vig5-FirstWomenPG.pdf.

University of Toronto Monthly. "Honour the Dead by Helping the Living, Ontario Society for Occupational Therapy Curative Workshop." *University of Toronto Monthly,* 1923.

– "Occupational Therapy." *University of Toronto Monthly,* September 1929.

– "The Ontario Society of Occupational Therapy." *University of Toronto Monthly,* February 1930.

– "The Ontario Society of Occupational Therapy." *University of Toronto Monthly,* March 1930.

– "The Ontario Society of Occupational Therapy." *University of Toronto Monthly,* May 1930.

– "Occupational Therapy Course Lengthened." *University of Toronto Monthly,* September 1946.

Valverde, M. *The Age of Light, Soap, and Water: Moral Reform in English Canada, 1885–1925.* Toronto: McClelland & Stewart, 1991.

Vicinus, M. *Independent Women: Work and Community for Single Women, 1850–1920.* Chicago: University of Chicago Press, 1992.

Warsh, C.K. *Moments of Unreason: The Practice of Canadian Psychiatry and the Homewood Retreat, 1883–1923.* Montreal & Kingston: McGill-Queen's University Press, 1989.

Wasteneys, H. "A History of the University Settlement of Toronto, 1910–1958: An Exploration of the Social Objectives of the University Settlement and Their Implementation." PhD diss., University of Toronto, 1975.

Wathen, M.A., J.W. Chester, F.S. Patterson, M.M. Harris, W.D. Paton, F.S. Harrod, and L. Scott. *Weaving and Rug-Making Note-Book No. 2*. Department of Soldiers' Civil Re-establishment, 1918.

Watt, S. "Rights of Passage." *University of Toronto Bulletin*, 2004, 9.

Whalley Hammell, K. "Sacred Texts: A Sceptical Exploration of the Assumptions Underpinning Theories of Occupation." *Canadian Journal of Occupational Therapy* 76, no. 1 (2009): 6–13.

Wharton, E. *A Son at the Front*. DeKlab, IL: Northern Illinois University Press, 1995.

White, R. "The Urge towards Competence." *American Journal of Occupational Therapy* 25, no. 6 (1971): 271–4.

Wilcock, A. "Creating Self and Shaping the World." *Australian Occupational Therapy Journal* 46, no. 2 (1999): 77–88.

– *An Occupational Perspective of Health*. Thorofare, NJ: Slack, 1998.

– *Occupation for Health: A Journey from Prescription to Self Health*. Vol. 2. London: British Association of Occupational Therapists, 2002.

– *Occupation for Health: A Journey from Self-Health to Prescription*. Vol. 1 London: British Association and College of Occupational Therapy, 2001.

Wilde, O. *Extracts from Wilde's lecture on Art and the Handicraftsman: Reprinted from Essays and Lectures by Oscar Wilde*. London Methuen and Co., 1908.

Wilson, D., R. Stamp, and L.P. Audet. *Canadian Education: A History*. Toronto: Prentice Hall, 1970.

Wilson, S.J. *Women, Families, and Work*. 3rd edn. Canadian Sociology series. Toronto: McGraw-Hill Ryerson, 1981.

Wilton, P. "Spanish Flu Outdid WWI in Number of Lives Claimed." *Canadian Medical Association Journal* 148, no. 11 (1993): 2036–7.

Winnipeg General Hospital. *Winnipeg General Hospital Reports and Accounts, 1920*. Winnipeg: Winnipeg General Hospital, 1920.

– *Winnipeg General Hospital Reports and Accounts, 1923*. Winnipeg: Winnipeg General Hospital, 1923.

Wollons, R. *Kindergartens and Cultures: The Global Diffusion of an Idea*. London: Yale University Press, 2000.

Wood, W. "Weaving the Warp and Weft of Occupational Therapy: An Art and Science for All Times." *American Journal of Occupational Therapy* 49, no. 1 (1995): 44–52.

Worthington, J.R., and W. Moynihan. "What Is Occupational Therapy?," *This Little World* 1, no. 5 (1944): 8, 10.

Wright, B.A.P. *Physical Disability: A Psychosocial Approach*. New York: HarperCollins, 1983.

Wright, D. *The Professionalization of History in English Canada*. Toronto: University of Toronto Press, 1965.

Yerxa, E. "Some Implications of Occupational Therapy's History for Its Epistemology, Values, and Relation to Medicine." *American Journal of Occupational Therapy* 46, no. 1 (1992): 79–83.

– "Health and the Human Spirit for Occupation." *American Journal of Occupational Therapy* 52, no. 6 (1998): 412–18.

Yerxa, E., and G. Sharrott. "Liberal Arts: The Foundation for Occupational Therapy Education." *American Journal of Occupational Therapy* 40, no. 3 (1986): 153–9.

Young, C.R. *Engineering Education at Toronto 1851–1919*. Toronto: University of Toronto Press, 1958.

Young, G.S. "Obituaries: Dr. Alexander Primrose." *Canadian Medical Association Journal* 50, no. 4 (1944): 389–90.

INDEX